Managing the Oral Effects of Cancer Treatment: Diagnosis to Survivorship

Edited by

Marilyn L. Haas, PhD, CNS, ANP-BC
Deborah L. McBride, RN, MSN, CPON®

Oncology Nursing Society
Pittsburgh, Pennsylvania

ONS Publications Department
Interim Publisher and Director of Publications: Barbara Sigler, RN, MNEd
Managing Editor: Lisa M. George, BA
Technical Content Editor: Angela D. Klimaszewski, RN, MSN
Staff Editor II: Amy Nicoletti, BA
Copy Editor: Laura Pinchot, BA
Graphic Designer: Dany Sjoen

Library of Congress Cataloging-in-Publication Data
Managing the oral effects of cancer treatment : diagnosis to survivorship /
edited by Marilyn L. Haas and Deborah L. McBride.
         p. ; cm.
    Includes bibliographical references.
    ISBN 978-1-935864-03-5 (alk. paper)
    1. Cancer–Nursing. 2. Cancer–Treatment–Complications. 3. Antineoplastic
agents–Side effects. 4. Oral manifestations of general diseases. 5.
Radiotherapy. I. Haas, Marilyn. II. McBride, Deborah L. III. Oncology Nursing
Society.
    [DNLM: 1. Neoplasms–nursing. 2. Neoplasms–therapy. 3. Antineoplastic
Agents–adverse effects. 4. Oral Manifestations. 5. Radiotherapy–adverse
effects. WY 156]

    RC266.M355 2011
    616.99'40231–dc22

                                                                    2010052059

Printed in the United States of America

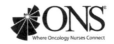

Oncology Nursing Society
Integrity • Innovation • Stewardship • Advocacy • Excellence • Inclusiveness

Contributors

Editors

Marilyn L. Haas, PhD, CNS, ANP-BC
Nurse Practitioner
Carolina Clinical Consultant and CarePartners Supportive and Palliative Services
Asheville, North Carolina
Chapter 10. Developing a Nursing-Centered "Spray and Weigh" Program

Deborah L. McBride, RN, MSN, CPON®
Assistant Professor of Nursing
Samuel Merritt University
Staff Nurse
Kaiser Permanente Oakland Medical Center
Oakland, California
Chapter 15. Special Considerations in Pediatric Populations

Authors

Mary J. Bacon, MA, CCC-SLP, BRS-S
Associate Professor/Clinical Educator
Communication Disorders and Sciences
Rush University Medical Center
Chicago, Illinois
Chapter 8. Speech, Voice, and Swallowing Problems: The Speech Pathologist's Role

Ingrid Bowser, MS, APRN-BC, AOCNP®, ADM-BC
Nurse Practitioner
Indiana University Health
Goshen Center for Cancer Care
Goshen, Indiana
Chapter 7. Pain Management

Susan D. Bruce, RN, MSN, OCN®
Oncology Clinical Nurse Specialist
Duke Raleigh Cancer Center
Raleigh, North Carolina
Chapter 3. Treatment of Side Effects

Patricia C. Buchsel, MSN, RN, OCN®, FAAN
Clinical Instructor
Seattle University College of Nursing
Seattle, Washington
Chapter 17. Oral Health Across the Continuum of Care: A Symptom Cluster Model

Carrie F. Daly, RN, MS, AOCN®
Oncology Nurse Manager/Advanced Practice Nurse
Radiation Oncology Department
Rush University Medical Center
Chicago, Illinois
Chapter 6. Xerostomia and Cytoprotection

Sarah D'Angelo, RN, BSc, BScN, MN, CON(C)
Advanced Practice Nurse Educator
Princess Margaret Hospital, University
  Health Network
Toronto, Ontario, Canada
*Chapter 4. Evidence-Based Practice: Tools to
  Measure Progress*

Vanna M. Dest, MSN, APRN, BC, AOCN®
Oncology Nurse Practitioner
CyberKnife Coordinator
Cancer Genetics Testing Coordinator
Hospital of Saint Raphael/Radiation Oncol-
  ogy Specialists of Southern Connecticut
New Haven, Connecticut
Chapter 1. Oral Health: The Basics

Catherine H.L. Hong, BDS, MS
Assistant Professor
Department of Preventive Dentistry
Faculty of Dentistry
National University of Singapore
Singapore
*Chapter 2. Fundamental Skills: Oral Assess-
  ment and Dental Hygiene*

Maureen B. Huhmann, DCN, RD, CSO
Assistant Professor
Department of Nutrition Sciences, School
  of Health Related Professions
University of Medicine and Dentistry of
  New Jersey
Cancer Institute of New Jersey
New Brunswick, New Jersey
Chapter 12. Paradigms of Eating

Sarah H. Kagan, PhD, RN, AOCN®
Lucy Walker Honorary Term Professor of
  Gerontological Nursing
School of Nursing
Clinical Nurse Specialist
Abramson Cancer Center
University of Pennsylvania
Philadelphia, Pennsylvania
*Chapter 14. Considerations for Older Cancer
  Survivors—Aging, Comorbidity, and
  Cancer Treatment*

Miranda J. Kramer, RN, MS, ACNP, CNS
Nurse Practitioner/Clinical Nurse Specialist
Assistant Clinical Professor, Physiological
  Nursing
University of California, San Francisco
San Francisco, California
Chapter 11. Sexuality and Quality of Life

Kristen W. Maloney, MSN, RN, AOCNS®
Clinical Nurse Specialist, Rhoads Three
  Nursing Unit—Medical Oncology
Hospital of the University of Pennsylvania
Philadelphia, Pennsylvania
*Chapter 14. Considerations for Older Cancer
  Survivors—Aging, Comorbidity, and
  Cancer Treatment*

Maurene McQuestion, RN, BA, BScN, MSc, CON(C)
Clinical Nurse Specialist, Advanced Practice
  Nurse
Princess Margaret Hospital, University
  Health Network
Toronto, Ontario, Canada
*Chapter 4. Evidence-Based Practice: Tools to
  Measure Progress*

Katherine Katen Moore, MSN, ANP-C, AOCN®
Associate Director, Student Health Services
Drew University
Madison, New Jersey
*Chapter 9. Complementary and Alternative
  Medicine and the Mouth*

Joel J. Napeñas, DDS
Director, General Practice Residency
Department of Oral Medicine
Carolinas Medical Center
Charlotte, North Carolina
*Chapter 2. Fundamental Skills: Oral Assess-
  ment and Dental Hygiene*

Maria Q.B. Petzel, RD, CSO, LD, CNSC
Senior Clinical Dietitian
Department of Clinical Nutrition
University of Texas MD Anderson Cancer
  Center
Houston, Texas
*Chapter 5. Nutrition Management Strate-
  gies for Oral Effects of Cancer Treatment*

Erika Schroeder, RN, MS, OCN®, CNL
Manager, Clinical Trials
Anne Arundel Health Systems Research
    Institute
Annapolis, Maryland
Chapter 13. Psychosocial Challenges

**Pamela Hallquist Viale, RN, MS, CS,
    ANP, AOCNP®**
Editor in Chief
*Journal of the Advanced Practitioner in
    Oncology*
Oncology Nurse Practitioner and Consul-
    tant
Goleta, California
*Chapter 16. Second Primary Cancers and
    Recurrence*

Mary Ellyn Witt, RN, MS, AOCN®
Clinical Research Nurse
Radiation Oncology
University of Chicago Medical Center
Chicago, Illinois
Chapter 13. Psychosocial Challenges

M. Renee Yanke, ARNP, MN, AOCN®
Oncology Program Manager, Oncology
    Advanced Practice Nurse
Whidbey General Hospital
Coupeville, Washington
*Chapter 9. Complementary and Alternative
    Medicine and the Mouth*

Disclosure

Editors and authors of books and guidelines provided by the Oncology Nursing Society are expected to disclose to the readers any significant financial interest or other relationships with the manufacturer(s) of any commercial products.

A vested interest may be considered to exist if a contributor is affiliated with or has a financial interest in commercial organizations that may have a direct or indirect interest in the subject matter. A "financial interest" may include, but is not limited to, being a shareholder in the organization; being an employee of the commercial organization; serving on an organization's speakers bureau; or receiving research from the organization. An "affiliation" may be holding a position on an advisory board or some other role of benefit to the commercial organization. Vested interest statements appear in the front matter for each publication.

Contributors are expected to disclose any unlabeled or investigational use of products discussed in their content. This information is acknowledged solely for the information of the readers.

The contributors provided the following disclosure and vested interest information:
Marilyn L. Haas, PhD, CNS, ANP-BC: MedPharma and Meniscus Educational Institute, honoraria
Carrie F. Daly, RN, MS, AOCN®: Roche, consultant; IMER, honoraria
Vanna M. Dest, MSN, APRN, BC, AOCN®: EUSA Pharma and Myriad Laboratories, honoraria
Pamela Hallquist Viale, RN, MS, CS, ANP, AOCNP®: Meniscus Educational Institute and Novartis, consultant; Amgen, Bristol-Myers Squibb, IMER, Meniscus Educational Institute, Merck, and Novartis, honoraria
M. Renee Yanke, ARNP, MN, AOCN®: Novartis, consultant, honoraria

Contents

Preface xv

Chapter 1. Oral Health: The Basics   1

Introduction 1
History of Oral Care 1
Epidemiology of Oral Diseases 2
Anatomy of the Oral Cavity 5
Common Oral Conditions 8
Oral Health and Overall General Health 11
Common Oral Manifestations of Systemic Medical Diseases 12
Oral Manifestations During Women's Reproductive Years 20
Maintenance of Oral Hygiene and Health 21
Conclusion 21
References 22

Chapter 2. Fundamental Skills: Oral Assessment and
Dental Hygiene   25

Introduction 25
History Taking 25
Diagnostic and Assessment Tools 32
Dental Care in Patients With Cancer 39
Barriers to Dental Care 43
Conclusion 44
References 44

Chapter 3. Treatment of Side Effects   47

Introduction 47
Oral Mucositis 47
Xerostomia and Hyposalivation 52
Chronic Graft-Versus-Host Disease 55
Dental Caries and Periodontal Disease 56

Taste Changes..57
Persistent Dysphagia 60
Trismus 60
Fungal Infections..62
Osteoradionecrosis...62
Osteonecrosis 63
Conclusion 64
References...64

Chapter 4. Evidence-Based Practice: Tools to Measure Progress   69

Introduction 69
Evidence-Based Practice..70
Types of Tools...71
Description and Critique of Specific Tools 78
Special Populations and Considerations...85
Naturopathic, Complementary, and Alternative Medicine 86
Conclusion 87
References...88

**Chapter 5. Nutrition Management Strategies for
Oral Effects of Cancer Treatment   93**

Introduction 93
Mucositis 94
Xerostomia..97
Dysgeusia and Hypogeusia..98
Dysphagia 99
Other Oral Effects of Treatment 99
Nutrition Support 100
Conclusion 101
References...101

Chapter 6. Xerostomia and Cytoprotection   103

Introduction 103
Sjögren Syndrome of the Oral Cavity...106
Review of Oral Cancers 107
Treatment for Oral Cancers...109
Advances in Radiation Therapy 111
Cytoprotection 114
Quality of Life 118
Conclusion 118
References...119

Chapter 7. Pain Management   125

Introduction 125
Causes of Oral Pain...125

Assessment 127
Interventions for Oral Pain 128
Other Treatments 135
Barriers to Pain Management 140
Conclusion 143
References 143

Chapter 8. Speech, Voice, and Swallowing Problems: The Speech Pathologist's Role   147

Introduction 147
Common Speech, Voice, and Swallowing Problems Related to Radiation
    Therapy and Chemotherapy for Oral and Oropharyngeal Cancers 148
Pretreatment Involvement of Speech Pathology 149
Speech Pathology Evaluations 149
Speech Pathology Treatment 151
Conclusion 154
References 155

Chapter 9. Complementary and Alternative Medicine and the Mouth   157

Introduction 157
Definitions 159
Evidence for Use 159
Interventions for Dysgeusia 160
Interventions for Oral Mucositis 160
Interventions for Orofacial Pain (Excluding Oral Mucositis) 168
Interventions for Xerostomia 168
Conclusion and Nursing Implications 170
References 171

Chapter 10. Developing a Nursing-Centered "Spray and Weigh" Program   175

Introduction 176
Oral Cavity Assessment 177
Symptom Assessment 182
Dental Health 183
Oral Hygiene at Home 183
Conclusion 183
References 184

Chapter 11. Sexuality and Quality of Life   185

Introduction 185
Factors in Sexuality 185

Patient Oral Symptoms and Their Effects on Sexuality and Intimacy..........................186
Assessing Sexual Health..188
Assessments and Interventions..189
Conclusion..191
References...191

Chapter 12. Paradigms of Eating   193

Introduction...193
Diet Following Chemotherapy..193
Bisphosphonate-Associated Osteonecrosis..194
Stem Cell Transplantation and Oral Development...194
Diet Following Radiation Therapy...196
Diet Following Surgery: Dysphagia...199
Conclusion..200
References...200

Chapter 13. Psychosocial Challenges   205

Introduction...205
Oral Complications of Survivorship..207
Financial Challenges...209
Assessment Tools..212
Screening Tools for Patients With Oral Complications..214
Additional Resources..217
Conclusion..218
References...218

Chapter 14. Considerations for Older Cancer Survivors—
Aging, Comorbidity, and Cancer Treatment   221

Introduction...221
Oral Health and the Aging Population...222
Oral Health Problems Among Older Adults..223
Considerations in Assessment and Intervention for Oral Effects in Older
    Survivors..231
Conclusion..232
References...232

Chapter 15. Special Considerations in Pediatric Populations   237

Introduction...237
Oral Complications Associated With Cancer Treatment in Children...........................238
Pediatric Oral Assessment Tools..242
Infections Associated With Cancer Treatment..242
Salivary Gland Dysfunction...244
Oral and Dental Management..244
Oral Care After Cancer Treatment...245

Conclusion 247
References 247

Chapter 16. Second Primary Cancers and Recurrence   251

Introduction 251
Scope of the Problem 251
Chemoprevention 255
Fear of Recurrence and Psychosocial Effect on Patients With Oral Cancer 256
Nursing Implications 257
Conclusion 258
References 259

Chapter 17. Oral Health Across the Continuum of Care:
A Symptom Cluster Model   263

Introduction 263
Major Advances in Treatment of Oral Problems in Cancer Treatments 264
Clinical and Functional Impairments 265
Prevention and Early Detection of Oral Complications 265
Oral Care Protocols 266
Symptom Clusters 271
Case Study in an Allogeneic Hematologic Stem Cell Transplant Recipient 272
Conclusion 276
References 276

Index   281

Recognizing that our patients travel many different paths during their oncology experience, oncology nurses are blessed to be their traveling companion. For my husband, who has traveled many of my professional paths, I now travel with him down his own cancer path. May this clinical information help us and others improve our care for patients dealing with oral oncology problems as they face their treatments.

—Marilyn Louise Younghouse Haas, PhD, CNS, ANP-BC

This book was inspired by my work caring for children with cancer. I hope it improves the care of both pediatric and adult patients who are dealing with the oral effects of cancer. I dedicate this book to my husband, Joe, the man whom I am blessed to have as a husband. I would like to thank him for his daily love and support.

—Deborah L. McBride, RN, MSN, CPON®

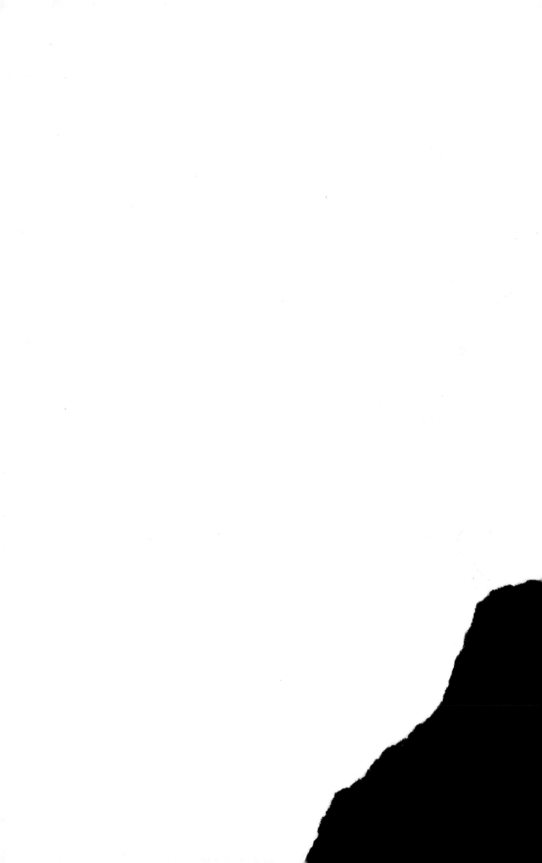

Preface

The mouth is a "mirror": the oral cavity can reflect the general health of a patient and reveal toxicities from oncology treatments.

Oral diseases may not be life threatening, but they can have systemic effects and greatly affect a person's quality of life. Oral cancers can be devastating, and the toxicities from oncology treatments can compound problems already experienced by patients who suffer from poor oral health and periodontal diseases. Concomitant high-dose radiation therapy and chemotherapy (targeted therapies) improves locoregional control of cancers but increases toxicities. Oral health becomes one of the primary responsibilities of the entire multidisciplinary team. Healthcare providers should employ interventions that prevent oral problems or anticipate oral side effects and be aggressive in treating the problems so as to not delay or interrupt therapy. Once the patient has completed therapy, follow-up over time is extremely important to maintain oral health.

This is the first oncology textbook available to guide physicians, nurse practitioners/physician assistants, and nurses who care for patients with cancer through the management of oral health problems. Comprehensive information about evidence-based principles and practice guidelines in caring for the oncology patient who has developed oral problems is presented. *Managing the Oral Effects of Cancer Treatment: Diagnosis to Survivorship* begins with an in-depth discussion about the fundamental skills of oral assessment and dental hygiene, treatment side effects as they relate to the oral cavity, management strategies, and insight into survivorship issues.

Initial chapters will discuss general overall oral health care, explain the necessary fundamental skills to perform a comprehensive oral assessment, and explain oral side effects from oncology treatments. Evidence-based tools to describe the progress back toward oral health will be shared. The second section will discuss management strategies to improve nutrition status, identify advantages of cytoprotection interventions, and gain control over pain issues. Speech therapy resources, complementary therapies, and an innovative mini-oral clinic will be discussed to improve the patient's tolerance with oncology treatments. Finally, the third section will provide in-depth insight into survivorship issues, sexuality, changing eating habits, psychosocial issues, older adult and pediatric challenges, recurrent cancers, and a symptom cluster model of care.

This textbook shares the efforts of many authors to synthesize scientific information to support patients toward better oral health care. Applying oral healthcare principles will improve the quality of care for patients with cancer.

CHAPTER 1

Oral Health: The Basics

Vanna M. Dest, MSN, APRN, BC, AOCN®

Introduction

Oral health is a crucial component of an individual's overall general health status and well-being. In 1948, the World Health Organization expanded the definition of health as a "complete state of physical, mental, and social well-being, and not just the absence of infirmity." The definition of oral health parallels the definition of health, and the two are regarded as inseparable. Oral health is a critical component of health care and must be incorporated into the delivery of care and within our community (Petersen, 2003, 2008).

History of Oral Care

The history of oral health began in the 1930s when researchers discovered that individuals drinking naturally fluoridated water had fewer dental caries than those who drank nonfluoridated water. During the World War II era, researchers conducted clinical trials, which led to the addition of fluoride to community water supplies. By the 1950s, the incidence of dental caries decreased, and by the 1970s, the incidence of tooth decay had also diminished (Petersen, 2003).

In 2000, the first Surgeon General's Report on Oral Health was released (U.S. Department of Health and Human Services [DHHS], 2000). This truly marked a milestone in the history of oral health care and how it would evolve in the years to come. The report described oral health issues as a "silent epidemic." This report addressed the magnitude of oral disease, access to care in various populations, and scientific evidence that linked oral disease to other underlying medical conditions. The report also described oral health as being more than just having healthy teeth but also the absence of chronic oral and maxillofacial pain, oral and pharyngeal cancers, oral soft tissue lesions, birth defects, and other diseases that affect the craniofacial complex. The craniofacial complex is responsible for many of the functions of the face and oral cavity, such as smiling, speaking, sighing, kissing, smelling, tasting, touching, chewing, and swallowing.

In 2003, the World Health Organization released a report on oral health. This report summarized the continued burden of oral health issues in the world despite the advances over the past decades. The strategies proposed included strengthening public health initiatives through prevention. In 2007, the 60th World Health Assembly took place, and the plan for oral health and integrated disease prevention was addressed. They confirmed the approach of the 2003 report as well as the development of oral health programs, especially in developing countries (Petersen, 2008).

The World Health Organization Global Oral Health Programme (2008) strives to increase awareness of oral health throughout the world and to integrate it as an important component of general health and quality of life. Oral-related diseases continue to be a major public health epidemic in high-income countries, and the burden of oral disease continues to escalate in underdeveloped and middle-income countries. The main thrust of oral disease prevention is aimed at promoting oral health. Oral health promotion must be integrated into chronic disease prevention and detection, as well as general health promotion, in hopes to increase early detection and prevention of oral health issues in addition to reduction of oral cancers. Risks to oral health and overall health are highly correlated. The Global Oral Health Programme policy proposed the development or adjustment of oral health programs at the national level (Petersen, 2008, 2009).

Epidemiology of Oral Diseases

Poor oral health and oral diseases are a major public health problem in America and worldwide (Douglass & Maier, 2008). They have a significant effect on individuals and communities, causing pain and suffering, impairment of function, and diminished quality of life. A core group of modifiable risk factors play a considerable role in oral health and include tobacco cessation, reduced alcohol consumption, optimal nutrition status, and maintenance of periodontal health. It is estimated that most adults show signs of periodontal or gingival disease, and about 14% of people ages 45–54 have severe periodontal disease. Furthermore, 23% of older adults (ages 65–74) have severe periodontal disease (U.S. DHHS, 2000). Most older adults take both prescribed and over-the-counter medications; at least one medication will cause an oral side effect (see Table 1-1). The most common side effect is xerostomia, or dry mouth. Most older adults lose their dental insurance when they convert to Medicare (Petersen, 2003).

Table 1-1. Medications: Causes of Oral Manifestations

Drug Classification	Specific Drug	Oral Manifestation
Analgesics	Aspirin	Hemorrhage, erythema multiforme
	Nonsteroidal anti-inflammatory drugs	Hemorrhage
	Barbiturates, codeine	Erythema multiforme
Anesthetics (local)	Benzocaine, lidocaine, procaine hydrochloride	Taste alterations
Antiarrhythmics	Procainamide	Lupus-like reaction
	Quinidine	Lichenoid mucosal reaction
Antibiotics	All	Oral candidiasis
	Erythromycin	Hypersensitivity reaction, stomatitis
	Penicillin	Hypersensitivity reaction, erythema multiforme, stomatitis
	Chloramphenicol, ciprofloxacin, clindamycin, dapsone, isoniazid, sulfa antibiotics, tetracyclines	Erythema multiforme
	Minocycline	Melanosis
	Chlorhexidine	Brown pigmentation of teeth and tongue
	Ampicillin, metronidazole, sulfasalazine, tetracyclines	Taste alterations
Anticoagulants	All	Hemorrhage
Anticonvulsants	Carbamazepine	Erythema multiforme, taste alterations
	Phenytoin	Erythema multiforme, gingival enlargement, taste alterations
Antidiarrheals	Bismuth	Dark pigmentation of tongue
Antihistamines	All	Xerostomia
Antihypertensives	All	Xerostomia
	Calcium channel blockers	Gingival enlargement
	Angiotensin-converting enzyme inhibitors	Stomatitis, pemphigus vulgaris
	Hydralazine	Lupus-like reaction, erythema multiforme
	Thiazide diuretics	Lichenoid mucosal reaction

(Continued on next page)

Table 1-1. Medications: Causes of Oral Manifestations *(Continued)*

Drug Classification	Specific Drug	Oral Manifestation
Antihypertensives *(Cont.)*	Minoxidil, verapamil	Erythema multiforme
	Amiloride, captopril, diltia-zem, enalapril, nifedi-pine	Taste alterations
Antilipidemics	Cholestyramine, clofibrate	Taste alterations
Antineoplastics	All	Oral candidiasis, oral hemorrhage, recurrent oral viral infections, stomatitis/mucositis, taste alterations
Antiparkinsonians	All	Xerostomia
	Levodopa	Taste alterations
Antipyretics/ anti-inflammatory agents	Allopurinol, colchicines, dexamethasone, hydro-cortisone, levamisole, salicylates	Taste alterations
Anti-reflux	All	Xerostomia
	Cimetidine	Erythema multiforme
Antithyroids	Carbimazole, methimazole, methylthiouracil, propyl-thiouracil	Taste alterations
Anxiolytics	Benzodiazepines	Xerostomia
Corticosteroids	All	Oral candidiasis, recurrent oral viral infections, stomatitis
Hypoglycemics	Sulfonylureas	Erythema multiforme
Immunosuppres-sants	Cyclosporine	Gingival enlargement
Muscle relaxants	All	Xerostomia
	Baclofen, chlorzoxazone	Taste alterations
Psychotropics	All	Xerostomia
	Phenothiazines	Oral pigmentation, tardive dyskinesia
	Lithium carbonate	Erythema multiforme, taste alterations

(Continued on next page)

Table 1-1. Medications: Causes of Oral Manifestations *(Continued)*		
Drug Classification	Specific Drug	Oral Manifestation
Vasodilators	Nitroglycerin	Taste alterations

Note. From "Oral Manifestations of Systemic Disease" (pp. 1495–1496), by J.A. Ship and E.M. Ghezzi in C.W. Cummings, P.W. Flint, L.A. Harker, B.H. Haughey, M.A. Richardson, K.T. Robbins, … J.R. Thomas (Eds.), *Cummings Otolaryngology: Head and Neck Surgery* (4th ed.), 2005, Philadelphia, PA: Elsevier Mosby. Retrieved from http://www.mdconsult.com. Copyright 2005 by Elsevier. Adapted with permission.

Anatomy of the Oral Cavity

The word *oral* means "mouth" in Latin and other languages. However, oral health encompasses not only the mouth but also the teeth, gingiva, and their supporting connective tissues, ligaments, and bone. The teeth are small, calcified, whitish structures found in the mouth. As a child, 20 primary teeth, also called deciduous or baby teeth, are present. All primary teeth are replaced with permanent teeth. As an individual reaches early adulthood, 32 permanent teeth are present in the mouth—16 in the maxilla and 16 in the mandible. The maxillary teeth are the maxillary central incisor, maxillary lateral incisor, maxillary canine, maxillary first molar, maxillary second molar, and maxillary third molar. The mandibular teeth are the mandibular central incisor, mandibular lateral incisor, mandibular canine, mandibular first molar, mandibular second molar, and mandibular third molar. The third molars are also referred to as wisdom teeth. The teeth have various components, including the enamel, dentin, cementum, and pulp. Tooth enamel is the hardest and most highly mineralized substance of the body. The normal color of enamel varies from light yellow to grayish white. Dentin is the substance between the enamel and the pulp chamber. It is a mineralized connective tissue that is softer than enamel but decays more rapidly and can lead to an increased incidence of dental caries. Cementum is a bony substance covering the root of the tooth. It serves as a medium for periodontal ligaments to ensure bone stability. The pulp is the central portion of the tooth that is filled with connective tissue. This tissue (pulp) consists of blood vessels and nerves and is commonly referred to as the nerve of the tooth (Rout & Brown, 2008).

The oral cavity is a complex organ that is composed of muscles, glands, teeth, and specialized sensory receptors. It includes the hard and soft palates, mucosal lining of the mouth and throat, the tongue, lips, salivary glands, masticator muscles, upper and lower jaws, and temporomandibular joint (TMJ) (see Figure 1-1). The oral cavity carries out three critical functions: intake of solids and liquids, communication/speech, and protec-

Figure 1-1. Anatomy of the Oral Cavity

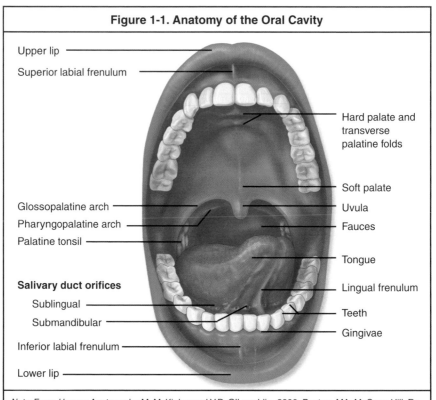

Note. From *Human Anatomy*, by M. McKinley and V.D. O'Loughlin, 2006, Boston, MA: McGraw-Hill. Retrieved from http://academic.kellogg.cc.mi.us/herbrandsonc/bio201_McKinley/f26-3a_oral_cavity_ante_c.jpg. Copyright by the McGraw-Hill Companies, Inc. Reprinted with permission.

tion of the host from noxious substances. The functions of the oral structures are sensory, motor, and specialized sensory in nature. Sensory function of the oral cavity is provided by the maxillary and mandibular branches of the trigeminal nerve (cranial nerve [CN] V) and the glossopharyngeal nerve (CN IX). Oral motor functions include mastication, swallowing, respiration, and speech.

Swallowing is a complex neuromuscular function involving the oral cavity, pharynx, larynx, and esophagus. Swallowing consists of four stages. First is the oral preparatory stage, which is mechanical and reduces food to a pulverized consistency, as well as mobilizing food on the floor of the mouth or against the hard palate with the lateral rolling motion of tongue. Second is the oral stage, which is also mechanical and is designed to move food from the front of the oral cavity to the pharynx. Next, the pharyngeal stage is physiologic, as coordination must exist between the lower brain stem and the respiratory system. During this phase, respiration must cease for a fraction of a second when the airway closes during pharyngeal swallowing. Last is the esophageal stage, which occurs when the food bolus has passed through the cricopharyngeal opening or upper esophageal sphincter. Normal esophageal transit may take 8–20 seconds. The duration of swallowing increases with age (Travers & Travers, 2005).

Specialized sensory functions include taste and its interaction with saliva. Taste, also referred to as gustation, is a function of direct chemoreception and is one of the five traditional senses. Taste is defined as the ability to detect the flavor of certain substances such as food, minerals, and poisons and is a sensory function of the central nervous system. Receptor cells located within the taste buds mediate taste perception. These receptor cells are located on the surface of the tongue, soft palate, epithelium of the pharynx, and epiglottis. The taste receptors detect chemical signals, leading to release of neurotransmitters, which transmit the signal to brain stem. The three cranial nerves responsible for taste are the facial nerve (CN VII) for the anterior two-thirds of the tongue, the glossopharyngeal nerve (CN IX) for the posterior one-third of the tongue, and the vagus nerve (CN X) for the epiglottis. The four most common taste sensations in the Western hemisphere are sweet, salty, sour, and bitter. In the Eastern hemisphere, piquance (i.e., the sensation provided by chili peppers) and savoriness (or *umami*) have also been identified as basic taste sensations. Most recently, three other taste categories have been identified: fatty acid, metallic, and water tastes. Any alteration in the release of neurotransmitters will lead to taste dysfunction (Smith & Margolskee, 2006). Common terms used for taste alterations include *ageusia* (complete loss of taste) and *dysgeusia* (persistent abnormal taste).

Saliva is an extremely important component of oral health and has five distinct functions, including lubrication and protection; buffering and clearance; maintenance of tooth integrity; antibacterial activity; and taste and digestion. Saliva is a sero-mucous substance that coats the structures of the oral cavity. It is a complex mixture of electrolytes and macromolecules secreted from major and minor salivary glands. The dominant salivary glands are the parotid, submandibular, and sublingual glands. The minor salivary glands coat the lip, tongue, palate, and pharynx. Saliva assists in the functions of speech, mastication, and swallowing. It is made up of several buffer systems such as bicarbonate and is slightly alkaline. The buffering and clearance properties of saliva are known to prevent dental caries. Saliva plays a role in remineralization, in which it replaces minerals lost from the crystalline matrix of the enamel. It also has an antibacterial function; it contains immunologic mediators such as IgA, IgG, and IgM, which aggregate bacteria and prevent it from adhering to the oral soft and hard palates. Saliva plays a major role in the preservation of taste. It assists in the solubilization of ingested food particles, the transport of taste substances to taste receptors, and the protection of those receptors. Saliva helps to bathe and hydrate the taste receptors (Brosky, 2007; Elluru & Kumar, 2005).

Common Oral Conditions

The most common oral care problems are dental caries and periodontal disease, gingivitis, and periodontitis. All are caused by numerous factors, including dental plaque, nutrition and dietary factors, oral hygiene, genetics, environment, and lifestyle behaviors (Wood, 2006).

Dental caries are the most common chronic illness during childhood. Early childhood caries is an infection with associated decay in the primary teeth of young children between the ages of one and six years old (Limbo, 2006). Objective findings include visible lesions in the teeth at the gum line, discoloration of tooth enamel, or uneven ridges or broken enamel (see Figure 1-2). The functions of primary teeth include proper chewing, aiding in speech and pronunciation, guiding proper eruption of the permanent teeth, and maintaining arch integrity.

If dental caries are untreated, they can result in irreversible damage to other teeth with associated pain, difficulty with eating and drinking, and infection. This can lead to complete erosion and disintegration of teeth, resulting in systemic infections (see Figure 1-3). Causes of dental caries include (a) frequent intake of fermentable carbohydrates, (b) acquisition of microbes such

Figure 1-2. Dental Caries

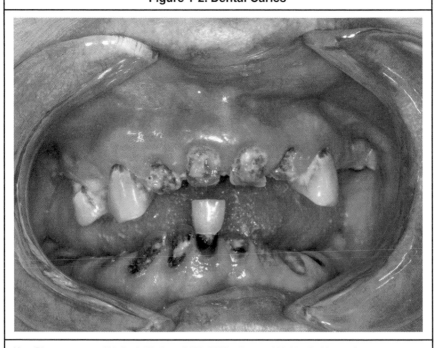

Note. Photo courtesy of Nathaniel Treister, DMD, DMSc, Boston, MA. Used with permission.

Figure 1-3. Tooth Erosion

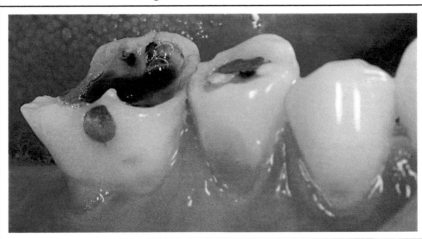

Note. Photo courtesy of Kevin Guze, MD, Harvard Medical School. Used with permission.

as *Streptococcus mutans*, *Streptococcus sobrinus*, and *Lactobacillus*, and (c) delayed early dental care.

The American Academy of Pediatrics (2003) issued a policy statement advocating that oral health evaluations, risk assessments, and parent education be initiated at six months of age and that establishment of dental practices within the home should be achieved by 12 months of age. Oral maintenance includes initiation of oral hygiene at infancy with oral cleaning after each feeding, at least twice-daily brushing or wiping of the teeth once they erupt through the gums, limited exposure to fermented carbohydrates, awareness of medications with added sweeteners, inclusion of caries risk assessment, and early dental referral. Preventive care measures have been proved to reduce the incidence of oral disease. Preventive measures include the use of varnishes, toothpastes, and rinses with fluoride; dental sealants; and increased awareness of the need for oral hygiene and biannual care (U.S. DHHS, 2000). The U.S. Preventive Services Task Force recommendations for prevention of dental caries include oral fluoride supplementation to preschool children older than six months of age whose water source is deficient in fluoride. Dental caries or missing teeth can make it difficult to bite and chew, leading to compromised oral function. In turn, the consequences of impaired nutrition status, risk of systemic diseases, altered body image, and decreased quality of life can occur (Wood, 2006).

Periodontal disease includes gingivitis and periodontitis, which are both plaque-induced inflammatory conditions that are considered infectious in nature. The inflammatory process significantly affects periodontal health. Dental plaque releases gram-positive and gram-negative bacteria that colonize on the tooth surface around the gingiva. These molecules penetrate the gingival tissues and elicit a host response leading to gingivitis (Gurenlian, 2009). Gingivitis is a reversible condition that begins when the bacteria in plaque cause gum inflammation (see Figure 1-4). Objective findings of gingivitis include redness, swelling, spontaneous bleeding, and the presence of pus. Signs of advanced disease may include periodontal pocketing or apical tissue migration along the tooth root. Periodontal pocketing is defined as an abnormal gingival sulcus where the gum comes in contact with a tooth and leads to edema, irritation, and inflammation. Recommendations for preventing gingivitis include daily brushing and flossing and regular dental care by a dentist or dental hygienist. If gingivitis is untreated or neglected, it can progress to periodontitis. Patients with periodontitis have increased levels of proinflammatory mediators, such as C-reactive protein, fibrinogen, interleukin-1, and interleukin-6 (Gurenlian, 2009). Periodontitis is an irreversible condition that ultimately destroys the mandible, leading to loss of teeth (see Figure 1-5) (Loesche, 2007).

Oral piercings of the tongue, cheeks, and lips can increase the risk of tooth chipping, gum recession, and periodontal disease (Silk & Romano-Clark, 2009). The use of tobacco can lead to tooth staining and gum disease, as well as an increased risk of certain cancers. Alcohol use can increase the risk of periodontal disease and dental caries and has a synergistic effect with tobacco use. Recreational drug use can increase the risk of oral conditions such as

---

Figure 1-4. Gingivitis

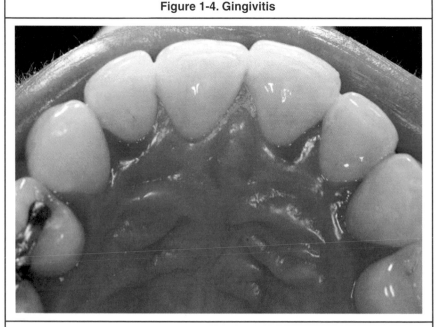

Note. Photo courtesy of Kevin Guze, MD, Harvard Medical School. Used with permission.

Figure 1-5. Periodontitis

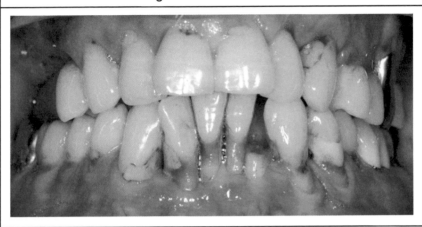

Note. Photo courtesy of Kevin Guze, MD, Harvard Medical School. Used with permission.

xerostomia, bruxism (tooth grinding), and severe tooth decay and erosion, also referred to as "meth mouth." When cocaine is applied to the gingivae, it can cause lip disease, tongue pain, gingivitis, and bruxism (Silk & Romano-Clark, 2009; Wood, 2006).

Oral Health and Overall General Health

The oral cavity has frequently been referred to as a window into a person's body. Research focus has shifted to investigate the potential impact of periodontal diseases on general health. Oral health and general state of health have many correlations. The biologic mechanism of this relationship is beginning to evolve (Gurenlian, 2009). Many systemic medical conditions present as oral manifestations. The burden of oral diseases and oral manifestations of other medical conditions is significant. Systemic diseases that have oral manifestations include disorders of the bone, cardiovascular disease, cerebrovascular disease, collagen-vascular conditions, skin disorders, endocrine conditions such as diabetes, genetic disorders, gastrointestinal disorders, hematologic diseases, infections, liver diseases, neoplastic processes, neurologic conditions, pulmonary diseases such as chronic obstructive pulmonary disease, and renal disease. Medications also can cause oral manifestations in patients (Blende, 2008; Hughes, 2007; Loesche, 2007; Ship & Ghezzi, 2005).

Oral health and its relationship to other medical conditions are significant in the care of patients and can influence the plan of care, overall outcome, and nursing care. With the burden of other medical conditions, poor oral health, and utilization of various medications throughout the health/illness continuum, the diagnosis of cancer exacerbates and complicates the overall care of patients. Healthcare professionals must obtain a history of medical, surgical, and oral conditions as part of a thorough assessment of oral manifestations. The manifestations of cancer and its treatment may exacerbate oral health issues. The next section will discuss the various oral manifestations associated with medical conditions.

Common Oral Manifestations of Systemic Medical Diseases

Bone Disorders

Many arthritic conditions can cause oral manifestations. Rheumatoid arthritis is a progressive destruction of articular and periarticular structures, including the TMJ. The signs and symptoms of TMJ disease are clicking, locking, crepitation, tenderness to palpation of the preauricular area, and pain during mandibular movement, although TMJ disease has many other causes (Delozier, 2008; Kelsey & Lamster, 2008; Ship & Ghezzi, 2005). Osteoarthritis has fewer oral manifestations but is related to one's inability to perform certain activities, including oral hygiene, secondary to pain and mobility (Ship & Ghezzi, 2005).

Cardiac Disease

Cardiac disease, such as ischemic heart disease, myocardial infarction, and hypertension, may have oral manifestations. Angina-like pain can often be characterized as referred pain to the neck, clavicle, and mandible. The differential diagnosis may include dental caries, periodontal disease, TMJ disease, musculoskeletal pain, neuropathic pain, and myocardial infarction. Several epidemiologic studies have shown an association between heart disease and dental and periodontal diseases (Beck, Offenbacher, Williams, Gibbs, & Garcia, 1998; Hughes, 2007; Loesche, 2000). The treatment of cardiac disease with medications also has a deleterious effect on oral hygiene. Antihypertensives have been shown to cause salivary dysfunction, especially diuretics, calcium channel blockers, and beta-blockers. In addition, calcium channel blockers have been shown to cause gingival enlargement; angiotensin-converting enzyme inhibitors and calcium channel blockers can cause taste disturbances; and thiazide diuretics can cause lichenoid mucosal reactions. For patients undergoing cardiac transplantation, immunosuppressive therapies that are noted in the development of oral opportunistic infections, such as herpes simplex and oral candidiasis, are used (Ship & Ghezzi, 2005). Cyclosporine, an immunosuppressive agent, has been reported to cause gingival enlargement in as many as 13%–85% of patients (Meraw & Sheridan, 1998). Patients receiving anticoagulation therapy may present with hemorrhagic lesions of the oral mucosa (Ship & Ghezzi, 2005).

Cerebrovascular Diseases

Cerebrovascular accident (CVA) can lead to permanent oral sensory and motor deficits. This is manifested by poor tongue function and lip seal, difficulty with eating and drinking, and altered use and fit of dentures. These can lead to nutrition deficiencies and diminished quality of life caused by impaired food and fluid intake. These motor, sensory, and cognitive alterations can cause deleterious effects on oral health and function. The oral-facial deficits are determined by the location of the cerebrovascular event in the brain. CVA that occurs within the left cerebral cortex can cause right-sided paralysis and difficulty with auditory memory, speech, language, and swallowing. Right-cortex CVA can cause left-sided paralysis with subsequent neglect of the affected side, pharyngeal dysfunction with the potential for aspiration, and difficulty with memory and performing certain tasks. Oral-facial motor and sensory impairment can lead to improper dental and denture hygiene with food accumulation or pocketing around teeth. This is a risk factor for dental and periodontal diseases and oral microbial infections. Excessive drooling can lead to angular cheilitis (Blende, 2008; Jimenez, Krall, Garcia, Vokonas, & Dietrich, 2009; Ship & Ghezzi, 2005). Angular cheilitis is erythematous, cracked lesions located in the corners of the lips (see Figure 1-6).

Figure 1-6. Angular Cheilitis

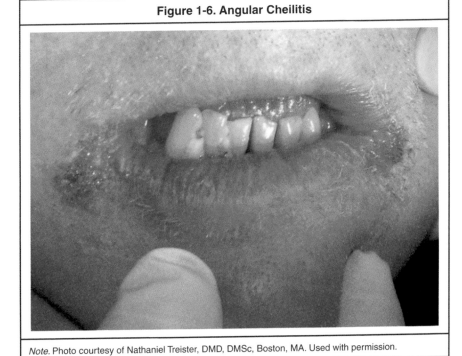

Note. Photo courtesy of Nathaniel Treister, DMD, DMSc, Boston, MA. Used with permission.

Anticoagulation therapy in patients who have had a stroke can produce hemorrhage, petechiae, ecchymosis, or purpura of all mucosal tissues, including the oral cavity. Periodontal disease and tooth loss have been associated with increased risk of stroke. Infectious oral disease is thought to initiate the proliferation of inflammatory cells and clotting factors, which increases the risk for atherosclerotic and thromboembolic events (Blende, 2008; Joshipura, 2002).

Collagen-Vascular Disorders

Many autoimmune disorders cause oral manifestations. The most common is Sjögren syndrome, which is associated with inflammation of the epithelial tissues, resulting in xerostomia and salivary gland dysfunction. It has two forms. The primary form involves the salivary and lacrimal glands and leads to decreased production of saliva and tears. The secondary form commonly occurs with other autoimmune diseases such as rheumatoid arthritis, lupus, scleroderma, polymyositis, and polyarteritis nodosa. Xerostomia, or dry mouth, leads to an increased risk for the development of dental caries, oral microbial infections, dysphagia, dysgeusia, impaired eating, and problems with dentures (Ship & Ghezzi, 2005).

Lupus is another autoimmune disorder, in which 25% of patients will develop superficial, erythematous ulcers within the oral cavity (Ship & Ghezzi, 2005). They generally occur on the lips and oral mucosa.

Scleroderma can cause fibrosis of the masticatory muscles secondary to collagen deposits. Patients may experience difficulty opening their mouth, as well as immobility of the tongue and dysphagia. Scleroderma is often associated with other autoimmune disorders such as Sjögren syndrome. Xerostomia is another common oral manifestation in these patients (Ship & Ghezzi, 2005).

Dermatomyositis-polymyositis is another autoimmune disease that affects the muscles of the tongue and upper esophagus, leading to difficulty with phonation, chewing, and dysphagia. A medical complication of dysphagia is aspiration pneumonia. Sarcoidosis is a systemic granulomatous condition that can cause masses (granulomas) on the tongue, lips, mandible, and maxilla (Ship & Ghezzi, 2005).

Dermatologic Conditions

Many dermatologic autoimmune conditions affect oral health. Lichen planus, a chronic, mucocutaneous autoimmune disorder, causes plaque-like, bullous, atrophic, erosive lesions. These lesions can occur on the buccal mucosa, gingiva, and tongue. Another autoimmune condition is pemphigus vulgaris. This is characterized by bullous lesions developing into vesicles. The most common locations are the palate, buccal mucosa, and tongue (Ship & Ghezzi, 2005).

A common finding with any hypersensitivity reaction is erythema multiforme, which causes blistering oral and skin lesions. Symptoms include acute development of vesicles with a subsequent rupture causing painful ulcers of the clinical mucosa, lips, palate, and tongue (Ship & Ghezzi, 2005).

Endocrine Disorders

Many endocrine conditions can cause oral problems, including diabetes mellitus, adrenal abnormalities, and diseases of the pituitary, thyroid, and parathyroid glands. Patients with diabetes mellitus are known to have an increased incidence of oral diseases. Some clinical studies have suggested that patients with controlled diabetes have the same incidence of oral disease as the general population. Periodontal disease is the most common oral disease seen in the diabetic population. It has been shown that patients with poor glycemic control have increased incidence and progression of periodontal disease. With poorly controlled diabetes, patients exhibit sensory and peripheral neuropathies, which can lead to taste and smell alterations (Kunzel, Lalla, & Lamster, 2007; Ship & Ghezzi, 2005; Skamagas, Breen, & LeRoith, 2008).

Hypoadrenalism or Addison disease can cause oral manifestations including diffuse, cutaneous pigmentation of the skin and mucous membranes. Patients with hyperadrenalism or Cushing disease may exhibit oral infections, such as oral candidiasis, or muscle weakness, which will manifest through difficulty with speaking and eating and dysphagia. Diseases of the pituitary gland, such as acromegaly (a chronic hypersecretion of growth hormone), can cause overgrowth of the bony and soft tissue in the oral-facial region. Other complications include tooth separation and malocclusion secondary to alveolar enlargement of the maxilla and mandible. Oral-facial changes include frontal bossing (an unusually prominent forehead), nasal bone hypertrophy, mandibular prognathism, and enlargement of the paraspinal sinuses. Overgrowth of soft tissue can occur in the oral mucosa and salivary gland tissues, tonsils, and lips.

Disease of the thyroid gland can cause problems with oral health. Patients with hypothyroidism are likely to have macroglossia, which is thickening of the tongue, pronounced lips, and delayed tooth eruption. Patients with hyperthyroidism or Graves disease can develop hyperplasia of the tonsillar and oropharyngeal regions (Roggow, 2009; Ship & Ghezzi, 2005).

Genetic Disorders

Although genetic disorders are relatively rare, they can affect oral health. Turner syndrome, also referred to as gonadal dysgenesis, is a condition characterized by absence of a sex chromosome in females, leading to physical abnormalities, amenorrhea, and sterility, as well as palate abnormalities. Marfan syndrome is an autosomal dominant trait leading to a genetic disorder of the connective tissue and causes hard palate defects such as cleft lip and palate. Gaucher disease is a genetic disease in which lipids accumulate in cells and certain organs. In particular, radiolucent lesions in the jaw are seen. Osteopetrosis is a rare inherited disorder that is characterized by the inability of osteoclasts to resorb bone, thereby leading to hardened bones. This is often seen in the mandible and maxilla (Ship & Ghezzi, 2005).

Gastrointestinal Disorders

Recurrent oral aphthous ulcers (canker sores) are common in patients with Crohn disease, inflammatory bowel disease, and ulcerative colitis. Patients with gastroesophageal reflux disease (GERD) may develop erosions in the oral cavity and gingivae secondary to acid. Severe GERD can lead to erosion of tooth enamel. Disorders resulting from vitamin deficiencies can affect oral health. For example, patients with celiac disease or gluten-sensitive enteropathy can develop aphthous ulcers. Vitamin A deficiency can manifest as dyskeratotic changes of the skin and mucous membranes, angular cheilitis, and alterations in the dentin and enamel of developing teeth. Riboflavin (vitamin B_2) deficiency can also cause angular cheilitis. Folate (vitamin B_{12}) deficiency can cause aphthous ulcers. Pellagra, or niacin deficiency, can cause tongue swelling. Vitamin C deficiency (scurvy) can cause petechiae in the mouth, leading to gingival hyperplasia and stomatitis. Vitamin D deficiency will complicate calcium metabolism and can contribute to mandible osteopenia or osteoporosis. Vitamin K deficiency leads to hemorrhagic diathesis, which often presents with oral hemorrhagic bullae. These bullae are similar to the appearance of a blister. Zinc deficiency has been associated with taste alterations (Huber, 2008; Ship & Ghezzi, 2005; Wood, 2006).

Hematologic Disorders

Anticoagulation therapy can lead to hemorrhagic oral lesions such as petechiae, ecchymosis, and purpura in the oral cavity. Other conditions that can cause bleeding within the oral cavity include Von Willebrand disease and hemophilia A. Both are disorders involving factor VIII, which normally prevents or controls bleeding. Alterations in factor VIII can lead to hemorrhage (Ship & Ghezzi, 2005).

Alterations in white blood cells, as seen with leukemia, can cause oral mucosa changes. These changes include bleeding, ulceration, petechiae, and gingival hyperplasia. In immunocompromised patients, the development of bacterial, fungal, and viral infections is common. Chemotherapy also can cause mucositis and mucosal alterations. In addition, poor oral hygiene can result in gingival inflammation, bleeding, mucosal ulcerations, and dental disease. Graft-versus-host disease (GVHD) is common in the bone marrow and stem cell transplantation arena. Oral sequelae of GVHD include mucosal ulcerations, mucositis, xerostomia, and dysphagia (Ship & Ghezzi, 2005).

Anemia can cause pale oral mucosa, whereas vitamin B_{12} deficiency and iron-deficiency anemia can cause loss of tongue papillae and angular cheilitis. Plummer-Vinson syndrome is a complication of severe anemia that leads to oral soreness, dysphagia, and increases in oral and pharyngeal cancers (Ship & Ghezzi, 2005).

Infectious Diseases

The herpes family of viruses includes herpes simplex virus-1 (HSV-1) (predominantly oral), herpes simplex virus-2 (predominantly genital but can be oral), varicella zoster (chicken pox and shingles), Epstein-Barr virus (nasopharyngeal carcinoma, mononucleosis, and hairy leukoplakia), cytomegalovirus (opportunistic infection in the immunocompromised host), and Kaposi sarcoma–associated herpes virus (Centers for Disease Control and Prevention, 2010). The two most common that affect oral health are HSV-1 and varicella zoster. HSV-1 presents as oral stomatitis, whereas varicella zoster presents as acute painful oral-facial lesions. These infections usually occur during childhood and become reactivated secondary to immunosuppression, trauma, stress, sunlight, gastrointestinal disorders, and concurrent infection. People with HIV or AIDS may develop oral complications secondary to their immunocompromised state, as well as HIV-related malignancies (Epstein, 2007). The most common presenting oral conditions with AIDS are oral candidiasis, Kaposi sarcoma, and hairy leukoplakia (a white, flat patch that is caused by the Epstein-Barr virus). Periodontal disease is very common in HIV-infected patients. Cytomegalovirus is a common infection in the general and HIV population and occurs in about 90% of patients with HIV (Centers for Disease Control and Prevention, 2010; Ship & Ghezzi, 2005). Cytomegalovirus can cause oral ulcerations and esophagitis.

The most common oral fungal infection is *Candida albicans* (see Figure 1-7). This is associated with diabetes, immunosuppression, nutrition disturbances,

Figure 1-7. Oral Candidiasis

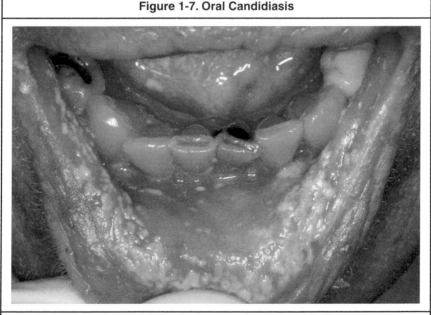

Note. Photo courtesy of Nathaniel Treister, DMD, DMSc, Boston, MA. Used with permission.

certain medications, salivary gland hypofunction, and poor oral and denture hygiene. The oral manifestations of candidiasis include pseudomembranous appearance (white, easily removable patches), erythematous or atrophic lesions, chronic hyperplastic/dentures stomatitis, which are lesions found underneath dentures, and angular cheilitis. The oral cavity is a common place for many kinds of bacteria that are responsible for causing oral and pharyngeal infections. Two bacteria, *Porphyromonas gingivalis* and *Treponema denticola*, play a major role in the development of periodontal disease. *Staphylococcus aureus* and *Staphylococcus viridians* play a role in the salivary gland infections. The development of new and recurrent dental caries is most commonly caused by *Streptococcus mutans* and *Lactobacillus* species (Ship & Ghezzi, 2005).

Oral disorders can be seen with sexually transmitted diseases. They are most commonly caused by *Neisseria gonorrhoeae* and *Treponema pallidum*. Common oral findings include stomatitis and pharyngeal infection with gonorrhea and chancre with syphilis. Primary syphilis can cause a chancre, and secondary syphilis can be associated with papular lesions, erythematous or grayish-white erosions, pharyngitis, lymphadenopathy, and parotid enlargement (Gennaro, Naidoo, & Berthold, 2008; Ship & Ghezzi, 2005).

Liver Disease

Chronic alcoholism has been shown to correlate with poor oral hygiene resulting in dental caries and periodontal disease. Alcohol has a deleterious effect on oral health and is related to decreased neutrophil, macrophage, and T-cell function. Many nutrition disturbances occur in alcoholism, which can cause glossitis and recurrent oral infections. Excessive alcohol intake and tobacco use have a synergistic effect and are major components in the development of oral cancers. Patients with cirrhosis commonly develop oral infections and have problems with wound healing. Patients receiving liver transplants are at risk for developing oral infections secondary to immunosuppressive agents (Ship & Ghezzi, 2005).

Malignant Neoplasms

Cancers of the oral cavity and oropharynx represent approximately 3% of all cancers in the United States. Approximately 90% of all head and neck cancers are squamous cell carcinoma and generally occur within the lips, floor of mouth, posterior lateral borders of the tongue, and posterior oropharynx (Jemal, Siegel, Xu, & Ward, 2010). Tobacco and alcohol use are responsible for up to 75% of oral cancers (Gonsalves, Wrightson, & Henry, 2008). The common presenting signs include nonhealing ulcerated leukoplakia and erythematous lesions. Cancer treatments either directly or indirectly affect oral health and function. These treatments are generally multimodal in nature, using a combination of surgery, chemotherapy, and/or radiation therapy. Surgery can be very complex and radical, leading to neck and facial disfiguration, dysphagia, altered speech and mastication, trismus, facial and oral paresthesias, salivary gland dysfunction, and diminished neck and shoulder mobility. The delivery of radiation therapy can result in mucositis, dysphagia, permanent salivary gland dysfunction, smell and taste dysfunction, oral microbial infections, and an increased risk of developing osteoradionecrosis. Common oral infections include herpes simplex, varicella zoster, and oral candidiasis. Most chemotherapeutic agents can cause mucositis, salivary hypofunction, smell and taste dysfunction, diminished appetite, and an increased susceptibility to oral microbial infections. Because of the significant morbidity of cancer treatment modalities, patients require frequent, long-term follow-up with dental professionals (Ship & Ghezzi, 2005).

Neurologic Diseases

The chronicity and deterioration that come with dementia are associated with the inability to perform activities of daily living and a loss of independence. This negatively affects the quality of oral hygiene. It is known that patients with dementia have a greater prevalence of dental plaque, gingival bleeding, and calculus secondary to poor oral hygiene. Common medications used in this population include antidepressants, which have anticholinergic effects, thus leading to salivary dysfunction (Ship & Ghezzi, 2005).

Another common neurologic disorder that causes oral manifestations is Parkinson disease. Esophageal dysmotility and dysphagia secondary to Parkinson disease are thought to be caused by increased amounts of acetylcholine within the brain. Another common finding is the inability to seal the lips, causing drooling. Anticholinergic medications, such as levodopa and selegiline, are used in the treatment of Parkinson disease. They cause salivary dysfunction and xerostomia. Tardive dyskinesia is an adverse effect of levodopa, which causes involuntary orofacial movements including lip smacking, grimacing, and tongue clearing. Loss of facial expression, difficulty with mastication, slowed speech, and tremors of the lips are seen (Ship & Ghezzi, 2005).

Myasthenia gravis is a neurologic autoimmune disorder that blocks or destroys acetylcholine receptor sites, resulting in episodic muscle weakness, which can lead to dysphagia, subsequent choking, nasal regurgitation, and voice changes. Bell's palsy is unilateral facial paralysis, which is fairly common and is caused by a defect of the facial nerve (CN V). It leads to distortion of the face with a lack of control of the muscles for facial expression and functional ability of the lips and cheek on the affected side. This can lead to decreased natural cleansing on the affected side and tooth decay. Multiple sclerosis is the loss of muscle coordination resulting from the demyelination of long nerves. This is commonly manifested by weakness of the tongue and loss of upper extremity use, leading to severely impaired oral hygiene. Trigeminal neuralgia is common in these patients and is characterized by excruciating unilateral pain throughout the lips, gingivae, and chin (Ship & Ghezzi, 2005).

Pulmonary Diseases

Tobacco smoking is the most common risk factor for pulmonary disease. Tobacco plays a major deleterious role in oral health. The use of tobacco can cause nicotinic stomatitis and oral fungal infections. Little is known regarding the direct effects of chronic obstructive pulmonary disease on oral health other than the use of corticosteroids, which increase the incidence of oral fungal infections. Another pulmonary complication is aspiration pneumonia, which is caused by aspiration of gastric or oropharyngeal secretions. Swallowing dysfunction is a common finding in patients with neuromuscular and cerebrovascular diseases. As a result, colonization of the oropharynx with gram-negative bacilli predisposes this patient population to pneumonia. Another major harbor of anaerobic infection is the gingival crevice (Ship & Ghezzi, 2005).

Tuberculosis is the major global epidemic that occurs because of the spread of *Mycobacterium tuberculosis*. Oral manifestations, although infrequent, may include a painful, deep, irregular ulcer on the dorsum of the tongue, as well as on the palate, lips, buccal mucosa, and gingivae (Ship & Ghezzi, 2005).

Renal Diseases

Patients with renal disease also may experience oral manifestations. Patients requiring dialysis, either hemodialysis or peritoneal dialysis, are more susceptible to salivary hypofunction, impaired wound healing, recurrent oral mucosal infections, dental caries, gingivitis, or periodontitis. These problems generally are caused by the chronic use of corticosteroids and other immunosuppressants. Another oral condition is uremic stomatitis. It presents as an erythematous thickening of the buccal mucosa with a pseudomembranous covering, ulcerative lesions, gingival and mucosal hemorrhage, and ecchymosis. This is directly correlated to an elevated blood urea nitrogen level. Gingival hyperplasia and oral fungal infections are common in renal transplant recipients. They also have a greater incidence of oral lesions such as candidiasis, leukoplakia, dysplasia, and cancer of the lip (Gonyea, 2009; Ship & Ghezzi, 2005; Summers, Tilakaratne, Fortune, & Ashman, 2007).

Oral Manifestations During Women's Reproductive Years

Women experience many changes throughout their reproductive years, which include various oral changes caused by circulating hormones. During puberty, females experience many intraoral changes, such as inflammatory hyperplastic gingival reactions, which are caused by food debris. Eating disorders are commonly diagnosed during puberty. Bulimia and anorexia are often associated with self-induced vomiting and chronic regurgitation of gastric contents, which can cause tooth enamel erosion. Other oral manifestations include traumatized oral and pharyngeal mucosal tissue, angular cheilitis, dehydration, and parotid gland enlargement.

During menses, oral changes may include swollen and erythematous gingival tissues, development of aphthous ulcers, activation of herpes, prolonged hemorrhage following oral surgery, and swollen salivary glands. Oral contraceptive use can cause oral changes such as gingival inflammation and increased risk of a form of osteitis after third molar extraction, also known as "dry socket."

Pregnancy gingivitis is characterized by erythematous gingival and interproximal tissues. This is the most common dental condition during pregnancy and occurs in approximately two-thirds of all pregnancies (Ship & Ghezzi, 2005). The symptoms usually appear during the first trimester and continue throughout the pregnancy. Maternal periodontal disease has been identified as a possible precursor to preeclampsia, preterm birth, and growth restriction (Ship & Ghezzi, 2005).

Menopause is associated with oral manifestations such as burning mouth syndrome and xerostomia. Perimenopausal and postmenopausal women can experience gingival stomatitis, which is characterized as pale, dry, shiny, and bleeding gingival tissues (Hughes, 2007; Ship & Ghezzi, 2005).

Maintenance of Oral Hygiene and Health

Good oral hygiene is essential in the prevention of oral diseases. These practices need to start at infancy and continue throughout one's lifetime. Brushing with fluoridated toothpaste is the most effective approach to the removal of plaque. The removal of plaque will reduce the risk of tooth decay and gum disease. Dental flossing is another essential component in the removal of plaque between the teeth and under the gumline. Oral health recommendations are to see a dental professional on a regular basis for an oral evaluation and dental cleaning prophylaxis. These healthcare practices are even more essential when one's life is compounded by a cancer diagnosis and treatment.

The goals of oral health care are to educate the public about oral health, prevention, and maintenance of oral hygiene and to improve outcomes by increasing dental benefits through insurance coverage.

Conclusion

Oral care is a major health initiative throughout the world. The World Health Organization and the Surgeon General's Report on Oral Health stress the importance of reducing risk factors associated with oral disease (Petersen, 2008; U.S. DHHS, 2000). When oral health is affronted by the development of cancer and the use of various treatment modalities such as surgery, radiation, and chemotherapy, the problems become exacerbated. Cancer and its treatment significantly affect oral health. Oral consequences of cancer treatment can subsequently cause treatment delays or dose reductions, leading to decreased locoregional control, decreased quality of life, and reduced survival (Rosenthal, 2007). The most common oral manifestations of cancer and its treatment will be discussed throughout this book. The oral manifestations can have a significant effect on treatment delivery, overall outcome, and quality of life. This book will focus on the issues of oral health in the oncology population, including the acute and chronic toxicities of various treatment modalities. In addition, this book will focus on oral assessment and dental hygiene, oral management strategies, and survivorship issues.

References

American Academy of Pediatrics. (2003). Oral health risk assessment timing and establishment of the dental home [Policy statement]. *Pediatrics, 111,* 1113–1115. doi:10.1542/peds.111.5.1113

Beck, J., Offenbacher, S., Williams, R., Gibbs, P., & Garcia, R. (1998). Periodontitis: A risk factor for coronary heart disease? *Annals of Periodontology, 3,* 127–141.

Blende, D. (2008). Your mouth: A window to your overall health. *Exceptional Parent Magazine, 38*(5), 44–47.

Brosky, M. (2007). The role of saliva in oral health: Strategies for prevention and management of xerostomia. *Journal of Supportive Oncology, 5,* 215–225.

Centers for Disease Control and Prevention. (2010). Cytomegalovirus and congenital CMV infection. Retrieved from http://www.cdc.gov/cmv/overview.html

Delozier, C. (2008). Inflammation: Its impact on oral health and the total body. *Access, 2*(7), 2–3.

Douglass, A.B., & Maier, R. (2008). Promoting oral health: The family physician's role. *American Family Physician, 78,* 814–815.

Elluru, R.G., & Kumar, M. (2005). Physiology of the salivary glands. In C.W. Cummings, P.W. Flint, L.A. Harker, B.H. Haughey, M.A. Richardson, K.T. Robbins, … J.R. Thomas (Eds.), *Cummings otolaryngology: Head and neck surgery* (4th ed., pp. 1293–1312). Philadelphia, PA: Elsevier Mosby. Retrieved from http://www.mdconsult.com

Epstein, J.B. (2007). Oral malignancies associated with HIV. *Journal of the Canadian Dental Association, 73,* 953–956.

Gennaro, S., Naidoo, S., & Berthold, P. (2008). Oral health and HIV/AIDS. *MCN: The American Journal of Maternal/Child Nursing, 33,* 50–57. doi:10.1097/01.NMC.0000305658.32237.7d

Gonsalves, W.C., Wrightson, A.S., & Henry, R.G. (2008). Common oral conditions in older persons. *American Family Physician, 78,* 845–852.

Gonyea, J. (2009). Oral health care for patients on dialysis. *Nephrology Nursing Journal, 36,* 327–328, 332.

Gurenlian, J.R. (2009). Inflammation: The relationship between oral health and systemic disease. *Dental Assistant, 78*(2), 8–40.

Huber, M.A. (2008). Gastrointestinal illnesses and their effects on the oral cavity. *Oral and Maxillofacial Surgery Clinics of North America, 20,* 625–634. doi:10.1016/j.coms.2008.06.005

Hughes, P. (2007). Women, aging and oral health needs. *Access, 21*(5), 1–13.

Jemal, A., Siegel, R., Xu, J., & Ward, E. (2010). Cancer statistics, 2010. *CA: A Cancer Journal for Clinicians, 60,* 277–300. doi:10.1002/caac.20073

Jimenez, M., Krall, E.A., Garcia, R.I., Vokonas, P.S., & Dietrich, T. (2009). Periodontitis and incidence of cerebrovascular disease in men. *Annals of Neurology, 66,* 505–512. doi:10.1002/ana.21742

Joshipura, K. (2002). The relationship between oral conditions and ischemic stroke and peripheral vascular disease. *Journal of the American Dental Association, 133*(Suppl. 1), 23S–30S.

Kelsey, J.L., & Lamster, I.B. (2008). Influence of musculoskeletal conditions on oral health among older adults. *American Journal of Public Health, 98,* 1177–1183. doi:10.2105/AJPH.2007.129429

Kunzel, C., Lalla, E., & Lamster, I. (2007). Dentists' management of the diabetic patient: Contrasting generalists and specialists. *American Journal of Public Health, 97,* 725–730. doi:10.2105/AJPH.2006.086496

Limbo, D. (2006). Oral health matters. *Viewpoint, 28*(6), 12–14.

Loesche, W. (2007). Dental caries and periodontitis: Contrasting two infections that have medical implications. *Infectious Disease Clinics of North America, 21,* 471–502. doi:10.1016/j.idc.2007.03.006

Loesche, W.J. (2000). Periodontal disease: Link to cardiovascular disease. *Compendium of Continuing Education in Dentistry, 21,* 463–466.

Meraw, S.J., & Sheridan, P.J. (1998). Medically induced gingival hyperplasia. *Mayo Clinic Proceedings, 73,* 1196–1199.

Petersen, P.E. (2003). *The World Oral Health Report 2003: Continuous improvement of oral health in the 21st century: The approach of the WHO Global Oral Health Programme.* Geneva, Switzerland: World Health Organization.

Petersen, P.E. (2008). World Health Organization global policy for improvement of oral health—World Health Assembly 2007. *International Dental Journal, 58,* 115–121.

Petersen, P.E. (2009). Oral cancer prevention and control—The approach of the World Health Organization. *Oral Oncology, 45,* 454–460. doi:10.1016/j.oraloncology.2008.05.023

Roggow, S. (2009). Thyroid disease and oral health. *Access, 23*(2), 31–33.

Rosenthal, D.I. (2007). Consequences of mucositis-induced treatment breaks and dose reductions on head and neck cancer treatment outcomes. *Journal of Supportive Oncology, 5*(9, Suppl. 4), 23–31.

Rout, J., & Brown, J.E. (2008). Dental and maxillofacial radiology. In A. Adam & A.K. Dixon (Eds.), *Grainger and Allison's diagnostic radiology: A textbook of medical imaging* (5th ed., pp. 1429–1460). Philadelphia, PA: Elsevier Churchill Livingstone. Retrieved from http://www.mdconsult.com

Ship, J., & Ghezzi, E. (2005). Oral manifestations of systemic disease. In C.W. Cummings, P.W. Flint, L.A. Harker, B.H. Haughey, M.A. Richardson, K.T. Robbins, ... J.R. Thomas (Eds.), *Cummings otolaryngology: Head and neck surgery* (4th ed., pp. 1493–1510). Philadelphia, PA: Elsevier Mosby. Retrieved from http://www.mdconsult.com

Silk, H., & Romano-Clarke, G. (2009). The seven tenets to teen oral health. *Contemporary Pediatrics, 26*(6), 50–59.

Skamagas, M., Breen, T.L., & LeRoith, D. (2008). Update on diabetes mellitus: Prevention, treatment, and association with oral diseases. *Oral Diseases, 14,* 105–114. doi:10.1111/j.1601-0825.2007.01425.x

Smith, D.V., & Margolskee, R.F. (2006). Making sense of taste. *Scientific American Special, 16*(3), 85–92.

Summers, S.A., Tilakaratne, W.M., Fortune, F., & Ashman, N. (2007). Renal disease and the mouth. *American Journal of Medicine, 120,* 568–573. doi:10.1016/j.amjmed.2006.12.007

Travers, J.B., & Travers, S.P. (2005). Physiology of the oral cavity. In C.W. Cummings, P.W. Flint, L.A. Harker, B.H. Haughey, M.A. Richardson, K.T. Robbins, ... J.R. Thomas (Eds.), *Cummings otolaryngology: Head and neck surgery* (4th ed., pp. 1409–1436). Philadelphia, PA: Elsevier Mosby. Retrieved from http://www.mdconsult.com

U.S. Department of Health and Human Services. (2000). *Oral health in America: A report of the Surgeon General.* Rockville, MD: U.S. Department of Health and Human Services, National Institutes of Health, and National Institute of Dental and Craniofacial Research.

Wood, N. (2006). Oral health: How to reduce risks of periodontitis. *Positive Health,* Issue 127, 20–35.

CHAPTER 2

Fundamental Skills: Oral Assessment and Dental Hygiene

Catherine H.L. Hong, BDS, MS, and Joel J. Napeñas, DDS

Introduction

Cancer is the second most common cause of mortality after cardiovascular disease in adults and unintentional injuries in children (Jemal, Siegel, Xu, & Ward. 2010). Fortunately, much progress has occurred in the medical treatment of malignancies, thus resulting in improved outcomes and subsequently higher survival rates. However, antineoplastic treatments are not without side effects; chemotherapy and radiation therapy, although effective in eradicating tumor cells, often negatively affect normal structures in the body. In some patients, problems also may develop as a result of the cancer itself. Healthcare professionals should educate patients of the acute and chronic effects of a cancer diagnosis and medical treatments on their oral health and should assist patients with lifestyle adjustments to cope with these issues.

The purposes of this chapter are to enable healthcare providers to become comfortable with directing and supervising patients' oral care during cancer therapy, to distinguish between normal and abnormal oral structures, and to involve oral healthcare specialists whenever necessary. The oral and dental manifestations other than dental disease of cancer therapies are discussed briefly, but their treatments are beyond the scope of this chapter.

History Taking

History taking is essential prior to commencement of medical or dental treatment. A well-taken medical and dental history provides valuable insights to patients' acute, chronic, and possibly undiagnosed problems, which may significantly influence the clinician's decision to provide a particular medical or dental treatment.

The following medical history information should be elicited routinely.
- Cancer diagnosis
- Goal of cancer treatment
- Type and schedule of treatment modality received and planned
- Hematologic and immunologic status
- Secondary medical diagnoses
- Medications
- Allergies

The dental history should include the following.
- Date of last dental visit
- Presence and description of oral pain or complaints (i.e., character, location, onset, intensity, duration, and exacerbating factors)
- History of dental trauma
- Dietary habits
- Use of prosthesis (removable or fixed appliances)

Armamentarium

Healthcare providers in both the inpatient and outpatient settings need only a few items to perform an oral assessment (see Figure 2-1). First is an adequate light source with the ability to direct light into the oral cavity. Relying on the external light sources in the room will not allow adequate visualization of the oral cavity. Several options for this include flashlights, head lamps, or even ophthalmoscopes.

A tongue blade is useful to retract soft tissue structures, such as the cheeks and tongue, in order to provide better visualization. In some instances, there is too much plaque, calculus, or food debris to properly assess the oral cavity; therefore, a means by which one can clean the oral mucosa and teeth intraorally is necessary when performing the oral examination. This may be done by having gauze sponges (2 × 2 inches or 4 × 4 inches) or disposable oral swabs or sponge toothettes available. Such methods of cleansing do not replace tooth brushing and flossing as the primary means by which one performs daily oral hygiene measures. Lastly, proper assessment requires having a mouth mirror available. These are available in both disposable and the standard reusable forms.

Clinical Examination

Many oncology treatment centers require patients to undergo a dental examination and treatment (if indicated) prior to initiating cancer therapy (Barker, Epstein, Williams, Gorsky, & Raber-Durlacher, 2005). The main objectives of the pre-therapy dental protocol are to identify and ideally eliminate

Figure 2-1. Armamentarium to Perform an Oral Examination

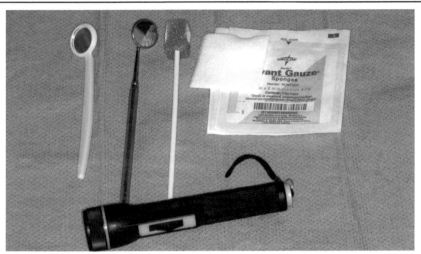

Components of an examination kit for an oral examination (clockwise from upper left)
- Mouth mirror with handle (either a disposable or reusable variety)
- Sponge toothette or 2 × 2 gauzes to remove debris
- Light source (flashlight)
- Tongue blade (not pictured)

all existing and potential sources of irritation (e.g., sharp tooth cusps, rough restorations) and infection (e.g., extraction of hopeless teeth) that may become problematic during and after cancer therapy (Brennan, Woo, & Lockhart, 2008; Hong & daFonseca, 2008).

In addition to the pretreatment dental examination, regular assessment of the oral cavity during and after antineoplastic therapy is also indicated because oral problems can occur at any time. Patients in active cancer therapy and those who have completed therapy experience varying degrees of immunosuppression, and a considerable concern is that a minor odontogenic infection can progress to overwhelming septicemia. Additionally, in the absence of a robust immune system, patients may present with an atypical appearance of an oral infection; they are also at increased risk for the development of secondary malignancies (Cohen, Curtis, Inskip, & Fraumeni, 2005; Curtis et al., 2005).

Extraoral examination: An extraoral examination includes a thorough inspection of the head and neck region for notable asymmetry, swelling, erythema, and skin lesions. The following head and neck structures should be palpated.
1. Neck muscles (trapezius muscle, sternocleidomastoid muscle) (see Figure 2-2)
2. Temporomandibular joints (see Figure 2-3)

Figure 2-2. Examination of Neck Muscles

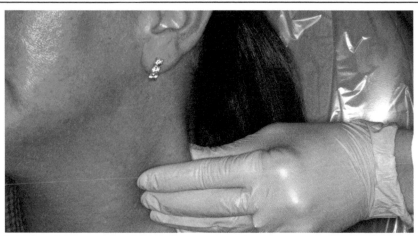

Palpation of the sternocleidomastoid muscle to look for hypertrophy or tenderness that may refer to or manifest as pain in the oral cavity.

Figure 2-3. Examination of the Temporomandibular Joint

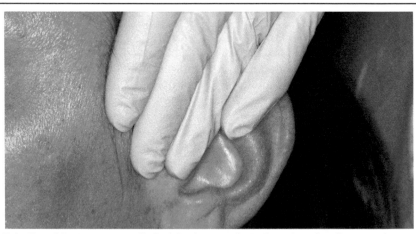

Palpation of the temporomandibular joint, just anterior to the external auditory canal. Tenderness to palpation at rest or upon opening or closing may indicate joint pathology (e.g., arthritis, disk displacement, synovitis, capsulitis).

3. Muscles of mastication (masseters, lateral pterygoid muscles, temporalis)
4. Major salivary glands (parotid, submandibular, and sublingual glands)
5. Lymph nodes (see Figure 2-4)

Intraoral examination: The intraoral examination encompasses a thorough inspection of the soft tissues (i.e., oral mucosa and periodontal appa-

Figure 2-4. Examination of Lymph Nodes

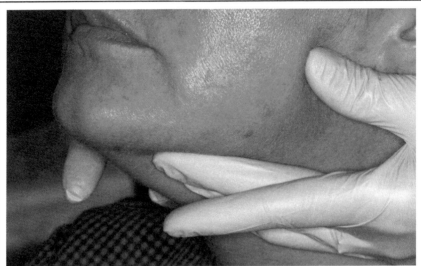

Palpation of the submandibular and submental region. Lymphadenopathy, manifested as swelling and tenderness to palpation, can be indicative of an oral infection. Nontender swelling of the lymph nodes can be indicative of metastatic spread of a head and neck malignancy.

ratus), hard tissues (i.e., teeth and jaw bone), quality and quantity of saliva, and any oral prostheses.

1. Soft tissue examination
   a. Oral mucosa: The lips, buccal mucosa, floor of the mouth, tongue, palate, and oropharynx should be inspected. The oral mucosa should appear pink and be devoid of erythema, red or white areas or patches, blisters, abscesses, swellings, erosions, ulcerations, and hemorrhages.
   b. Periodontium: Pink gingiva with minimal or no plaque or calculus accumulation is an indication of good periodontal health. In contrast, fiery red and swollen gingiva that bleeds easily is a sign of poor periodontal health. Other common indicators of poor periodontal health are heavy plaque and calculus accumulation, gingival abscesses, loose teeth, generalized dental pain, and halitosis (see Figure 2-5, photos a and b).
2. Hard tissue examination
   a. Dentition (see Figure 2-5, photo c): The teeth and dental restorations should be evaluated for the presence of pain to percussion and to hot and cold stimulus, sharp edges, decay, fractures, mobility, and swellings or draining fistulas on the adjacent soft tissue, which are possible indications of a tooth infection.

Figure 2-5. Dental Status (Dentition and Gingiva)

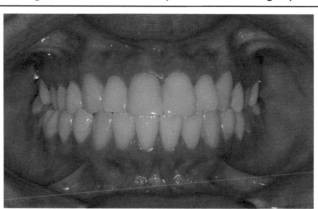

a. A healthy dentition. Teeth, gingiva, and periodontium are in good health.

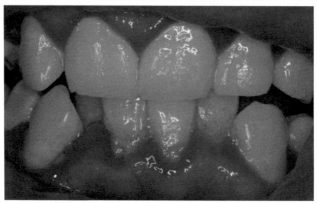

b. A patient with moderate gingival inflammation, as indicated by inflammation, erythema, and edema. Note the moderate plaque buildup that is contributing to the inflammation.

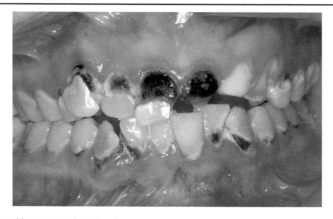

c. Patient with rampant dental caries.

    b. Maxilla and mandible: Asymmetry and areas of exposed bone in the maxilla and mandible should be noted. Maxillary and mandibular tori are benign areas of harmless bone growth and rarely require any clinical treatment. Maxillary tori occur on the palate and are more common than mandibular tori (see Figure 2-6). Mandibular tori are bilateral in 90% of the cases and commonly are found lingual to the premolars (Neville, Damm, Allen, & Bouquot, 2002).

3. Oral prostheses

    a. Removable complete or partial dentures should be checked for retention. All tissue surfaces contacting the dentures should be inspected for areas of infection or irritation. Preferably, any denture-related problems should be addressed before the initiation of cancer therapy. Patients should be reminded of the importance of proper care of these prostheses (i.e., removal of dentures during sleep time, cleaning of dentures, and storage of dentures in appropriate solutions). In patients who develop painful mouth ulcers from their cancer therapy, the use of dentures may be temporarily discontinued.

    b. Orthodontic appliances: It is difficult to maintain good oral hygiene around orthodontic appliances because of the tendency for these appliances to accumulate plaque. Some appliances also may irritate the gingival and oral mucosa. Therefore, removal of these appliances sometimes is indicated in cancer treatment protocols that carry a high risk for the development of moderate to severe mucositis.

Figure 2-6. Maxillary Torus

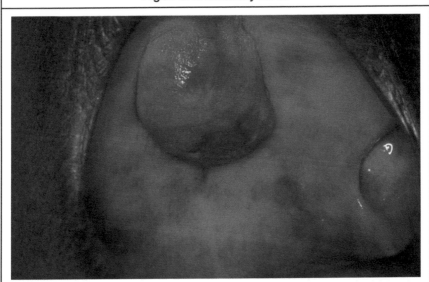

Note the large, firm torus on the palate that shows erythema (redness) and ulceration due to secondary irritation and trauma.

Diagnostic and Assessment Tools

Radiographic Examination

Dental radiography is a valuable adjunctive diagnostic tool for the confirmation of clinical findings and establishment of baseline measures. Dental radiographs provide images of areas in the hard tissue (e.g., periodontal bone loss, contact areas of teeth, and jaws) that otherwise cannot be assessed during a clinical oral examination. Ideally, all patients should have imaging of the entire dental apparatus, which typically consists of a full mouth series of intraoral radiographs and/or a panoramic radiograph (see Figure 2-7) prior to the initiation of antineoplastic therapy. All patients should have any intraoral prostheses removed while radiographs are taken.

Microbiology and Pathology

The decision to carry out microbiology or pathology testing is significant if its results will affect the patient during the course of the cancer treatment. Of utmost concern are active or potential sources of infection in the oral cavity and suspected involvement of the oral cavity by the malignancy. A number of oral hard and soft tissue disorders are bacterial, viral, or fungal in etiology. With respect to infections in the mouth, prompt diagnosis is critical in preventing progression to systemic infection in this immunocompromised patient population.

Bacterial testing is indicated if a localized bacterial infection in the mouth is not responsive to empirical therapy for odontogenic infections. Culture and

Figure 2-7. Panoramic Radiograph of the Mouth

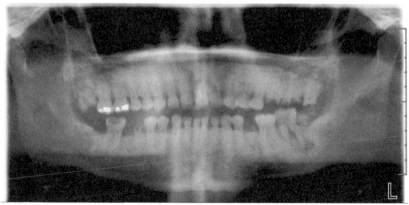

Panoramic radiograph is best for looking for maxillary and mandibular bony abnormalities and pathology. Note the grossly decayed and carious molars in all four quadrants. The radiolucency on the lower left jaw at the apex of the lower left molar is indicative of infection of that tooth.

antibiotic sensitivity testing of areas containing purulent drainage are helpful in determining the most appropriate antibiotic regimen.

Fungal infections from the genus *Candida* are the most common opportunistic fungal infections in neutropenic patients (DiNubile, Hille, Sable, & Kartsonis, 2005). Smears, swabs, and oral rinse samples can be used to diagnose suspected oral fungal infections. A smear can be taken by scraping the lesion with the edge of a flat plastic instrument and transferring the sample to a glass microscope slide. In the laboratory, smears can be stained with Gram stain or periodic acid–Schiff reagent and examined microscopically for the presence of *Candida*. A dry swab of the lesion and oral rinse samples can be cultured for fungal species identification.

Identification of suspected viral infections of the mouth, such as herpes simplex, can be accomplished by applying a dry sterile swab to a lesion. To prevent false-negative results, the swab must be applied to a newly formed vesicle or blister. Culturing of viruses is performed using tissue culture cells. Bacterial and viral culturing also may be performed on soft tissue samples obtained by biopsy, whereas yeasts may be identified through microscopic evaluation of the tissue.

An incisional tissue biopsy is indicated if unusual lesions are present in the soft tissue and the clinician is unsure of the origin of the lesions. Biopsy should be pursued in the following instances: oral ulcers that persist for two to three weeks after the suspected cause is eliminated; red and white lesions on the oral mucosa or gingiva that are persistent; suspected neoplasms; or any other unidentified tissue masses. The tissue specimen should be fixed immediately by placing it in 5%–10% formalin solution (Ellis & Alexander, 2008).

Assessing Oral Complications

Validated scoring systems exist that provide an objective, semiquantitative way of measuring clinical oral parameters. For the measure of dental disease, a scale quantifies the number of decayed, filled, and missing teeth, whereas the degree of periodontal disease can be graded based on the clinical periodontal probing depths. These measures are not routinely performed by the healthcare provider.

With respect to xerostomia, a patient's subjective complaint of oral dryness may or may not correspond with an actual decrease in salivary flow rates. Thus, a number of methods have been described for objective measurement of unstimulated whole saliva (UWS) and stimulated whole saliva (SWS) flow rates that require no specialized equipment, are controlled and reproducible, and can be performed in any setting (Navazesh, 1993). A UWS below 0.12–0.16 ml/min and an SWS flow rate below 0.5 ml/min are considered indicative of hyposalivation (Heintze, Birkhed, & Björn, 1983).

A number of different scoring systems exist for oral mucositis; however, no system is universally accepted. Such scoring systems are important in assessing the impact of therapy on patient morbidity and quality of life. Commonly used scoring systems include those from the World Health Organization (WHO) (Miller, Hoogstraten, Staquet, & Winkler, 1981), the National Cancer Institute

(NCI) Common Terminology Criteria for Adverse Events (CTCAE) (NCI Cancer Therapy Evaluation Program, 2009; Trotti et al., 2000), and the Radiation Therapy Oncology Group (RTOG) scales (Cox, Stetz, & Pajak, 1995) (see Table 2-1). The WHO and NCI CTCAE scales take into account objective clinical findings, subjective feelings of pain, and the need for parenteral nutrition, with the WHO scale ranging from 0 through 4 and the NCI CTCAE scale ranging from 1 through 5. The RTOG scale is scaled from 0 through 4 and takes into account clinical appearance and the need for analgesic use. Although simple to perform, each rating scale has the distinct disadvantage of being imprecise in terms of extent of involvement (i.e., isolated patch versus entire buccal mucosa), etiology of objective findings (i.e., chemotherapy-induced versus candidiasis), and subjective complaints (i.e., inability to eat due to pain versus dryness).

Differential Diagnosis

The oral pathologies that could be present in patients in any stage of their cancer therapy are listed in Table 2-2. This table will assist clinicians in formulating the most probable differential diagnosis based on the various clinical presentations of the oral mucosa (see Figures 2-8 through 2-11).

Table 2-1. Commonly Used Scoring Systems for Assessing Oral Mucositis			
Grade	WHO	NCI CTCAE	RTOG
0	No change	–	No change over baseline
1	Soreness/ erythema	Asymptomatic or mild symptoms; intervention not indicated	Injection; may experience mild pain not requiring analgesic
2	Erythema, ulcers; can eat solids	Moderate pain; not interfering with oral intake; modified diet indicated	Patchy mucositis that may have a serosanguineous discharge; may experience pain requiring analgesics
3	Ulcers; requires liquid diet only	Severe pain; interfering with oral intake	Confluent fibrinous mucositis; may include severe pain requiring narcotics
4	Alimentation not possible	Life-threatening consequences; urgent intervention indicated	Ulceration, hemorrhage, or necrosis
5	–	Death	–

NCI CTCAE—National Cancer Institute Common Terminology Criteria for Adverse Events; RTOG—Radiation Therapy Oncology Group; WHO—World Health Organization

Note. Based on information from Cox et al., 1995; Miller et al., 1981; National Cancer Institute Cancer Therapy Evaluation Program, 2009.

Table 2-2. Differential Diagnosis of Oral Mucosal Lesions Presenting in Patients With Cancer

Oral Presentation	Differential Diagnosis

Erythematous/ red lesions of the oral mucosa (see Figure 2-8)	• Infectious process
	  – Fungal infection (e.g., erythematous candidiasis)
	  – Viral infection (e.g., herpes simplex infection)
	  – Bacterial infection
	• Systemic process
	  – Graft-versus-host disease
	  – Petechiae, hematoma, purpura due to clotting disorders
	• Reactive process
	  – Mucositis related to cancer therapy
	  – Oral hypersensitivity reactions (e.g., allergic contact stomatitis)
	  – Recurrent aphthous stomatitis
	  – Reactions to trauma (e.g., petechiae, hematoma, purpura)
	• Premalignant and malignant process
	  – Oral erythroplakia
	  – Squamous cell carcinoma

White lesions of the oral mucosa (see Figure 2-9)	• Infectious process
	  – Fungal infection (e.g., pseudomembranous candidiasis)
	  – Viral infection (e.g., human papillomavirus infections [common wart], hairy leukoplakia)
	• Systemic process: Graft-versus-host disease
	• Reactive process
	  – Frictional irritation (e.g., hyperkeratosis from chronic cheek biting)
	  – Trauma (e.g., thermal or chemical burn)
	  – Oral hypersensitivity reactions (e.g., allergic contact stomatitis, lichenoid drug/contact reaction)
	  – Recurrent aphthous stomatitis
	• Premalignant and malignant process
	  – Oral leukoplakia
	  – Oral cancer (e.g., squamous cell carcinoma)

Ulceration (see Figure 2-10)	• Infectious process
	  – Deep fungal infection (e.g., histoplasmosis, blastomycosis)
	  – Viral infection (e.g., herpes simplex, cytomegalovirus)
	  – Bacterial infection (e.g., necrotizing ulcerative gingivitis and periodontitis)
	• Systemic process
	  – Mucositis related to cancer therapy
	  – Acute or chronic graft-versus-host disease
	• Reactive process
	  – Trauma (e.g., thermal or chemical burn)
	  – Oral hypersensitivity reactions (e.g., allergic contact stomatitis)
	  – Recurrent aphthous stomatitis
	• Premalignant and malignant process
	  – Oral leukoplakia or erythroplakia
	  – Oral cancer (e.g., squamous cell carcinoma)
	  – Cancer metastases

(Continued on next page)

Table 2-2. Differential Diagnosis of Oral Mucosal Lesions Presenting in Patients With Cancer *(Continued)*	
Oral Presentation	**Differential Diagnosis**

Lumps and bumps (see Figure 2-11)	• Infectious process
	   – Odontogenic infection (e.g., sinus tract formation, gingival or periodontal abscesses)
	   – Viral infection (e.g., human papillomavirus infections [common wart], hairy leukoplakia)
	• Reactive process to trauma
	   – Epulis (e.g., pyogenic granuloma, irritation fibromas)
	   – Minor salivary gland cyst
	• Malignant process
	   – Oral cancer (e.g., squamous cell carcinoma, lymphoma, Kaposi sarcoma)
	   – Cancer metastases (e.g., leukemic infiltrates)

Figure 2-8. Red Lesions of the Oral Cavity

This patient on chemotherapy shows multiple pinpoint red macules on the gingival and labial mucosa. The macules are petechiae secondary to chemotherapy-induced thrombocytopenia.

Figure 2-9. White Lesions of the Oral Cavity

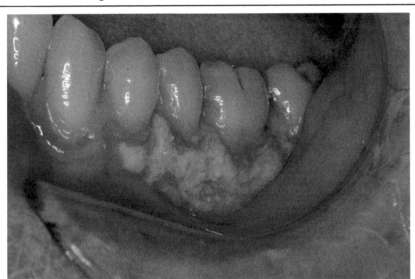

This post–bone marrow transplant patient is showing leukoplakic lesions in the lower left gingiva due to graft-versus-host disease.

Figure 2-10. Ulceration Within the Oral Cavity

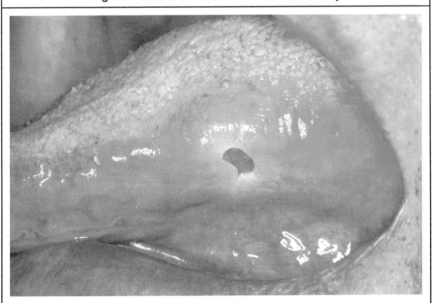

This ulcer on the left lateral tongue was most likely induced by trauma and irritation.

Figure 2-11. Lumps and Bumps Within the Oral Cavity

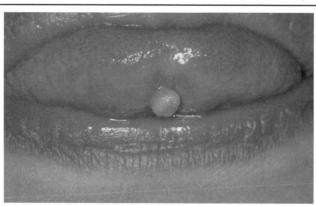

a. This pediatric patient has a papule on the mid ventral tongue that was a mucocele (minor salivary gland cyst).

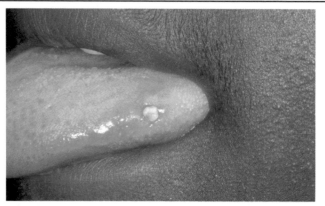

b. Papule on the left lateral tongue that was due to human papillomavirus.

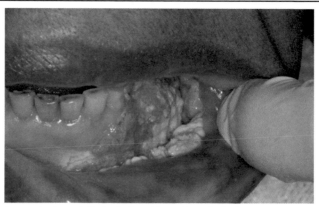

c. Large lesion on the lower left gingival and buccal vestibule that was a squamous cell carcinoma.

Dental Care in Patients With Cancer

Streptococcus viridans group bacteria, a normal inhabitant of the oral cavity, have emerged as a frequent cause of bloodstream infections with the potential to result in morbid septicemia in neutropenic patients (Huang et al., 2007; Marron et al., 2000). Based on findings of an increased incidence of *Streptococcus viridans* bacteremia in individuals with poor oral hygiene, it seems rational that patients should continue their routine oral hygiene practices during cancer therapy (Graber et al., 2001; Kennedy et al., 2003; Lockhart et al., 2009). However, it is not an appropriate time to introduce patients to new oral cleansing devices during cancer therapy. For example, in patients who do not routinely floss their teeth, flossing may cause trauma and bleeding to the gingival tissue and inadvertently cause bacteremia. Patients who are thrombocytopenic may continue brushing their teeth, but this should be performed in an atraumatic fashion. Parents or caregivers should supervise young children to ensure atraumatic tooth brushing. Extra-soft bristle toothbrushes, sponge toothbrushes, or sponge toothettes are much less effective than soft bristle toothbrushes in removing plaque and generally are not recommended except during times of severe oral mucositis (Addems, Epstein, Damji, & Spinelli, 1992; Ransier, Epstein, Lunn, & Spinelli, 1995). Regular toothpaste may burn and irritate the mucosa, and its use may need to be discontinued until mucosal ulceration resolves. The use of mouth rinses containing alcohol should be avoided.

Nausea and vomiting are common in patients going through chemotherapy. Rinsing with water or bland mouth rinses such as baking soda and water after each emesis episode is highly recommended to prevent the acidic contents of the stomach from eroding the tooth structure and increasing their susceptibility to dental decay (Belfield & Dwyer, 2004).

Dental Care After Cancer Therapy

Following cancer therapy, patients often experience or are at high risk for the following dental problems: permanent oral dryness or xerostomia as a result of salivary gland damage or chronic graft-versus-host disease; radiation caries; postradiation jaw osteonecrosis (PRON), usually with head and neck radiation doses greater than 6,000 centigray; trismus causing difficulty in performing everyday functions such as routine oral hygiene practices (i.e., tooth brushing and flossing) and receiving dental treatment; and taste changes (Ransier et al., 1995) (see Table 2-3).

Xerostomia and Dental Caries

In patients whose salivary glands are irreversibly damaged by head and neck radiation or as a result of chronic graft-versus-host disease, dry mouth or xerostomia may be an issue that they have to cope with for the rest of their

Table 2-3. Oral Manifestations of Cancer Therapy

Oral Manifestations	During Cancer Therapy		After Cancer Therapy		
	Head and Neck Radiation	Chemotherapy	Head and Neck Radiation	Chemotherapy	Allogeneic Bone Marrow Transplantation
Oral mucositis/stomatitis	Y	Y (specific chemotherapy agents)*	N	N	Y (in patients with acute or chronic graft-versus-host disease [GVHD])
Opportunistic infections • Bacterial (*Pseudomonas*) • Viral (cytomegalovirus, Epstein-Barr, herpes simplex, varicella zoster) • Fungal (*Candida albicans*)	Y	Y	Y (consequence of dry mouth)	Y (in patients with persistent immunosuppression)	Y (in patients with persistent immunosuppression)
Oral bleeding	N	Y	N	N	N
Nausea and vomiting	N	Y	N	N	N
Xerostomia	Y	Y (transient)	Y (if salivary glands were in radiation field)	N	Y (complication of chronic GVHD)
Post-treatment caries	N/A	N/A	Y (in patients with xerostomia)	N	Y (in patients with xerostomia as a result of chronic GVHD)

(Continued on next page)

Table 2-3. Oral Manifestations of Cancer Therapy (Continued)

Oral Manifestations	During Cancer Therapy		After Cancer Therapy		
	Head and Neck Radiation	Chemotherapy	Head and Neck Radiation	Chemotherapy	Allogeneic Bone Marrow Transplantation
Post-treatment trismus	N/A	N/A	Y	N	Y (complication of chronic GVHD)
Postradiation osteonecrosis	N/A	N/A	Y (dose > 60 Gy)	N/A	N/A
GVHD	N/A	N/A	N/A	N/A	Y
Secondary malignancies	N/A	N/A	Y	Y (unlikely)	Y
Anomalies in craniofacial and dental development in pediatric patients	N/A	N/A	Y (dose dependent)	Y	Y

* 5-fluorouracil, melphalan, methotrexate, cisplatin, doxorubicin, bleomycin, actinomycin, etoposide, docetaxel

lives. Patients with significant salivary gland hyposalivation are at risk for opportunistic fungal infections, oral mucosal trauma due to friction, taste changes, speaking difficulties, and dental decay. Two medications, cevimeline and amifostine, are currently approved for radiation-induced xerostomia in adults. The use of topical agents such as bland mouth rinses (e.g., 0.9% saline or sodium bicarbonate solution), mucosal coating agents, salivary substitutes, sugar-free candy, and frequent sipping of water may relieve oral dryness (Amerongen & Veerman, 2003; Vissink, Burlage, Spijkervet, Jansma, & Coppes, 2003). Because of their risk for dental decay, it is imperative for patients to adopt a meticulous oral hygiene regimen, such as fluoride supplementation, regular and frequent visits to the dentist, and adherence to a noncariogenic diet.

Postradiation Osteonecrosis

The mean incidence of PRON is 5%–15%, and it may occur spontaneously or be triggered by a traumatic episode (i.e., irritation during normal masticatory function or by a prosthesis, dental extractions) or an infection (Vissink, Jansma, Spijkervet, Burlage, & Coppes, 2003). The treatment of PRON frequently involves removal of necrotic bone and improving the vascularity of irradiated bone with hyperbaric oxygen therapy (Vissink, Burlage, et al., 2003).

Trismus

The severity of trismus (i.e., decreased or limited mouth opening) depends on the extent of tumor invasion, surgical procedures, and the dose and field of radiation therapy. Oral stretching exercises and physical therapy during radiation and continuing for three to six months after radiation often are recommended in patients at high risk for developing trismus. Commercial physical therapy devices are available for these purposes; however, their superiority over traditional mouth opening exercises is uncertain (Dijkstra, Kalk, & Roodenburg, 2004).

Management of Dental Infections During Cancer Therapy

The clinical signs of inflammation, such as erythema, swelling, and purulence, are highly variable and sometimes may be absent in immunosuppressed patients. The incidence of opportunistic oral mucosal infections (i.e., fungal, bacterial, and viral) appears to be higher than odontogenic infections during cancer therapy, and it has been difficult to assess whether this is a true reflection of the incidences or a result of reporting bias (Peterson, 1990) (see Table 2-2). However, in the presence of dental or oral pain with evidence of dental pathology (e.g., large restorations, periapical radiolucency, gross decay), it is reasonable to suspect that the pain is originating from an odontogenic infection. It is important to recognize (though not necessarily diagnose) the presence of an abnormal oral appearance or infection and convey this to the physician or oral healthcare specialist for further evaluation and treatment.

The management of dental infections during active cancer treatment is dependent on several factors, most importantly the patient's degree of bone marrow suppression. Invasive dental treatments, such as extractions, incisions, and drainage, typically are not performed in severely pancytopenic patients, and empiric therapy with broad-spectrum antibiotics is often the treatment of choice. The decision to carry out definitive dental treatment should be discussed with the patient's physicians with regard to the appropriate timing for the procedure and the need for adjunctive measures (e.g., pretreatment with antibiotics and/or blood products).

Barriers to Dental Care

The diagnosis of cancer is devastating and overwhelming for patients and their families, and it is not surprising that the medical diagnosis takes priority over all other health issues. Most patients are ignorant of the merits of good oral hygiene and the implications of having poor oral health during their medical treatment. Members of the oncology team must educate patients and family members of the rationale for a pre-therapy dental evaluation and treatment (if indicated), the importance of maintaining good oral hygiene, and the need for aggressive preventive care (e.g., frequent visits to dentist, adherence to noncariogenic diet) during and after cancer therapy.

Even though dental examination and treatment are often part of the workup prior to cancer therapy, the cost is seldom covered by medical insurance, and many patients cannot afford the costs of both medical and dental treatment. In a 2000 Institute of Medicine report titled *Extending Medicare Coverage for Preventive and Other Services*, the committee gave a recommendation based on limited evidence that dental care to prevent or eliminate acute oral infections for patients with leukemia prior to chemotherapy can prevent or reduce subsequent episodes of septicemia and prevent or reduce the oral complications of treatment (Patton, White, & Field, 2001). This recommendation was derived largely from the opinions of respected authorities based on clinical experience, descriptive studies, and reports of expert committees (level of evidence AIII). However, given the potential for significant morbidity and mortality from infection in this population, the report concluded that it was reasonable for Medicare to cover a dental examination, teeth cleaning, and treatment of acute infections in patients with leukemia prior to chemotherapy (Patton et al., 2001). Currently, Medicare only covers the cost of oral examinations for kidney transplant candidates and the extraction of teeth before head and neck radiation therapy.

Some dental professionals are not comfortable treating patients with cancer because of the array of medical problems either from the cancer itself or from their medical therapy. Therefore, these patients are often referred to state institutions or tertiary-level hospitals to receive care. For some patients, this may involve time away from work and the added cost of travel to these institutions.

Conclusion

The oral health of patients with cancer is of the utmost importance, as oral manifestations are prevalent because of the treatment of cancer and the actual disease itself, and oral conditions may affect treatment of the disease and the patient's quality of life. Constant care and attention to the oral cavity is required of all healthcare providers involved in the treatment of these patients. Therefore, it is imperative that all members of the healthcare team have the skills to perform a basic oral assessment, assist patients in maintaining optimal oral care, and identify when patients require additional treatment from their oral healthcare provider.

References

Addems, A., Epstein, J.B., Damji, S., & Spinelli, J. (1992). The lack of efficacy of a foam brush in maintaining gingival health: A controlled study. *Special Care in Dentistry, 12,* 103–106.

Amerongen, A.V.N., & Veerman, E.C.I. (2003). Current therapies for xerostomia and salivary gland hypofunction associated with cancer therapies. *Supportive Care in Cancer, 11,* 226–231. doi:10.1007/s00520-002-0409-5

Barker, G.J., Epstein, J.N., Williams, K.B., Gorsky, M., & Raber-Durlacher, J.E. (2005). Current practice and knowledge of oral care for cancer patients: A survey of supportive health care providers. *Supportive Care in Cancer, 13,* 32–41. doi:10.1007/s00520-004-0691-5

Belfield, P.M., & Dwyer, A.A. (2004). Oral complications of childhood cancer and its treatment: Current best practice. *European Journal of Cancer, 40,* 1035–1041. doi:10.1016/j.ejca.2003.09.041

Brennan, M.T., Woo, S.B., & Lockhart, P.B. (2008). Dental treatment planning and management in the patient who has cancer. *Dental Clinics of North America, 52,* 19–37. doi:10.1016/j.cden.2007.10.003

Cohen, R.J., Curtis, R.E., Inskip, P.D., & Fraumeni, J.F., Jr. (2005). The risk of developing second cancers among survivors of childhood soft tissue sarcoma. *Cancer, 103,* 2391–2396. doi:10.1002/cncr.21040

Cox, J.D., Stetz, J., & Pajak, T.F. (1995). Toxicity criteria of the Radiation Therapy Oncology Group (RTOG) and the European Organization for Research and Treatment of Cancer (EORTC). *International Journal of Radiation Oncology, Biology, Physics, 31,* 1341–1346. doi:10.1016/0360-3016(95)00060-C

Curtis, R.E., Metayer, C., Rizzo, J.D., Socié, G., Sobocinski, K.A., Flowers, M.E.D., ... Deeg, H.J. (2005). Impact of chronic GVHD therapy on the development of squamous-cell cancers after hematopoietic stem-cell transplantation: An international case-control study. *Blood, 105,* 3802–3811. doi:10.1182/blood-2004-09-3411

Dijkstra, P.U., Kalk, W.W.I., & Roodenburg, J.L.N. (2004). Trismus in head and neck oncology: A systematic review. *Oral Oncology, 40,* 879–889. doi:10.1016/j.oraloncology.2004.04.003

DiNubile, M.J., Hille, D., Sable, C.A., & Kartsonis, N.A. (2005). Invasive candidiasis in cancer patients: Observations from a randomized clinical trial. *Journal of Infection, 50,* 443–449. doi:10.1016/j.jinf.2005.01.016

Ellis, E., III, & Alexander, R.E. (2008). Principles of differential diagnosis and biopsy. In J.R. Hupp, E. Ellis III, & M.R. Tucker (Eds.), *Contemporary oral and maxillofacial surgery* (5th ed., pp. 423–448). St. Louis, MO: Elsevier Mosby.

Graber, C.J., de Almeida, K.N.F., Atkinson, J.C., Javaheri, D., Fukuda, C.D., Gill, V.J., … Bennett, J.E. (2001). Dental health and viridans streptococcal bacteremia in allogeneic hematopoietic stem cell transplant recipients. *Bone Marrow Transplantation, 27,* 537–542. doi:10.1038/sj.bmt.1702818

Heintze, U., Birkhed, D., & Björn, H. (1983). Secretion rate and buffer effect of resting and stimulated whole saliva as a function of age and sex. *Swedish Dental Journal, 7,* 227–238.

Hong, C.H., & daFonseca, M. (2008). Considerations in the pediatric population with cancer. *Dental Clinics of North America, 52,* 155–181. doi:10.1016/j.cden.2007.10.001

Huang, W.T., Chang, L.Y., Hsueh, P.R., Lu, C.Y., Shao, P.L., Huang, F.Y., … Huang, L.M. (2007). Clinical features and complications of viridans streptococci bloodstream infection in pediatric hemato-oncology patients. *Journal of Microbiology, Immunology, and Infection, 40,* 349–354.

Jemal, A., Siegel, R., Xu, J., & Ward, E. (2010). Cancer statistics, 2010. *CA: A Cancer Journal for Clinicians, 60,* 277–300. doi:10.3322/caac.20073

Kennedy, H.F., Morrison, D., Tomlinson, D., Gibson, B.E.S., Bagg, J., & Gemmell, C.G. (2003). Gingivitis and toothbrushes: Potential roles in viridans streptococcal bacteraemia. *Journal of Infection, 46,* 67–70. doi:10.1053/jinf.2002.1084

Lockhart, P.B., Brennan, M.T., Thornhill, M., Michalowicz, B.S., Noll, J., Bahrani-Mougeot, F.K., & Sasser, H.C. (2009). Poor oral hygiene as a risk factor for infective endocarditis-related bacteremia. *Journal of the American Dental Association, 140,* 1238–1244.

Marron, A., Carratalà, J., González-Barca, E., Fernández-Sevilla, A., Alcaide, F., & Gudiol, F. (2000). Serious complications of bacteremia caused by viridans streptococci in neutropenic patients with cancer. *Clinical Infectious Diseases, 31,* 1126–1130. doi:10.1086/317460

Miller, A.B., Hoogstraten, B., Staquet, M., & Winkler, A. (1981). Reporting results of cancer treatment. *Cancer, 47,* 207–214.

National Cancer Institute Cancer Therapy Evaluation Program. (2009). *Common terminology criteria for adverse events* [v.4.03]. Retrieved from http://evs.nci.nih.gov/ftp1/CTCAE/CTCAE_4.03_2010-06-14_QuickReference_8.5x11.pdf

Navazesh, M. (1993). Methods for collecting saliva. *Annals of the New York Academy of Sciences, 694,* 72–77. doi:10.1111/j.1749-6632.1993.tb18343.x

Neville, B.W., Damm, D.D., Allen, C.M., & Bouquot, J.E. (2002). *Oral and maxillofacial pathology* (2nd ed.). Philadelphia, PA: Saunders.

Patton, L.L., White, B.A., & Field, M.J. (2001). Extending Medicare coverage to medically necessary dental care. *Journal of the American Dental Association, 132,* 1294–1299.

Peterson, D.E. (1990). Pretreatment strategies for infection prevention in chemotherapy patients. *NCI Monographs, 1990*(9), 61–71.

Ransier, A., Epstein, J.B., Lunn, R., & Spinelli, J. (1995). A combined analysis of a toothbrush, foam brush and a chlorhexidine-soaked foam brush in maintaining oral hygiene. *Cancer Nursing, 18,* 393–396.

Trotti, A., Byhardt, R., Stetz, J., Gwede, C., Corn, B., Fu, K., … Curran, W. (2000). Common toxicity criteria: Version 2.0. An improved reference for grading the acute effects of cancer treatment: Impact on radiotherapy. *International Journal of Radiation Oncology, Biology, Physics, 47,* 13–47. doi:10.1016/S0360-3016(99)00559-3

Vissink, A., Burlage, F.R., Spijkervet, F.K.L., Jansma, J., & Coppes, R.P. (2003). Prevention and treatment of the consequences of head and neck radiotherapy. *Critical Reviews in Oral Biology and Medicine, 14,* 213–225. doi:10.1177/154411130301400306

Vissink, A., Jansma, J., Spijkervet, F.K.L., Burlage, F.R., & Coppes, R.P. (2003). Oral sequelae of head and neck radiotherapy. *Critical Reviews in Oral Biology and Medicine, 14,* 199–212. doi:10.1177/154411130301400305

CHAPTER 3

Treatment of Side Effects

Susan D. Bruce, RN, MSN, OCN®

Introduction

Oral side effects are a common complication resulting from cancer treatment and can be quite challenging for oncology nurses to manage. These side effects manifest as acute and chronic side effects. Acute side effects occur during cancer treatment and usually resolve within six to eight weeks after completion of treatment. Chronic side effects occur 6–12 months after completion of treatment and can last for an undefined period of time. Acute side effects can significantly affect patients' ability to complete treatment without delays, as well as their quality of life. Multiple factors, such as location of the cancer, treatment modality, and the patient's pretreatment oral hygiene, can contribute to the development of oral complications.

This chapter will discuss some of the more common oral side effects and their incidence, pathophysiology, evidence-based management, and impact on the patient's quality of life. Oral complications are difficult to manage and require a multidisciplinary approach by all members of the healthcare team providing care to the patient. The importance of educating patients and their families cannot be overemphasized. The saying "it takes a village" is certainly applicable in the management and successful treatment of patients experiencing these symptoms.

Oral Mucositis

Oral mucositis (OM) is defined as an inflammatory, ulcerative process resulting from the systemic effects of cytotoxic chemotherapy and the local effects of radiation therapy (Avritscher, Cooksley, & Elting, 2004; Brown & Wingard, 2004). OM can occur anywhere throughout the gastrointestinal tract, but for the purposes of this chapter, OM will be confined to the oral cavity, oropharynx, and hypopharynx. OM is one of the most challenging side effects to manage and is responsible for unplanned treatment interruptions and dose reductions, which can ultimately reduce the probability for cure. OM is a dose-limiting toxicity for treatment and can be accompanied by the risk of life-threatening bacteremia and sepsis (Spielberger et al., 2004). Patients with OM frequently have issues with pain management, which can limit adequate nutrition and fluid intake, often resulting in unwillingness to continue the prescribed treatment plan. Patients who are unable to maintain an adequate daily caloric and fluid intake may need to have a feeding tube placed to support them through the treatment and post-treatment phases.

The incidence of OM is 90%–100% for patients with head and neck cancer who are undergoing chemotherapy and/or radiation therapy, 80% in patients receiving intensive high-dose chemotherapy regimens in preparation for bone marrow transplantation, and 40% in patients receiving standard-dose chemotherapy (National Cancer Institute, 2008). OM is the most significant adverse symptom of cancer therapy reported by patients. The duration of OM is typically 5–14 days for patients undergoing chemotherapy and 6–8 weeks for patients who have completed radiotherapy.

Risk factors for OM can be categorized as treatment-related or patient-related (see Figure 3-1). Many of the patient-related risk factors are not modifiable, such as age, sex, and genetics. Others, such as diet, oral hygiene, smoking, and alcohol use, are modifiable risk factors with appropriate patient education and patient motivation. Individuals older than 50 are more likely to develop OM that is of increased severity and longer duration, possibly because of a physiologic decline in renal function, which could alter chemotherapy excretion (Raber-Durlacher et al., 2000). More women than men ex-

---

Figure 3-1. Risk Factors for Oral Mucositis

Treatment-Related	Patient-Related
• Type of cancer • Mucotoxic and multi-cycle chemotherapy agents • Radiation dose and fractionation schedule • Radiation to the head and neck • Chemoradiation • Myeloablative therapy and stem cell transplantation • Total body irradiation • Graft-versus-host disease prophylaxis • Neutropenia • Xerostomia • Biologic agents	• Age • Sex • Comorbidities • Baseline oral dentition and hygiene • Nutrition status • Alcohol and tobacco use • Salivary gland dysfunction • Oral trauma and irritation • Dental appliances • Dehydration • Hepatic or renal impairment

Note. Based on information from Bensinger et al., 2008; Polovich et al., 2009.

perienced an increased incidence and severity of OM when receiving fluoro-uracil-based chemotherapy (Sloan et al., 2000, 2002).

Therapy-related risk factors are dependent on treatment modalities, drug doses, and schedules. OM results from various chemotherapy agents. Some of the most mucotoxic chemotherapy agents are methotrexate, 5-fluoroura-cil, cisplatin, cytarabine, and etoposide (McGuire, 2002). The method of delivery can affect OM, as seen with 5-fluorouracil, where a higher incidence of OM occurs with continuous infusion versus bolus administration. Dose intensity affects OM. Wardley et al. (2000) discovered that 99% of patients undergoing high-dose chemotherapy prior to stem cell transplantation experienced OM, most often grade 3 or 4. Radiation therapy contributes to the development of OM based on the location of the tumor, dose per fraction, total dose, and fractionation schedule. Concurrent treatment with chemotherapy, particularly in patients with head and neck cancer, significantly increases the risk of OM.

OM was once thought to be an isolated event. Mucosal injury is the collective consequence of a number of concurrent and sequential biologic processes (Rubenstein et al., 2004). Sonis (2004) identified five distinct phases of OM: (1) initiation, (2) message generation, (3) signaling and amplification, (4) ulceration, and (5) healing (see Figure 3-2). During the initiation phase, exposure to chemotherapy or radiation therapy generates the release of reactive oxygen species that damage DNA and results in cell, tissue, and blood vessel damage to the mucosa. In the upregulation and message-generating phase, chemotherapy or radiation therapy activates the release of pro-

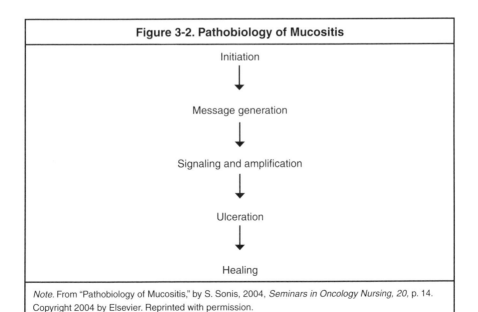

Figure 3-2. Pathobiology of Mucositis

Initiation
↓
Message generation
↓
Signaling and amplification
↓
Ulceration
↓
Healing

Note. From "Pathobiology of Mucositis," by S. Sonis, 2004, *Seminars in Oncology Nursing, 20,* p. 14. Copyright 2004 by Elsevier. Reprinted with permission.

inflammatory cytokines, resulting in tissue injury and programmed cell death (apoptosis). It is in this phase that the oral mucosa begins to thin, and erythema and pain become apparent. The signaling and amplification phase is the continued release of cytokines, which indirectly trigger other pathways that alter the tissues in the mucosa. During the ulceration phase, tissue damage has penetrated the epithelium and submucosa, resulting in visible ulceration, pain, and other symptoms. Angiogenesis is stimulated during the ulceration phase. In the last phase, healing, signals from the extracellular tissues stimulate epithelial proliferation until the mucosa reaches its normal thickness and is healed. Despite the healing, the patient remains at risk for future injury and recurrence.

The first symptom of OM is a feeling of discomfort with some redness and slight swelling of the lining of the mouth (Tipton, 2009). This is usually followed several days later by the development of small sores and ulceration. Other signs and symptoms of OM include changes in taste and ability to swallow, pain with swallowing and talking, changes in the color of the oral mucosa evidenced by pallor or erythema, and changes in the moisture of the oral mucosa. Visible signs of OM occur within four to five days of standard chemotherapy, three to five days after the conditioning regimen in stem cell transplant recipients, and during the second week of head and neck irradiation (Keefe et al., 2007).

Pain is considered the hallmark symptom of OM. McGuire et al. (1998) found that 75% of patients with OM complain of oral pain. The severity of pain varies from patient to patient and often depends on the treatment modalities used. The associated pain has a varied duration (one to two weeks for patients receiving chemotherapy and up to several months for patients undergoing radiation therapy) and remits when the underlying tissue damage resolves (Epstein & Schubert, 2004). OM is much more than a "sore mouth," and oncology nurses are well positioned to advocate for patients and manage this most debilitating symptom. Unfortunately, little evidence-based literature exists on management strategies for OM pain. The current pain management strategies for OM include topical anesthetics, systemic analgesics, and emerging therapies. Topical anesthetics, such as viscous lidocaine, are used for mild to moderate pain. Taken prior to meals, viscous lidocaine provides temporary relief of pain. Another disadvantage to the use of viscous lidocaine is that the numbing effect can allow patients to unknowingly further traumatize their mouth. Other topical agents include "magic" mouthwashes and sucralfate suspension, but they have no proven efficacy in the management of OM pain. Gelclair® (EKR Therapeutics, Inc.) is a bioadherent oral gel that has been indicated for use in the management of OM pain. Initial evidence indicates that Gelclair provides rapid and durable oral pain relief by forming an adherent barrier over the oral mucosa that shields the exposed or sensitized nerves (Peterson, Beck, & Keefe, 2004). The U.S. Food and Drug Administration (FDA) approved Gelclair as a medical device and requires a prescription. Caphosol® (EUSA Pharma [USA], Inc.) is a supersaturated calcium phosphate oral rinse that lubricates the mucosa and theoretically helps maintain the integrity of the oral cavity. Caphosol requires a prescription as a medical device. In a study conducted by Haas and Mercedes (2008), preliminary data suggested that Caphosol had a significant positive impact on the occurrence and severity of OM in patients receiving chemotherapy, radiation therapy, and concurrent chemoradiation. Patients and physicians reported low pain medication use and high levels of satisfaction with Caphosol. They found that 13% did not develop OM, 36% had grade 1 (mild) OM, 33% had grade 2 (moderate) OM, 16% had grade 3 (severe) OM, and 2% had grade 4 (life-threatening or disabling) OM (Haas & Mercedes, 2008). Papas et al. (2003) conducted a randomized trial of 95 patients looking at prevention of OM in stem cell transplant recipients. The results showed favorable effects when Caphosol was used in combination with fluoride as compared to the control group that used fluoride only.

Systemic analgesics have been the cornerstone of pain management for patients with OM experiencing moderate to severe oral pain. Systemic analgesics have been the best-studied approach for the management of severe OM pain. The World Health Organization recommends morphine sulfate as the opioid of choice for the management of severe pain (Ripamonti & Dickerson, 2001). Elting et al. (2003) found that although 37% of patients identified significant pain with OM, only 8% of patients received opioids. Patients who cannot be managed on oral opioids will need other options, such as narcotic patches, patient-controlled analgesia (PCA), or continuous-infusion opioids. PCA as a mode of delivery has been used for patients with severe OM pain in the bone marrow transplantion setting. Other agents, such as capsaicin (the active ingredient in chili peppers), ketamine (an anesthetic agent) as an oral rinse, benzydamine hydrochloride (a nonsteroidal rinse), cytoprotection with amifostine, and hematopoietic growth factors, have been used, but none have proved to be beneficial in the management of OM pain.

No evidence-based standards of care currently exist for the prevention and treatment of OM. The only evidence-based preventive strategies include the use of palifermin (Kepivance®, Biovitrum AB) to prevent OM in the setting of hematopoietic stem cell transplantation, oral cryotherapy used in conjunction with bolus 5-fluorouracil, melphalan, and edatrexate, which is an investigational antimetabolite agent (Bensinger et al., 2008). The management of OM is based on supportive care and palliation of symptoms. Palifermin is a human recombinant keratinocyte growth factor that is FDA-approved for the prevention of OM in autologous stem cell transplant recipients receiving high-dose chemotherapy or total body irradiation (Bensinger et al., 2008; Harris, Eilers, Cashavelly, Maxwell, & Harriman, 2007; Multinational Association of Supportive Care in Cancer, 2005). Palifermin is administered by an IV bolus daily three days prior to the preparatory regimen and three days after transplantation. It is well tolerated with minimal side effects that include altered taste, transient skin rash, and the sensation of a thickened tongue.

OM is a management challenge especially in the hematopoietic stem cell transplantation setting. These patients receive high-dose, myeloablative chemotherapy as a conditioning regimen. OM becomes so severe for these patients that they often require parenteral narcotics for pain control and total parenteral nutrition (TPN) if oral intake cannot be maintained. OM can be the most debilitating complication of transplantation. When these patients experience neutropenia, severe OM puts them at risk for developing septicemia. Sonis et al. (2001) found that the extent and severity of OM in hematopoietic stem cell transplant recipients were positively correlated with the use of TPN and injectable narcotic therapy, the risk of significant infection and death, and total hospital days and charges.

Xerostomia and Hyposalivation

Xerostomia is the term used for the symptom of oral dryness. Xerostomia is one of the most debilitating consequences of cancer therapy to the head and neck region. It starts as early as the first week of radiotherapy and can be a life-long problem. Xerostomia can contribute to OM, dysphagia, dental caries, changes in taste, and increased risk of fungal infections. In a quality-of-life study of patients who received radiation therapy for head and neck cancer, the most common complaint (95%) was dry mouth and was reported to be moderate or severe by 70% of the patients (Epstein, Robertson, Emerton, Phillips, & Stevenson-Moore, 2001).

To understand xerostomia and its impact, it is important to understand normal salivary function. Three major salivary glands (parotid, sublingual, and submandibular) produce 80% of the saliva (Chong & Armstrong, 2004). The nervous system regulates the salivary glands, and they respond within two to three seconds as a result of a conditioned reflex (sight, smell, and taste of food). The remainder of salivary flow comes from 600–1,000 minor salivary glands located throughout the mouth. Normal salivary glands produce 1–1.5 liters of saliva daily (Chong & Armstrong, 2004). Approximately three-quarters of a teaspoon of saliva is produced per minute, and chewing gum can stimulate about one tablespoon of saliva per minute. The importance of saliva cannot be emphasized enough. Saliva is necessary for the lubrication of food during chewing and swallowing. It prepares food for swallowing by keeping the oral cavity moist while softening the food for swallowing. Saliva helps cleanse the mouth of any remaining food particles. Another important function of saliva is that of protecting the mouth against bacterial or fungal infections. Saliva coats the teeth with minerals necessary for protecting them from cavities. Keeping the mouth moist helps prevent irritation that can occur while speaking. Lack of moisture can contribute to redness, swelling, and pain of the mucous membranes.

The parotid glands produce the serous component in saliva, whereas the minor salivary glands produce the mucous component. The serous salivary tissues are more sensitive to the effects of radiation, resulting in more ropey, tenacious saliva that is diminished in amount. Patients may have more difficulty handling these tenacious secretions with their dry oral mucosa. Researchers hypothesize that radiation exposure does not damage the salivary glands but rather the blood vessels or nerves supplying the glands (Logemann et al., 2001). Patients, often within 12 hours of their first radiation treatment, will experience parotiditis, which is a transient, painless enlargement of one or more of the salivary glands in the treatment field. The swelling disappears within a day or two, and over-the-counter anti-inflammatory agents alleviate any discomfort. Radiation contributes to OM as a result of the rapidly dividing epithelial cells and the high proliferation of these cells. If OM becomes severe enough, patients will need a break from their treatment to allow the damaged oral mucosa to heal.

Good oral hygiene is the foundation for oral health and can be difficult for patients with xerostomia. Permanent xerostomia causes discomfort, altered taste acuity, poor oral hygiene, and accelerated dental decay (Chong & Armstrong, 2004). It is essential for the nurse to educate patients and families on the importance of a strict oral care regimen and the complications that can result from not following it. A strict oral hygiene regimen needs to become a life-long routine for these patients, particularly after radiation treatment. The basic care for patients with xerostomia is outlined in Table 3-1.

Current management of xerostomia is mainly palliative and provides only short-lived relief. Treatment can be local or systemic. The biggest disadvantages of local treatments are that they provide temporary relief and may require frequent use or application, which is often cumbersome for the patient. Patients often are encouraged to suck on sugar-free hard candies or chew sugar-free gum to stimulate saliva. Gums containing xylitol, such as Biotene® (GlaxoSmithKline), Orbit® (Wrigley Co.), or Xylifresh® (BioScience), provide anti-cariogenic properties that help prevent cavities. Artificial saliva products are

Table 3-1. Oral Care Regimen for Patients With Xerostomia	
Basic Oral Care	**Additions for Patients With Xerostomia**
Oral care (before and after meals and at bedtime)	Brush teeth with nonabrasive fluoride toothpaste.
Flossing (daily)	Use unwaxed, nonshredding dental floss.
Oral assessment (daily)	Inspect mouth for oral lesions and infections.
Mouthwashes (nonalcohol), such as Biotene® (GlaxoSmithKline)	Use to loosen debris and moisten the mouth.
Fluoride treatment (daily at bedtime)	Use custom-made trays for 5 minutes. Do not eat or drink for 30 minutes after application.
Note. Based on information from Bruce, 2004.	

another option for patients. These agents help keep the oral mucosa lubricated, and use is encouraged before meals and at bedtime. These agents, however, fail to provide any antibacterial protection (Miller & Kearney, 2001). Some patients find saliva substitutes to have an unpleasant taste. Saliva stimulants are another class of treatment agents that can help increase production of saliva. The most common agent is pilocarpine (Salagen®, Eisai Inc.). It is a systemic agent that works through the cholinergic nervous system to stimulate any residual functioning of salivary gland tissue. The manufacturer's recommended dose is one 5 mg tablet three to four times a day. The dose can be adjusted to 15–30 mg per day, with no more than two tablets taken per dose (Eisai Inc., 2009). The duration of effect is two to four hours. It is important when starting patients on this drug to inform them that it may take 90 days to notice an effect. The primary side effects associated with pilocarpine are excessive sweating and runny nose; therefore, the patient must drink at least two to three liters of fluid a day to stay hydrated. Some patients find the side effects intolerable and will abandon treatment with the drug.

Amifostine (Ethyol®, MedImmune, LLC) is a cytoprotective agent that has been used in the management of xerostomia. It is indicated for use in patients undergoing postoperative radiation therapy for squamous cell cancer of the head and neck when significant portions of the parotid glands are in the treatment field. In a pivotal trial conducted by Brizel et al. (2000), amifostine significantly reduced the overall incidence of grade 2 or higher acute xerostomia from 78% to 51% ($p < 0.0001$). They found that patients who received amifostine produced significantly more saliva than patients treated with radiotherapy alone. Cytoprotection will be discussed in more detail in Chapter 6.

Cevimeline hydrochloride (Evoxac®, Daiichi Sankyo, Inc.) received FDA approval in 2000 for the treatment of dry mouth in patients with Sjögren syndrome (an autoimmune disease characterized by salivary dysfunction and dry mouth). Evoxac is a cholinergic agonist that binds to muscarinic receptors and significantly improves salivary flow for patients suffering from dry mouth associated with Sjögren syndrome. Evoxac is pharmacologically similar to pilocarpine hydrochloride because both drugs stimulate residual salivary gland tissues that are still functioning despite damage induced by radiation (Bruce, 2004). A study conducted by Chambers et al. (2007) looked at the efficacy of cevimeline treatment for radiation-induced xerostomia in patients with head and neck cancer. These patients received cevimeline hydrochloride 45 mg three times a day for 52 weeks. Overall, the global efficacy showed that cevimeline hydrochloride improved dry mouth in 59.2% of the study subjects. Most patients (68.6%) experienced mild to moderate expected treatment-related adverse events. Most frequent was increased sweating (47.5%), followed by dyspepsia (9.4%), nausea (8.2%), and diarrhea (6.3%), with 17.6% of study subjects discontinuing study medication because of adverse events. Evoxac is not currently FDA-approved for use in patients with xerostomia, so use in these patients is strictly off-label.

Acupuncture has been reported in Western medical literature back to 1981 as a treatment for xerostomia. Nearly a decade ago, Johnstone, Niemtzow, and Riffenburgh (2002) reported that 34%–40% of patients with xerostomia seek nontraditional medical treatment, and that number has grown since then. The basis for acupuncture is the balance and flow of qi (pronounced "chee") and the belief that the body's symptoms are distress signals of an imbalance in the qi. Eastern philosophy claims that xerostomia relief is achieved by removing the blockage of qi. Acupuncture is being used more to complement conventional medical care. Although the mechanism of action is not clearly understood, it is theorized that the autonomic stimulation by the needles used in acupuncture is at least partially responsible for the effect. It is claimed that acupuncture regulates the balance of fluid in the body, preventing too little or too much flow (Johnstone et al., 2002).

Acupuncture for the relief of xerostomia consists of the placement of eight needles. Special acupuncture needles are placed at a single point in the distal radial aspect of the index fingers and three points in each ear. Patients are asked to suck on a piece of sugar-free candy to help "milk" the salivary glands. The visits last 30–60 minutes and are scheduled weekly for four to six weeks or until a response is reported. Monthly to bimonthly visits are encouraged for those patients who achieve some benefit. No adverse reactions have occurred from acupuncture, but possible side effects are hematoma at the acupuncture site and fatigue that occurs initially with the first several treatments. Early studies show that acupuncture can improve salivary function in patients with xerostomia (Blom & Lundeberg, 2000).

Chronic Graft-Versus-Host Disease

Allogeneic bone marrow transplant recipients commonly have oral complications related to their disease or its treatment. They experience many of the same complications experienced by patients receiving chemotherapy and radiation, including xerostomia, mucositis, dental caries, and infections. Graft-versus-host disease (GVHD) is a complication specific to the transplantation setting. GVHD is a significant cause of morbidity and mortality in bone marrow transplant (BMT) recipients. It is estimated that 40%–70% of patients develop acute GVHD or chronic GVHD after undergoing allogeneic BMT, despite the prophylactic regimen used (França, Domingues-Martins, Volpe, Filho, & de Araújo, 2001). Chronic GVHD occurs 100 days or more after the transplantation procedure and may take the form of oral manifestations. Oral manifestations are observed in about 80% of patients who have extensive forms of chronic GVHD (França et al., 2001). Lesions known as lichenoid lesions can affect the mucosal surfaces with predominantly reticular and papular forms, while tongue lesions are more plaque-like. Some studies have reported that the presence of oral lichenoid lesions shows a statistically significant relationship with a chronic GVHD diagnosis

(Nakamura et al., 1996). Ulcerative lesions are common and are mainly localized in the buccal mucosa, the palate, and the dorsal part of the tongue. These ulcers usually are covered with a gray or yellow pseudomembrane and accompanied by erythema. Prophylactic regimens that are used to prevent oral manifestations of GVHD include the removal of traumatic factors and severely diseased teeth, as well as definitive oral rehabilitation before BMT (França et al., 2001). To alleviate GVHD's oral manifestations, patients should use a basic protocol that includes meticulous oral hygiene, topical steroids (dexamethasone or betamethasone mouthwash), effective analgesia (lidocaine), and artificial saliva or a saliva stimulant (Woo, Lee, & Schubert, 1997). GVHD is a complex process that emphasizes the value of a multidisciplinary team that includes a dentist to assist with the management of oral complications experienced by this patient population.

Dental Caries and Periodontal Disease

Patients with head and neck cancer are particularly at risk for dental caries and periodontal disease before undergoing treatment for their cancer. Many of these patients have existing issues with their oral hygiene prior to diagnosis, and cancer treatment would further compound the problems. For these patients, it is of the utmost importance that they receive a full comprehensive dental evaluation by a dentist and/or oral surgeon. The patient should be evaluated for preexisting gum disease and teeth that are in poor repair and need extraction. A routine cleaning should be performed, as well as any restorative dental work before beginning treatment, especially radiation therapy. Any dental extractions will require 10–14 days to ensure that adequate healing has occurred prior to starting radiation therapy (National Institute of Dental and Craniofacial Research, 2010). Any invasive dental work will need to be completed 7–10 days before the start of myelosuppressive chemotherapy to ensure that healing occurs before the patient becomes neutropenic or thrombocytopenic (National Institute of Dental and Craniofacial Research, 2010). The oral complications experienced as a result of chemotherapy will be dependent on the chemotherapy drugs used, the dosage, and the degree of preexisting dental disease.

Oral assessment and care are essential components of nursing care for patients with head and neck cancer both during and after treatment. The oral cavity should be assessed at weekly treatment visits and as problems arise. Patients should be instructed to report pain, tenderness, a burning sensation, and any other symptoms that may signal the need for further evaluation. Upon completion of radiotherapy, patients will need life-long and aggressive dental follow-up. Rather than the usual six-month follow-up examinations, these patients will require more frequent follow-up—every three to four months—to monitor for oral complications. The development of dental caries may begin as soon as three to six months after completion of therapy. Patients receiving radiotherapy will have custom fluoride trays made for daily, life-long treatment with fluoride gel to help prevent dental decay. Patients who have received radiotherapy should avoid elective oral surgery on irradiated bone due to the risk of osteoradionecrosis. It will be important for the dentist to know whether the mandible and maxilla were in the treatment field, the total dose of radiation delivered, and whether the vascularity of the mandible has been compromised by surgery.

Taste Changes

Taste changes are one of the most overlooked symptoms experienced by patients undergoing cancer treatment. *Taste* can be defined as the chemical sensation related to specialized receptors selectively stimulated by molecules and ions of solutions in contact with them (Redda & Allis, 2006). Patients with head and neck cancer who are undergoing treatment are most affected by taste changes. Complaints of taste disorders have been reported in 75% of patients with head and neck cancer undergoing radiation therapy, and 93% of these patients complain of long-term xerostomia (Yamashita et al., 2009). Approximately two out of three patients with cancer (68%) receiving chemotherapy report altered sensory perception, such as decreased or lost taste acuity or a metallic taste (Ravasco, 2005; Wickham et al., 1999). In a study of 42 patients who had received at least two cycles of chemotherapy (identified to be associated with taste changes), the taste changes patients reported most frequently were metallic taste (78%), no sense of taste (68%), and bitter taste (57%) (Rehwaldt et al., 2009).

Taste buds are pear-shaped organs found primarily on the tongue but also located on the soft palate, pharynx, larynx, uvula, upper third of the esophagus, lips, and cheeks. They are the receptor cells that are responsible for mediating the sense of taste. Each taste bud consists of 50–100 receptor cells that have an average life span of 10–11 days (Schiffman & Gatlin, 1993). The sense of taste is stimulated with the ingestion of food and serves as the main stimulus for the formation of saliva in the oral cavity, which is necessary for taste perception. Changes in taste are often one of the earliest side effects experienced with radiation therapy. Taste changes may occur before the development of OM. Taste changes associated with radiation therapy have been reported as early as two to three days after the onset of radiation, with doses as small as 200–400 cGy (Sandow, Hejrat-Yazdi, & Heft, 2006). The degeneration of taste buds typically occurs six to seven days after radiation and can be associated with damage to either intragemmal nerve cells, taste cells, or both (Nelson, 1998). Damage to the oral mucosa and taste buds is strongly related to radiation dose, fraction size, volume of irradiated tissue, and technique (Redda & Allis, 2006). These taste changes can vary from having no taste at all to experiencing an unpleasant metallic taste or bitter sensation. Lack of taste contributes to a loss of desire to eat and results in anorexia and weight loss in a group of patients that often are nutritionally challenged at the time of diagnosis. Loss of taste after radiation therapy was found to be most pronounced after 2 months with gradual improvement at 6 and 12–24 months, with further recovery in the period after 24 months, but taste loss could persist for one to two years after treatment (Maes et al., 2002).

Risk factors associated with taste changes include normal aging, malnutrition, poor dentition and oral hygiene, alcohol and tobacco use, oral infections, xerostomia and mucositis, vitamin and zinc deficiency, antineoplastic agents, location of the tumor, and treatment with radiation therapy. A variety of medical conditions may cause taste changes, such as diabetes, chronic renal disease, hypothyroidism, and malignancies in other sites (esophagus, lung, lymphomas, breast, and central nervous system) (Redda & Allis, 2006). Common antineoplastic agents known to affect taste include cisplatin, carboplatin, cyclophosphamide, doxorubicin, 5-fluorouracil, levamisole, and methotrexate. The taste changes accompanied by these agents usually are temporary and diminish once the drug is completed.

The main strategies for managing taste loss include protecting the healthy tissue from radiation damage, dietary measures, and zinc supplements. Recent advances in radiation treatment techniques can help shield and reduce the exposure of radiation to the tongue and salivary glands. These recent advances include three-dimensional conformal radiation therapy and intensity-modulated radiotherapy, more commonly known as IMRT. A third way to protect the oral and salivary tissues is with the use of the cytoprotective agent amifostine. Amifostine is a thiol compound that protects normal organs from the oxidative effects resulting from chemotherapy and radiotherapy. Amifostine has been widely used in the prevention of xerostomia in patients with head and neck cancer receiving radiation therapy to the salivary glands. Cytoprotective agents will be further discussed in Chapter 6.

IMRT is one of the state-of-the-art advances in radiotherapy that has occurred in the past decade or so. The use of IMRT allows for higher doses of radiation to be delivered to cancer cells in a targeted way. The advantage of IMRT is that it is more precise than conventional radiotherapy and spares the surrounding healthy tissues from radiation. IMRT uses computer-generated images in the planning and delivery of very focused radiation beams to the cancer target. The beams are designed to conform as closely as possible to the shape of the tumor. Radiotherapy using IMRT is delivered by a linear accelerator using a special piece of equipment called a multileaf collimator. The multileaf collimator has finger-like projections that open and close to shape the radiation beam being delivered to the tumor. The multileaf collimator can be rotated around the patient from various angles designed in the treatment plan to deliver a high dose to the tumor while sparing the healthy tissues. The conventional three-beam approach delivers radiation from the left, right, and front, making IMRT a much more desirable option.

Dietary measures for reducing taste abnormalities in patients with cancer are limited and do not resolve the recurring issues with these abnormalities.

Published recommendations (Ravasco, 2005; Vissink, Burlage, Spijkervet, Jansma, & Coppes, 2003) include

- Avoiding the use of metal flatware to reduce the risk of metallic taste
- Reducing the consumption of foods that taste metallic or bitter, such as red meat, coffee, and tea
- Increasing the consumption of high-protein, mildly flavored foods, such as chicken, fish, dairy products, and eggs
- Adding seasonings and spices to enhance flavors if hypogeusia (decreased taste) or hyposmia (decreased sense of smell) is experienced
- Serving foods at cold temperatures to reduce unpleasant flavors and odors
- Practicing good oral hygiene, including frequent tooth brushing and use of mouthwash
- Using sialogogues (agents that stimulate salivary secretion), such as sugar-free gum or sour-tasting hard candy
- Using saliva substitutes and lubricating solutions containing mucin and carboxymethylcellulose.

The relationship between zinc and taste perception has been studied with various conclusions (Vissink et al., 2003). Although clinical evidence suggests that exogenous zinc sulfate administration successfully improves taste and smell disorders (Henkin, Martin, & Agarwal, 1999; Takeda et al., 2004), others have not supported the same conclusions (Halyard et al., 2007). Ripamonti et al. (1998) conducted a double-blinded, randomized study evaluating the effects of zinc sulfate administration versus placebo in the management of taste alterations caused by radiotherapy. A total of 18 patients in this study who had external beam radiotherapy to the head and neck region were randomized to receive either zinc sulfate or placebo tablets three times a day from the onset of subjective perceptions of taste alterations. Researchers found the administration of zinc sulfate significantly slowed the worsening of taste and improved taste acuity. The results also showed that administering 25 mg of zinc sulfate four times a day was sufficient to normalize serum levels, taste perception, and taste bud anatomy. Others have demonstrated an association between taste alterations and low serum zinc levels (Henkin, 1972; Wright, King, Baer, & Citron, 1981). The results of these studies suggested that zinc sulfate merited further study in patients with cancer. Halyard et al. (2007) conducted a multi-institutional, double-blind, placebo-controlled trial to provide definitive evidence of zinc's palliative efficacy in taste alterations in patients with head and neck cancer undergoing radiation therapy. This study is the largest ever reported evaluating zinc sulfate in the treatment or prevention of taste alterations. A total of 169 patients were randomized to receive zinc sulfate 45 mg orally three times a day versus placebo. The zinc sulfate as prescribed in this trial did not prevent taste alterations in the patients who participated while undergoing radiation therapy to the oral pharynx. This is a rich area for nursing research because taste alteration continues to be an underrecognized symptom experienced by patients with no definitive treatment recommendations. See also Chapter 9.

Persistent Dysphagia

Dysphagia is experienced by many patients receiving head and neck irradiation, and it can be persistent, ultimately affecting the patient's quality of life in a negative manner. *Dysphagia* is defined as difficulty swallowing (Carper, 2007). It can affect the patient's ability to eat, thus resulting in the consumption of fewer calories than are required to sustain treatment and healing. There are multiple causes of treatment-related dysphagia, which include tone atrophy, vocal cord palsy, pharyngeal constriction, surgical resection or damage caused by the tumor itself that impedes the swallowing process, mucositis or esophagitis, and radiation fibrosis (Carper, 2007).

An estimated 25% or more of patients with nasopharyngeal cancer will have significant dysphagia with endoscopically determined aspiration occurring during the act of swallowing (Wu, Hsiao, Ko, & Hsu, 2000). Up to 34% of patients who undergo chemotherapy and irradiation for head and neck cancer experience severe dysphagia; moderate dysphagia has been reported in up to 43% of these patients; and mild dysphagia has been reported in 25% of patients (Nguyen et al., 2006).

A multidisciplinary approach is needed for the management of persistent dysphagia. Referral to a speech pathologist is necessary for a swallowing evaluation and determination of the risk for aspiration. The speech pathologist can provide various swallowing and oral motor exercises that can assist with swallowing. After the speech evaluation is completed, a dietitian can be instrumental in making recommendations on how best to ensure caloric intake given the patient's identified needs. The patient may require a feeding tube, particularly if aspiration occurs. Pain management should be aggressive to maximize comfort and ensure that the patient is able to maintain hydration and caloric intake.

Trismus

Trismus is a late side effect from radiation therapy to the oral cavity and is seen in patients treated for nasopharyngeal cancer, cancer of the base of the tongue, salivary gland cancer, and tumors of the maxilla. *Trismus* is defined as the contraction of the muscles of mastication, but the term is commonly used to refer to any restriction in ability to open the mouth (Carper, 2007). The incidence of trismus in patients with head and neck cancer receiving radiotherapy is 10%–40% (Oral Cancer Foundation, 2001–2010). Trismus occurs gradually and becomes progressive over time. This occurs when the connective tissue becomes tight and short, resulting in limited range of motion in the mandibular or temporomandibular region. It can have a significant impact on the patient's ability to chew and digest food, speak, and perform oral hygiene. Trismus puts the patient at risk for aspiration.

Radiation doses of greater than 60 Gy directed to the temporomandibular joint, pterygoid muscles, or the masseter muscles are most likely to cause injury leading to trismus (Carper, 2007). Patients who have been previously irradiated and are receiving treatment for recurrence are at higher risk for trismus. Trismus begins toward the end of treatment and gradually increases over several weeks and months. It develops over time and at a slow rate, so it is important to be proactive in monitoring the patient. Nurses should measure in millimeters the distance that patients can open their mouth. Ideally this should be done at or near the end of treatment as a baseline measurement and periodically during the follow-up period. It is important to teach patients to contact their physician or nurse at the onset of any difficulty opening their mouth or chewing foods and to not wait until their next regularly scheduled appointment. A simple test to teach patients for how to determine early signs of trismus is the "three-finger test" (Oral Cancer Foundation, 2001–2010). If the patient can insert three fingers into the mouth, the mouth opening is considered functional. If not, restriction is more likely. Prompt and early treatment will help restore function and prevent complications from trismus from occurring.

Trismus manifests clinically with patient complaints of difficulty opening their mouth or difficulty chewing. Patients with trismus may present with xerostomia, mucositis, and pain, thereby presenting with the associated symptoms of ear pain, jaw pain, and headache. The severity of trismus varies widely, with some patients having no limitation in opening their mouth and others who are restricted to 4–5 mm. Factors affecting the severity of the restriction include the placement of the radiation fields, total dose received, and the patient's ability to tolerate treatment. Patients with trismus are at risk for developing fibrosis of the muscles of the oral cavity. Trismus may go unnoticed in patients with feeding tubes who are not taking in oral nutrition and are not chewing on a regular basis.

Treatment for trismus is conservative. The goal of treatment is to minimize the degree of trismus and promote the return of normal jaw functioning. To prevent trismus, patients should be instructed to exercise their mouth regularly with chewing exercises. An example exercise for patients is to open the mouth as wide as possible, hold this position for a few seconds, and then repeat this multiple times throughout the day. Commercial devices are available that can be used to accomplish this activity, such as the Therabite Jaw Motion Rehabilitation System® (Atos Medical Corp.), E-Z Flex® (Fluid Motion Biotechnologies), and Dynasplint® Trismus System (Dynasplint Systems, Inc.). These devices help stretch the muscles of mastication but can be costly and may require a prescription or certificate of medical necessity to obtain. A simple, inexpensive way to achieve the same goal is to use a stack of tongue blades, increasing the number of stacked tongue blades to stretch the opening of the mouth. It is important to instruct the patient to do this stretching exercise but not to the point of pain or discomfort.

Fungal Infections

Fungal infections are another common oral complication experienced by patients with cancer undergoing treatment. Oral candidiasis, also known as "thrush" or "yeast," is the most frequent fungal infection experienced by patients. Risk factors for the development of candidiasis include poor salivation, ill-fitting dentures, continued tobacco or alcohol use, medications such as steroids, and the location of the cancer, particularly head and neck.

Oral candidiasis may appear as soft white patches covering part or all of the tongue, lips, gums, or buccal mucosa. These curd-like patches can be scraped off the tongue and mucosal areas. Patients often report a metallic taste, increased difficulty with swallowing, or a burning sensation. This requires further evaluation by the nurse or physician, as it may signal the onset of candidiasis. Candidiasis infection can exacerbate OM.

These infections usually respond well to fluconazole (Diflucan®, Pfizer Inc.) or other systemic antifungal agents. In severe cases of candidiasis, Diflucan can be administered intravenously initially and then transitioned to oral therapy. Clotrimazole troches are difficult to use in patients with head and neck cancer because their diminished saliva production makes it hard to dissolve the troche. Fungal reinfection may occur and should be treated as early as possible.

Osteoradionecrosis

Osteoradionecrosis (ORN) is a major late side effect and complication of radiotherapy. ORN is a condition of impaired healing and soft tissue necrosis of the jawbone (Carper, 2007). The soft tissue and bone necrosis fail to heal and usually do not respond to local treatment over a period of six months. Radiation causes hypoxia in the tissues of normal cells, causing an imbalance between cell death and collagen lysis and exceeding the homeostatic mechanism of cell replacement and collagen synthesis. The wound will not heal, as the increased metabolic demands far exceed the oxygen and vascular supply.

ORN occurs most commonly in the mandible after head and neck irradiation. It can occur in 5%–15% of patients receiving radiotherapy and typically presents after tooth extraction from the mandible (Viale & Lin, 2005). The clinical presentation of ORN may include oral or jaw pain, facial pain, exposed necrotic bone or pathologic fracture of the mandible, and purulent drainage.

Contributing factors that lead to the development of ORN are the total radiation dose, the field and fraction size, and the volume of mandible treated to a high dose (Bruner, Haas, & Gosselin-Acomb, 2005). Numerous risk factors exist for ORN (Jereczek-Fossa & Orecchia, 2002), including
- Poor oral hygiene
- Alcohol and tobacco use
- Bone inflammation
- Poor-fitting oral/dental prosthesis

- Poor overall nutrition status
- Premorbid state of dentition
- Dental trauma
- Proximity of tumor to the bone
- Dental extractions after radiotherapy to the jaw.

ORN has been treated over the years with variable success rates. Hyperbaric oxygen (HBO) therapy, although considered controversial by some, is a treatment modality that provides increased oxygen tension at the tissue level. This is accomplished by placing patients in a pressure-tolerant dive chamber where they can breathe 100% oxygen. The dive chamber is pressurized at 2.4 atmospheres absolute, and depending on the protocol, patients remain inside for one hour (David, Sàndor, Evans, & Brown, 2001). This is thought to increase vascular density, which stimulates angiogenesis, leading to the repair of tissue damaged by radiation (Corman, McClure, Pritchett, Kozlowski, & Hampson, 2003). Hyberbaric oxygen therapy has been found to enhance healing in a variety of radiation-injured tissues (Marx, Ehler, Tayapongsak, & Pierce, 1990).

Conservative treatment includes saline irrigation, diligent oral hygiene, antibiotics during periods of infection, analgesics, and topical antiseptics. Despite adherence to conservative treatment, it can take three to six months for the ORN wound to close. For some patients, surgery may be required whereby the necrotic tissue is removed, followed by primary closure of the wound. In severe cases of ORN, partial mandibulectomy may be required. HBO is used before surgery for up to as many as 20 daily treatments. Surgery is then followed by 10 daily postoperative HBO treatments to maximize healing.

Osteonecrosis

Bisphosphonate therapy has been used in the treatment for patients with metastatic bone disease and has reduced the skeletal complications (pain and pathologic fracture) from bone metastases. Bisphosphonates, such as pamidronate and zoledronate, have been used to treat hypercalcemia of malignancy. It was recently reported that bisphosphonates are capable of causing osteonecrosis of the jaws (Melo & Obeid, 2005). This unrecognized complication is seen in patients receiving treatment with the nitrogen-containing bisphosphonates (pamidronate and zoledronate). Patients present with lesions resembling those seen in ORN and may have exposed necrotic bone. It is proposed that the antiangiogenic properties of bisphosphonates, along with alteration in bone metabolism mediated by osteoclast inhibition, provide a plausible explanation for the development of bisphosphonate-related osteonecrosis of the jaws (Ruggiero, Mehrotra, Rosenberg, & Engroff, 2004).

Osteonecrosis, unlike ORN, does not respond to HBO therapy. In bisphosphonate-related osteonecrosis, the alteration in bone metabolism is such that revascularization alone is insufficient to alter the course of the lesions because bisphosphonates are not metabolized appreciably and have the potential to remain in the bone indefinitely (Russell et al., 1999). Attempts to increase the vascularity of the affected bone are unsuccessful in the long term. Bisphosphonate-induced osteonecrosis is commonly seen in the maxilla.

Oncology nurses are in a position to recognize and possibly prevent bisphosphonate-related osteonecrosis. Patients most at risk are those with multiple myeloma, breast cancer, or prostate cancer. Nurses performing oral assessments should be alert for soft tissue inflammation, pain, swelling, foul-tasting drainage, or bone exposure, particularly at the site of a previous dental extraction. Preventive dentistry measures cannot be overemphasized. A thorough dental examination with any tooth extractions, allowing for adequate healing time, needs to be performed prior to beginning bisphosphonate therapy. Meticulous oral care is essential.

Conclusion

Oral complications that result from cancer treatment can significantly affect a patient's quality of life, as many of these complications can be life-long problems. These problems can be devastating and debilitating to patients. A multidisciplinary approach is vital to manage oral complications and ensure that the best possible supportive and evidence-based care is provided. Oncology nurses are key members of the team and play a pivotal role in the coordination of care and education of patients and their families. Patients need to play an active role in their care to ensure compliance. The goal is to help patients return to a satisfying and productive life while managing the impact of problems in the most optimal manner. Although significant strides have been achieved in the treatment of various cancers and other supportive care issues, advances in the arena of oral complications have lagged behind. This area needs more research and is particularly ripe for nursing research.

References

Avritscher, E.B., Cooksley, C.D., & Elting, L.S. (2004). Scope and epidemiology of cancer therapy-induced oral and gastrointestinal mucositis. *Seminars in Oncology Nursing, 20,* 3–10.

Bensinger, W., Schubert, M., Ang, K.K., Brizel, D., Brown, E., Eilers, J.G., ... Trotti, A.M., III. (2008). NCCN task force report: Prevention and management of mucositis in cancer care. *Journal of the National Comprehensive Cancer Network, 6*(Suppl. 1), S1–S21.

Blom, M., & Lundeberg, T. (2000). Long-term follow-up of patients treated with acupuncture for xerostomia and the influence of additional treatment. *Oral Diseases, 6,* 15–24.

Brizel, D., Wasserman, T.H., Henke, M., Strnad, V., Rudat, V., Monnier, A., ... Sauer, R. (2000). Phase III randomized trial of amifostine as a radioprotector in head and neck cancer. *Journal of Clinical Oncology, 18,* 3339–3345.

Brown, C.G., & Wingard, J. (2004). Clinical consequences of oral mucositis. *Seminars in Oncology Nursing, 20,* 16–21.

Bruce, S.D. (2004). Radiation-induced xerostomia: How dry is your patient? *Clinical Journal of Oncology Nursing, 8,* 61–67. doi:10.1188/04.CJON.61-67

Bruner, D.W., Haas, M.L., & Gosselin-Acomb, T.K. (Eds.). (2005). *Manual for radiation oncology nursing practice and education* (3rd ed.). Pittsburgh, PA: Oncology Nursing Society.

Carper, E. (2007). Head and neck cancers. In M.L. Haas, W.P. Hogle, G.J. Moore-Higgs, & T.K. Gosselin-Acomb (Eds.), *Radiation therapy: A guide to patient care* (pp. 84–117). St. Louis, MO: Elsevier Mosby.

Chambers, M.S., Jones, C.U., Biel, M.A., Weber, R.S., Hodge, K.M., Chen, Y., … Haddad, R. (2007). Open-label, long-term study of cevimeline in the treatment of postirradiation xerostomia. *International Journal of Radiation Oncology, Biology, Physics, 69,* 1369–1376. doi:10.1016/j.ijrobp.2007.05.02

Chong, L.M., & Armstrong, J.G. (2004). Tumors of the salivary glands. In S. Leibel & T.L. Phillips (Eds.), *Textbook of radiation oncology* (2nd ed., pp. 699–729). Philadelphia, PA: Saunders.

Corman, J.M., McClure, D., Pritchett, R., Kozlowski, P., & Hampson, N.B. (2003). Treatment of radiation induced hemorrhagic cystitis with hyberbaric oxygen. *Journal of Urology, 169,* 2200–2202. doi:10.1097/01.ju.0000063640.41307.c9

David, L.A., Sàndor, G.K.B., Evans, A.W., & Brown, D.H. (2001). Hyperbaric oxygen therapy and mandibular osteoradionecrosis: A retrospective study and analysis of treatment outcomes. *Journal of the Canadian Dental Association, 67,* 384.

Eisai Inc. (2009, January). *Salagen®* [Package insert]. Retrieved from http://www.eisai.com/pdf_files/201370-B%20Salagen%20Outsert.pdf

Elting, L.S., Cooksley, C., Chambers, M., Cantor, S.B., Manzullo, E., & Rubenstein, E.B. (2003). The burdens of cancer therapy: Clinical and economic outcomes of chemotherapy-induced mucositis. *Cancer, 98,* 1531–1539. doi:10.1002/cncr.11671

Epstein, J.B., & Schubert, M.M. (2004). Managing the pain in mucositis. *Seminars in Oncology Nursing, 20,* 30–37.

Epstein, J.B., Robertson, M., Emerton, S., Phillips, N., & Stevenson-Moore, P. (2001). Quality of life and oral function in patients treated with radiation therapy for head and neck cancer. *Head and Neck, 23,* 389–398. doi:10.1002/hed.1049

França, C.M., Domingues-Martins, M., Volpe, A., Filho, R.S.P., & de Araújo, N.S. (2001). Severe oral manifestations of chronic graft-vs.-host disease. *Journal of the American Dental Association, 132,* 1124–1127.

Haas, M., & Mercedes, T. (2008). Improving quality of life in head/neck chemoradiation patients when using a supersaturated electrolyte oral rinse [Poster Abstract No. 3306]. *Oncology Nursing Forum, 35,* 977.

Harris, D.J., Eilers, J.G., Cashavelly, B.J., Maxwell, C.L., & Harriman, A. (2009). ONS PEP resource: Mucositis. In L.H. Eaton & J.M. Tipton (Eds.), *Putting evidence into practice: Improving oncology patient outcomes* (pp. 201–213). Pittsburgh, PA: Oncology Nursing Society.

Henkin, R.I. (1972). Prevention and treatment of hypogeusia due to head and neck irradiation. *JAMA, 220,* 870–871.

Henkin, R.I., Martin, B.M., & Agarwal, R. (1999). Decreased parotid saliva gustin/carbonic anhydrase VI secretion: An enzyme disorder manifested by gustatory and olfactory dysfunction. *American Journal of the Medical Sciences, 318,* 380–391.

Jereczek-Fossa, B., & Orecchia, R. (2002). Radiotherapy-induced mandibular bone complications. *Cancer Treatment Reviews, 28,* 65–74. doi:10.1053/ctrv.2002.0254

Johnstone, P.A.S., Niemtzow, R.C., & Riffenburgh, R.H. (2002). Acupuncture for xerostomia: Clinical update. *Cancer, 94,* 1151–1156. doi:10.1002/cncr.10348

Keefe, D.M., Schubert, M.M., Elting, L.S., Sonis, S.T., Epstein, J.B., Raber-Durlacher, J.E., … Peterson, D.E. (2007). Updated clinical guidelines for the prevention and treatment of mucositis. *Cancer, 109,* 820–831. doi:10.1002/cncr.22484

Logemann, J.A., Smith, C.H., Pauloski, B.R., Rademaker, A.W., Lazarus, C.L., Colangelo, L.A., … Newman, L.A. (2001). Effects of xerostomia on perception and performance of swallow function. *Head and Neck, 23,* 317–321. doi:10.1002/hed.1037

Maes, A., Huygh, I., Weltens, C., Vandevelde, G., Delaere, P., Evers, G., & Van den Bogaert, W. (2002). De Gustibus: Time scale of loss and recovery of tastes caused by radiotherapy. *Radiotherapy and Oncology, 63,* 195–201.

Marx, R.E., Ehler, W.J., Tayapongsak, P., & Pierce, L.W. (1990). Relationship of oxygen dose to angiogenesis induction in irradiated tissue. *American Journal of Surgery, 160,* 519–524.

McGuire, D.B. (2002). Mucosal tissue injury in cancer therapy. More than mucositis and mouthwash. *Cancer Practice, 10,* 179–191. doi:10.1046/j.1523-5394.2002.104009.x

McGuire, D.B., Yeager, K.A., Dudley, W.N., Peterson, D.E., Owen, D.C., Lin, L.S., & Wingard, J.R. (1998). Acute oral pain and mucositis in bone marrow transplant and leukemia patients: Data from a pilot study. *Cancer Nursing, 21,* 385–393.

Melo, M.D., & Obeid, G. (2005). Osteonecrosis of the jaws in patients with a history of receiving bisphosphonate therapy: Strategies for prevention and early recognition. *Journal of the American Dental Association, 136,* 1675–1681.

Miller, M., & Kearney, N. (2001). Oral care for patients with cancer: A review of the literature. *Cancer Nursing, 24,* 241–254.

Multinational Association of Supportive Care in Cancer. (2005). Summary of evidence-based clinical practice guidelines for care of patients with oral and gastrointestinal mucositis. Retrieved from http://data.memberclicks.com/site/mascc/Guidelines_mucositis.doc

Nakamura, S., Hiroki, A., Shinohara, M., Gondo, H., Ohyama, Y., Mouri, T., ... Niho, Y. (1996). Oral involvement with chronic graft-versus-host disease after allogeneic bone marrow transplantation. *Oral Surgery, Oral Medicine, Oral Pathology, Oral Radiology, and Endodontics, 82,* 556–563.

National Cancer Institute. (2008). Oral complications of chemotherapy and head/neck radiation (PDQ®) [Health professional version]. Retrieved from http://www.cancer.gov/cancertopics/pdq/supportivecare/oralcomplications/healthprofessional

National Institute of Dental and Craniofacial Research. (2010). *The dental provider's oncology pocket guide.* Retrieved from http://www.nidcr.nih.gov/OralHealth/Topics/CancerTreatment

Nelson, G.M. (1998). Biology of taste buds and the clinical problem of taste loss. *Anatomical Record, 253,* 70–78. doi:10.1002/(SICI)1097-0185(199806)253:3<70::AID-AR3>3.0.CO;2-I

Nguyen, N.P., Moltz, C.C., Frank, C., Karlsson, U., Nguyen, P.D., Vos, P., ... Sallah, S. (2006). Dysphagia severity following chemoradiation and postoperative radiation for head and neck cancer. *European Journal of Radiology, 59,* 453–459. doi:10.1016/j.ejrad.2006.03.019

Oral Cancer Foundation. (2001–2010). What is trismus? Retrieved from http://www.oralcancerfoundation.org/dental/trismus.htm

Papas, A.S., Clark, R.E., Martuscelli, G., O'Loughlin, K.T., Johansen, E., & Miller, K.B. (2003). A prospective, randomized trial for the prevention of mucositis in patients undergoing hematopoietic stem cell transplantation. *Bone Marrow Transplantation, 31,* 705–712. doi:10.1038/sj.bmt.1703870

Peterson, D.E., Beck, S.L., & Keefe, D.M. (2004). Novel therapies. *Seminars in Oncology Nursing, 20,* 53–58.

Polovich, M., Whitford, J.M., & Olsen, M. (Eds.). (2009). *Chemotherapy and biotherapy guidelines and recommendations for practice* (3rd ed.). Pittsburgh, PA: Oncology Nursing Society.

Raber-Durlacher, J.E., Weijl, N.I., Saris, M.A., de Koning, B., Zwinderman, A.H., & Osanto, S. (2000). Oral mucositis in patients treated with chemotherapy for solid tumors: A retrospective analysis of 150 cases. *Supportive Care in Cancer, 8,* 366–371. doi:10.1007/s005200050004

Ravasco, P. (2005). Aspects of taste and compliance in patients with cancer. *European Journal of Oncology Nursing, 9*(Suppl. 2), S84–S91. doi:10.1016/j.ejon.2005.09.003

Redda, M.G.R., & Allis, S. (2006). Radiotherapy-induced taste impairment. *Cancer Treatment Reviews, 32,* 541–547. doi:10.1016/j.ctrv.2006.06.003

Rehwaldt, M., Wickham, R., Purl, S., Tariman, J., Blendowski, C., Shott, S., & Lappe, M. (2009). Self-care strategies to cope with taste changes after chemotherapy [Online exclusive]. *Oncology Nursing Forum, 36,* E47–E56. doi:10.1188/09.ONF.E47-E56

Ripamonti, C., & Dickerson, E.D. (2001). Strategies for the treatment of cancer pain in the new millennium. *Drugs, 61,* 955–977.

Ripamonti, C., Zecca, E., Brunelli, C., Fulfaro, F., Villa, S., Balzarini, A., … De Conno, F. (1998). A randomized, controlled clinical trial to evaluate the effects of zinc sulfate on cancer patients with taste alterations caused by head and neck irradiation. *Cancer, 82,* 1938–1945. doi:10.1002/(SICI)1097-0142(19980515)82:10<1938::AID-CNCR18>3.0.CO;2-U

Rubenstein, E.B., Peterson, D.E., Schubert, M., Keefe, D., McGuire, D., Epstein, J., … Sonis, S.T. (2004). Clinical practice guidelines for the prevention and treatment of cancer therapy–induced oral and gastrointestinal mucositis. *Cancer, 100,* 2026–2046. doi:10.1002/cncr.20163

Ruggiero, S.L., Mehrotra, B., Rosenberg, T.J., & Engroff, S.L. (2004). Osteonecrosis of the jaws associated with the use of bisphosphonates: A review of 63 cases. *Journal of Oral Maxillofacial Surgery, 62,* 527–534. doi:10.1016/j.joms.2004.02.004

Russell, R.G., Rogers, M.J., Frith, J.C., Luckman, S.P., Coxon, F.P., Benford, H.L., … Fleisch, H.A. (1999). The pharmacology of bisphosphonates and new insights into their mechanisms of action. *Journal of Bone and Mineral Research, 14*(Suppl. 2), 53–65.

Sandow, P.L., Hejrat-Yazdi, M., & Heft, M.W. (2006). Taste loss and recovery following radiation therapy. *Journal of Dental Research, 85,* 608–611. doi:10.1177/154405910608500705

Schiffman, S.S., & Gatlin, C.A. (1993). Clinical physiology of taste and smell. *Annual Review of Nutrition, 13,* 405–436.

Sloan, J.A., Goldberg, R.M., Sargent, D.J., Vargas-Chanes, D., Nair, S., Cha, S.S., … Loprinzi, C.L. (2002). Women experience greater toxicity with fluorouracil-based chemotherapy for colorectal cancer. *Journal of Clinical Oncology, 20,* 1491–1498. doi:10.1200/JCO.20.6.1491

Sloan, J.A., Loprinzi, C.L., Novotny, P.J., Okuno, S., Nair, S., & Barton, D.L. (2000). Sex differences in fluorouracil-induced stomatitis. *Journal of Clinical Oncology, 18,* 412–420.

Sonis, S.T. (2004). Pathobiology of mucositis. *Seminars in Oncology Nursing, 20,* 11–15. doi:10.1053/S0749-2081(03)00134-7

Sonis, S.T., Oster, G., Fuchs, H., Bellm, L., Bradford, W.Z., Edelsberg, J., … Horowitz, M. (2001). Oral mucositis and the clinical and economic outcomes of hematopoietic stem-cell transplantation. *Journal of Clinical Oncology, 19,* 2201–2205.

Spielberger, R., Stiff, P., Bensinger, W., Gentile, T., Weisdorf, D., Kewalramani, T., … Emmanouilides, C. (2004). Palifermin for oral mucositis after intensive therapy for hematologic cancers. *New England Journal of Medicine, 351,* 2590–2598. doi:10.1056/NEJMoa040125

Takeda, N., Takaoka, T., Ueda, C., Toda, N., Kalubi, B., & Yamamoto, S. (2004). Zinc deficiency in patients with idiopathic taste impairment with regard to angiotensin converting enzyme activity. *Auris, Nasus, Larynx, 31,* 425–428. doi:10.1016/j.anl.2004.09.006

Tipton, J.M. (2009). Mucositis. In L.H. Eaton & J.M. Tipton (Eds.), *Putting evidence into practice: Improving oncology patient outcomes* (pp. 193–200). Pittsburgh, PA: Oncology Nursing Society.

Viale, P.H., & Lin, A. (2005). Exposed bone in oral cavities. *Clinical Journal of Oncology Nursing, 9,* 355–357. doi:10.1188/05.CJON.355-357

Vissink, A., Burlage, F.R., Spijkervet, F.K., Jansma, J., & Coppes, R.P. (2003). Prevention and treatment of the consequences of head and neck radiotherapy. *Critical Reviews in Oral Biology and Medicine, 14,* 213–225. doi:10.1177/154411130301400306

Wardley, A.M., Jayson, G.C., Swindell, R., Morgenstern, G.R., Chang, J., Bloor, R., … Scarffe, J.H. (2000). Prospective evaluation of oral mucositis in patients receiving myeloablative conditioning regimens and haemopoietic progenitor rescue. *British Journal of Haematology, 110,* 292–299. doi:10.1046/j.1365-2141.2000.02202.x

Wickham, R.S., Rehwaldt, M., Kefer, C., Shott, S., Abbas, K., Glynn-Tucker, E., … Blendowski, C. (1999). Taste changes experienced by patients receiving chemotherapy: A review of current knowledge. *Oncology Nursing Forum, 26,* 697–706.

Woo, S.B., Lee, S.J., & Schubert, M.M. (1997). Graft-vs.-host disease. *Critical Reviews in Oral Biology and Medicine, 8,* 201–216. doi:10.1177/10454411970080020701

Wright, A.L., King, J.C., Baer, M.T., & Citron, L.J. (1981). Experimental zinc depletion and altered perception for NaCl in young adult males. *American Journal of Clinical Nutrition, 34,* 848–852.

Wu, C.H., Hsiao, T.Y., Ko, J.Y., & Hsu, M.M. (2000). Dysphagia after radiotherapy: Endoscopic examination of swallowing in patients with nasopharyngeal carcinoma. *Annals of Otology, Rhinology and Laryngology, 109,* 320–325.

Yamashita, H., Nakagawa, K., Hosoi, Y., Kurokawa, A., Fukuda, Y., Matsumoto, I., ... Abe, K. (2009). Umami taste dysfunction in patients receiving radiotherapy for head and neck cancer. *Oral Oncology, 45,* e19–e23. doi:10.1016/j.oraloncology.2008.04.001

CHAPTER 4

Evidence-Based Practice: Tools to Measure Progress

Maurene McQuestion, RN, BA, BScN, MSc, CON(C),
and Sarah D'Angelo, RN, BSc, BScN, MN, CON(C)

Introduction

Oral effects of treatment are some of the most distressing consequences resulting from high-dose chemotherapy or radiation to the head and neck region. Strong correlations exist between individuals' oral health and their general health, wellness, and quality of life (Watt, 2005). A healthy oral cavity is a comfortable mouth that is able to maintain nutrition, protect against infection, and contribute to an individual's overall feeling of wellness (Coleman, 1995). Optimal oral assessment and care are of particular importance to patients with cancer because the rapidly dividing cells of the oral mucosa are highly vulnerable to the damaging and toxic effects of chemotherapy and radiation regimens. Oral changes can be both acute and chronic in nature (Holmes & Mountain, 1993), with the most common changes being mucositis, taste alterations, pain, dysphagia, xerostomia, trismus, odynophagia, and fungal infections (Knöös & Östman, 2010). Oral effects of treatment can have a negative impact on pain, body image, appetite, the ability to eat, maintaining nutrition and weight, hydration, speech, and communication, as well as economic costs and quality of life.

The comprehensive and ongoing measurement of the oral effects of cancer and its treatment is important for a number of reasons. Within research and clinical trials, measurement based on the use of tools shown to be reliable and valid ensures that there is methodological rigor within a study, that a study can be replicated, and that comparisons of findings across studies can be made. Within clinical practice, the consistent and precise description and classification of oral changes is critical for the assessment of local side effects, complications, and patient morbidity, as well as quality of life, treatment-related clinical decision making, and timely intervention (McGuire, Rubenstein,

& Peterson, 2004). The use or lack of use of appropriate tools has both direct and indirect effects on the care of the patient. Regular assessment of patients' concerns or symptoms supports the early identification of problems, which leads to early and appropriate intervention. This can affect several outcomes, including adherence to treatment, planned and unplanned treatment interruptions, dose reductions of single- or combined-modality therapies, pain, analgesic use, weight loss, hospital admissions, and the need for feeding tubes (Russo, Haddad, Posner, & Machtay, 2008; Trotti, Bellm, et al., 2003). Accurate assessment of the oral cavity and mucosal changes is an essential component of nursing care (Blot, Vandijck, & Labeau, 2008). Despite this recognition, Stone et al. (2007) identified that across transplantation centers in Europe, wide variation existed in the use of oral assessment tools and in the frequency of conducting assessments, ranging from daily to three times a day. While the majority of nurses in the study initiated assessments at the start of treatment, others only assessed patients after mucositis developed or the patient developed problems with swallowing or eating, despite their identification of the impact of mucositis on the use of opioids and parenteral nutrition. This variation in practice also occurs in centers across North America.

Evidence-Based Practice

Evidence-based practice "defines care that integrates current best scientific evidence with clinical expertise, knowledge of pathophysiology, knowledge of psychosocial issues, and decision-making preferences of patients" (Rutledge & Grant, 2002, p. 1). Guidelines related to assessment and intervention do not currently include or identify recommendations about the most appropriate assessment tools to use in clinical practice (Keefe et al., 2007). Quinn et al. (2008) reviewed 57 papers based on specific inclusion criteria and identified 11 recommendations for the assessment of oral mucositis in adults receiving cancer treatment. Included in the review was the identification of 14 different assessment tools, assessing various dimensions of physical changes, functional changes, and anatomic sites as well as several other elements. Despite the recommendations about routine oral assessment, from baseline prior to treatment and throughout and following treatment, no one tool was specifically recommended. In addition, although processes have been established to review and adapt clinical practice guidelines to the local context and practice setting (Harrison, Légaré, Graham, & Fervers, 2010), these processes do not specify how to choose a particular assessment and documentation tool for practice. A separate review or guideline would be required to determine which tools address the recommended domains or parameters of assessment identified in the practice guidelines prior to making any recommendations regarding particular tools for implementation into practice. This would build on the work of Quinn et al. (2008). Clinicians need to be aware of the various tools available in the literature in order to make the best decisions for implementation into their clinical setting.

Types of Tools

A variety of tools exist to measure multiple aspects of oral changes related to cancer treatment. These tools cover both screening and assessment. Screening tools are used as an initial quick assessment, which should then lead to a more in-depth assessment of specific concerns. Assessment tools are designed to elicit information, categorize a concern or symptom, and document the findings. Additionally, assessment tools may capture objective or subjective data and be administered by the clinician or completed by the patient. Tools also may be developed for use independent of a treatment modality or specific to chemotherapy or radiation treatment. They may be used for research purposes in clinical trials or as a tool in routine clinical practice, either as a one-time measurement or for serial measurements to assess changes and clinical progress. Tools need to be reliable, validated, easy to use, reproducible, and applicable across patient populations. Many studies include investigator-developed assessment tools without any psychometric testing being completed, thereby making it difficult to make meaningful conclusions from the study findings and compare results across studies (Chen, 2008).

The types of tools used to assess oral changes can be categorized in multiple ways. Types of tools used in oncology include (a) general profile instruments that include items related to oral effects of treatment (e.g., Quality of Life, QOL SF-36®), (b) condition- or disease-specific tools (e.g., Functional Assessment of Cancer Therapy–Head and Neck Cancer [FACT-H&N], the Rotterdam Symptom Checklist, Eilers' oral assessment tool), and (c) symptom-specific tools (e.g., the Oral Mucositis Assessment Scale [OMAS], the Oral Mucositis Index [OMI-20], the Xerostomia Questionnaire [XQ]). For the purposes of this chapter, a broad overview of types of tools will be provided followed by a more detailed summary and critique of some of the condition- or disease-specific and symptom-specific tools that are more commonly recognized and useful in clinical practice settings.

General Profile Instruments

Broad-based general profile instruments may assess quality of life as well as multiple symptoms or concerns affecting quality of life but do not focus on specific issues related to a disease or population. Although this allows for comparison across different groups of patients, the tools may not be sensitive enough to detect changes related to an intervention or change in practice in relation to a specific item on the scale (e.g., mucositis).

Condition- or Disease-Specific Tools

Broad-based tools specific to cancer have been designed to assess multiple symptoms or concerns and encompass several domains of assessment that include specific items related to the oral effects of treatment. The scales are often organized by disease site and then subdivided by symptoms, side effects, or toxicities (acute or late) related to the treatment of that type of cancer. Within this set of tools, specific sections address oral assessment. The National Cancer Institute Cancer Therapy Evaluation Program (NCI CTEP, 2009) Common Terminology Criteria for Adverse Events (CTCAE), the Canadian Cancer Society Research Institute tools, the Radiation Therapy Oncology Group (RTOG) scale, and the European Organisation for Research and Treatment of Cancer (EORTC, EORTC/RTOG, EORTC-H&N) toxicity scales include items of oral assessment. They have been designed to be simple and include a combination of variables that measure signs, symptoms, and functional changes, but the individual and total scores attached to specific symptoms vary across the different tools. Many of the tools have been developed for research purposes and do not lend themselves to comparative evaluation in clinical practice (Parulekar, Mackenzie, Bjarnason, & Jordan, 1998). Additional tools measuring multiple symptoms inclusive of oral changes include the FACT, FACT-H&N, the Quality of Life Questionnaire (QLQ, EORTC QLQ-C30, EORTC QLQ-H&N35), and the MD Anderson Symptom Inventory–Head and Neck (MDASI-HN) (Rosenthal et al., 2007). The latter scales are designed to be self-administered rather than by the clinician or researcher. Examples of the tools that include items related to oral assessment are identified in Table 4-1.

Tools Specific to Oral Symptoms

Tools that have been developed to measure unique concerns specific to oncology oral symptoms such as mucositis, xerostomia, or trismus may be included in broad tools designed by large organizations involved in clinical trials, such as NCI, EORTC, and RTOG as identified previously.

Conversely, tools or scales have been developed that combine objective, functional, and symptom measurements focusing on overall oral assessment, such as the Oral Exam Guide (Beck, 1979) or the Oral Assessment Guide (OAG) (Eilers, Berger, & Petersen, 1988).

A third group of more detailed objective tools have been developed to assess specific symptoms such as mucositis or xerostomia. Examples of objective measures as assessed by the clinician or researcher include the OMAS and the OMI-20, both of which measure 20 or more mucosal changes and signs, and the World Health Organization (WHO) index for mucositis and the Western Consortium for Cancer Nursing Research (WCCNR) Stomatitis Staging System, which are both being designed for clinical practice. The XQ and the Salivary Hypofunction Questionnaire (Fox, Busch, & Baum, 1987) are examples of tools designed specifically for the symptom of oral dryness. Symptom-specific oral tools have been used across patient populations, as well as with patients with a specific type of cancer or treatment, such as head and neck cancer or stem cell transplantation.

Table 4-1. Categories of Assessment Tools: General, Condition- or Disease-Specific, and Symptom-Specific Tools

Assessment Tool	Grading/Scoring	Domains or Components Measured	Reliability and Validity	Limitations
General Profile Tools	Patient self-report tool to assess oral symptoms or problems and their impact on quality of life (QOL)			
European Organiza-tion for Research and Treatment of Cancer (EORTC) Quality of Life Questionnaires (EORTC QLQ-C30, EORTC QLQ-H&N35 for head and neck cancer)	EORTC QLQ-C30: 28 items scored using a Likert scale from 1 (not at all) to 4 (very much) and 2 questions relat-ed to overall health and QOL rated on a 1–7 scale EORTC QLQ-H&N35: 30 items scored using a Likert scale from 1 (not at all) to 4 (very much) and 5 yes/no questions All scores are trans-formed to a 0–100 scale.	EORTC QLQ-C30 asks ques-tions to determine QOL—ability to perform activities of daily living and pursue hobbies, appetite, nausea, and pain. EORTC QLQ-H&N35 asks questions related to pain in mouth when eating and not eating, problems with teeth, alterations in sense of smell, alterations in ap-pearance, use of pain medi-cation, and weight loss.	EORTC QLQ-H&N35 has been extensive-ly tested in 12 coun-tries and successfully translated into 9 lan-guages and is regard-ed as the most com-prehensive assess-ment tool for QOL as-sessments in relation to oral changes in pa-tients with head and neck cancer (Bjordal et al., 1999).	• Assesses multiple vari-ables within tool (e.g., QOL and symptoms) • Does not focus on specific issues related to a disease or population of patients • May not be sensitive enough to detect changes related to an intervention in relation to a specific item on the tool (e.g., mucositis)

(Continued on next page)

Table 4-1. Categories of Assessment Tools: General, Condition- or Disease-Specific, and Symptom-Specific Tools (*Continued*)

Assessment Tool	Grading/Scoring	Domains or Components Measured	Reliability and Validity	Limitations
Condition- or Disease-Specific Tools	Within these sets of tools, specific items or sections address oral assessment. Tools include a combination of variables that measure signs, symptoms, and functional changes. Difficult to make comparisons across tools due to variation in scoring systems.			
Oral Assessment Guide (Eilers & Epstein, 2004)	Grades 1–3 Use of individual domain scores instead of total score provides a more detailed oral change data.	Eight domains: voice/talking, lips, tongue, mucous membranes, gingiva, teeth/dentures, saliva, and ability to swallow Easy to use in the clinical setting with minimal training required Has been translated into Swedish language and adapted for the pediatric setting	Face, content, and construct validity, inter-rater reliability (0.92) High inter-rater reliability (71%–80%) for radiation side effects Moderate association between radiation dose and side effects shown	• Observational assessment guided by verbal descriptors • Addresses the whole oral cavity; not ideal for detecting specific oral changes • Does not assess pain well • Weights each category equally; may not be consistent with priorities of the patient
National Cancer Institute (NCI) Common Terminology Criteria for Adverse Events (CTCAE) (Colevas & Setser, 2004; NCI Cancer Therapy Evaluation Program, 2009)	26 categories of toxicity events for different symptoms Scoring for clinical examination as well as functional and symptom assessment Grades 0–5 (0 = no alteration to 4 = disabling or life threatening and 5 = death)	Mucositis and stomatitis within gastrointestinal category, specific to a disease site regardless of causation (chemotherapy, radiation, graft-versus-host)	Designed for and used extensively in medical oncology clinical trials for assessment of toxicities associated with chemotherapy	Research tool using objective observer assessment only; does not address patient impact or distress related to mucositis

(Continued on next page)

Table 4-1. Categories of Assessment Tools: General, Condition- or Disease-Specific, and Symptom-Specific Tools (Continued)

Assessment Tool	Grading/Scoring	Domains or Components Measured	Reliability and Validity	Limitations
Radiation Therapy Oncology Group (RTOG) tools	Grades 0–4 with increasing severity	Severity measures of toxicity of radiation subdivided by acute versus late toxicity	No reliability and validity data available	Uses observer assessment only; does not include patient's perception of symptom or functional impact of treatment
EORTC, the EORTC/ RTOG, EORTC-H&N	Adoption of NCI CTCAE scoring	Objective and functional assessment	See NCI section.	See NCI section.
MD Anderson Symptom Inventory (MDASI, MDASI-HN for head and neck cancer) (Rosenthal et al., 2007)	0–10 scale ranging from symptom not present to as bad as can be imagined; Tool available in paper, electronic, and interactive voice response formats	Multisymptom patient-reported screening tool for severity of multiple symptoms (13 in general tool and 22 in HN tool) experienced in the previous 24 hours, caused by disease or treatment, and interfering with daily life	Reliability and validity testing on MDASI HN tool validated and compared to the Functional Assessment of Cancer Therapy–Head and Neck tool; MDASI-HN better at predicting severity of mucositis induced by radiation	Only 1 item specific to mouth/throat sores

(Continued on next page)

Table 4-1. Categories of Assessment Tools: General, Condition- or Disease-Specific, and Symptom-Specific Tools *(Continued)*

Assessment Tool	Grading/Scoring	Domains or Components Measured	Reliability and Validity	Limitations
Symptom-Specific Tools (Mucositis or Xerostomia)				
Oral Mucositis Assessment Scale (OMAS) (Sonis et al., 1999)	100 mm visual analog scale (VAS) plus a categorical scale of subjective outcomes (e.g., ability to eat)	Measures more than 20 mucosal changes and signs Has been used in chemotherapy and radiation 8-item assessment of anatomical locations, plus pain and dysphagia	High inter-rater reliability and validity (validated for chemotherapy and radiation)	• Primarily a research tool • Requires some training for appropriate use and scoring
Oral Mucositis Index (OMI-20)	Grading on 0–3 scale for changes from normal to severe for 8 anatomic regions plus assessment of tissue changes, oral pain, and dryness using a VAS	Measures more than 20 mucosal changes and signs; used mostly with bone marrow transplant recipients Good correlation shown between OMAS score for mucosal changes and VAS mucositis pain score	Content and construct validity reported; internal consistency (0.90–0.94); test-retest reliability ($r = 0.31$–0.73, $p < 0.0001$)	Caution is advised in interpretation of scores because multiple comparisons are used.
World Health Organization Index for Mucositis (McGuire et al., 2004)	5-point grading scale, 0–4 (no side effect for the inability to eat); scale easy to use	Tool was designed for and used extensively in clinical practice. Severity of mucositis based on patient impact rather than an oral examination.	No reliability and validity data reported	• Grading does not capture range of oral changes. • Descriptors are ambiguous.

(Continued on next page)

Table 4-1. Categories of Assessment Tools: General, Condition- or Disease-Specific, and Symptom-Specific Tools *(Continued)*

Assessment Tool	Grading/Scoring	Domains or Components Measured	Reliability and Validity	Limitations
Western Consortium for Cancer Nursing Research Staging System for Stomatitis (Olson et al., 2004)	Staging system scores 0–3 for lesions, color, and bleeding Sums of scores for lesions, color, and bleeding to identify mild (1–4), moderate (5–7), or severe (8–9) stomatitis	3 descriptors assessed (reduced from the original 8) Tool was designed for clinical practice and developed specifically for stomatitis/mucositis.	Good to high correlation for inter-rater reliability Good correlation with the OAG Quick and easy to use	Does not capture subjective and functional impact of mucositis
Xerostomia Questionnaire (XQ) (Eisbruch et al., 2001)	0–10 scale for total score up to 100; higher scores reflect worse xerostomia	Specifically assesses oral dryness 8 questions—4 addressing oral dryness when eating and 4 addressing dryness when not eating Translated into Taiwanese (XQ-T)	Test-retest correlations 0.82 (p < 0.01) High internal consistency (0.86) XQ-T shown reliable and valid; content reliability = 0.97	

Description and Critique of Specific Tools

The NCI CTCAE and RTOG scales for mucositis and xerostomia, the OAG, the OMAS, the OMI-20, the revised WCCNR scale, the XQ, and the Salivary Hypofunction Questionnaire are cited frequently in the literature, use a few variables, and have empirical evidence to support their use by nurses in various clinical settings. Nursing is interested in a holistic perspective that encompasses the toxicity of treatment but also the patients' subjective experience and the impact on functional outcomes. Each of these scales will be discussed in more detail.

National Cancer Institute and European Organisation for Research and Treatment of Cancer Toxicity Scales

The NCI CTCAE, EORTC, and the RTOG scales are commonly used tools in research and clinical practice and include scales to assess the acute as well as late effects of treatment by disease site. The original NCI CTCAE, then called the Common Toxicity Criteria, developed in 1982, was designed to assess toxicities associated with chemotherapies and was developed through a cooperative collaboration of the American oncology groups. A later version (2.0) was developed in 1998 following international collaboration and became the international standard for use in clinical trials. In 2003, version 3.0 was updated as the CTCAE. The later version included criteria across treatment modalities and merged criteria for early and late events into one system (Chen et al., 2006; Trotti, Colevas, et al., 2003; Williams, Chen, Rubin, Finkelstein, & Okunieff, 2003).

The CTCAE scales in version 4.0 reflect 26 categories of toxicity events organized by anatomy and physiology and are the standard criteria for terminology for capturing routine and adverse event data in clinical trials in North America (Colevas & Setser, 2004; NCI CTEP, 2009). The scales are observer ratings and assess toxicity specific to nausea, vomiting, anorexia, constipation, diarrhea, and mucositis, as well as several other specific symptoms, graded on a scale of 0 to 5, with 0 being no alteration, 1 being mild, 4 being the most severe, disabling, or having life-threatening consequences, and 5 indicating death. Within the category of gastrointestinal adverse events, mucositis/stomatitis is used for mucositis caused by radiation, chemotherapy, or graft-versus-host disease. The scales are specific to the location of disease and assessment (e.g., anus, esophagus, oral cavity) and address scores for clinical examination as well as functional and symptomatic changes. Mucositis scores for clinical examination range from erythema through patchy to confluent ulcerations and bleeding, with grade 4 involving necrosis and life-threatening complications. Functional and symptom assessment scores for mucositis of the oral cavity range from no stomatitis to increasing degrees of ulceration and impact on swallowing to severe stomatitis (Cella et al., 2003; Jaroneski,

2006). Dry mouth (xerostomia) and dysgeusia (taste alteration) are two additional scales that capture changes within the oral cavity in the gastrointestinal category. Although this tool was initially developed for use with clinical trials, it has evolved into use in clinical practice in some centers across the United States. It has been incorporated into the Oncology Nursing Society *Radiation Therapy Patient Care Record* publication (Catlin-Huth, Haas, & Pollock, 2002), but this resource has not been updated to reflect changes with the CTCAE.

EORTC has adopted the U.S.-based toxicity criteria from the CTCAE and includes objective assessment as well as the functional impact of treatment.

Radiation Therapy Oncology Group Toxicity Scales

The RTOG Acute Radiation Morbidity Scoring Criteria was initially developed in 1982, at the same time that NCI created the Common Toxicity Criteria. It was later revised and integrated into the CTCAE system. Similar to the CTCAE scales, the RTOG scales are severity measures of toxicity and are subdivided based on the time of occurrence of the event and identified as acute (less than 90 days) or late (more than 90 days from beginning of radiation). The severity scores are based on observer assessments and address only anatomic changes related to radiation treatment. They do not include aspects about the impact on a patient's perception of a symptom or the functional impact of treatment (i.e., pain, difficulty swallowing caused by oral changes). In many centers across North America, the severity scales have been integrated into computer programs that are used for treatment planning and delivery as well as for documentation of routine monitoring and symptom management (e.g., MOSAIQ® by Elekta AB).

Oral Assessment Guide

In an effort to guide and standardize oral assessment, a number of approaches have been undertaken in research and clinical practice. Ginsberg (1961) introduced a subjective functional and observational approach to the assessment of oral changes and identified key functional capabilities that affected overall oral health. These included mucous membrane moisture, airway patency, and the frequency with which the nurse administered oral hygiene care.

Building on the work of Ginsberg (1961), Passos and Brand (1966) developed an oral assessment tool in an effort to standardize oral assessments conducted as part of a research study designed to evaluate and compare the effectiveness of three oral rinsing agents. The daily worksheet for recording physical and oral conditions consisted of three broad categories: (a) physical data, (b) eight domains reflecting oral condition (saliva, tongue, palate, mucous membranes, teeth, odor, lips, and nares), and (c) patient comments. A numeric score ranging from 1 (normal) to 3 (abnormal) was assigned to each of the eight domains of oral conditions to indicate the severity of oral alterations. This score was then combined with the physical data score, which was collected through observational assessment to determine the total oral health, with a higher score indicating greater oral complications. Further modifications to the oral assessment tool were made by Beck (1979), who added gingiva, voice, and swallow as domains of assessment and removed odor and nares to complete the development of the Oral Exam Guide. Each domain was further expanded with verbal descriptors including texture, color, and moisture and then scored using a 1 to 4 scale, with 1 being normal or desirable and 4 being undesirable oral change. Total scores ranged between 15 and 60, with lower scores indicating more desirable oral health. Despite these early tools lacking reliability and validity and being initially tested in non-oncology populations, Beck conducted much of the ground-breaking work in bringing attention to the issue of oral changes in patients receiving chemotherapy.

Almost a decade later, in 1988, Eilers et al. developed the OAG based on a review of the literature with categories being validated through consensus by a group of nurses, in addition to content validity by experts. The tool has undergone psychometric testing indicating good inter-rater reliability (0.92). This new oral assessment tool incorporated eight oral domains: voice/talking, lips, tongue, mucous membranes, gingiva, teeth/dentures, saliva, and ability to swallow. Each domain is scored as a 1, 2, or 3, with normal findings assigned a 1 and severe oral changes assigned a score of 3, reflecting the degree of compromise of epithelial integrity or systemic functioning. The numeric score in each domain is then added together to produce a total oral health score. One of the weaknesses of the tool is that pain is not well assessed. Additionally, equal weightings of each category may not be consistent with the priorities of the patient. Although the OAG is detailed, it has had greater success with use in research studies than with implementation in routine clinical practice.

In 1993, in an effort to identify the most reliable and valid oral assessment tool for future studies on oral health, Holmes and Mountain used a heterogeneous cross-sectional study design to compare the three aforementioned oral assessment tools (Beck, 1979; Eilers et al., 1988; Passos & Brand, 1966). A comparison of total oral scores (sum of oral domains) reported by each researcher and nurse pair confirmed that each tool was reliable and had the ability to provide reproducible results when assessing gross oral changes. High inter-rater reliability and content validity was also evident when comparing domain scores. However, variation of oral descriptors in each of the domain subcategories made it difficult to precisely report the extent and severity of oral cavity changes (Holmes & Mountain, 1993). Additional reports suggested that the omission of domains such as infection and pain further compromise the value of each assessment tool because these symptoms are proven to have a significant impact on a patient's overall wellness (Holmes & Mountain, 1993). In light of the discrepancies and omissions, the OAG (Eilers et al., 1988) has shown to yield clinically significant results in a number of research studies examining oral changes in response to radiation and chemotherapy. Significant data have been reported using a translated (Swedish) version of the OAG (Andersson, Persson, Hallberg, & Renvert, 1999), as well as an OAG that has been adapted to include developmentally appropriate language for specific populations, such as pediatric patients (Chen, Wang, Cheng, & Chang, 2004). Currently, the Eilers et al. (1988) OAG is the recommended oral assessment tool for both clinical studies and practice because it is easy to use and does not require extensive training. The OAG provides assessors with a good indication of a patient's baseline oral condition and highlights gross oral abnormalities as they arise during and after treatment.

Mucositis Assessment Tools

Mucositis assessment tools have been developed for both research and clinical practice. They have been shown to be easy to use with minimal requirements for education; however, standardization in the implementation of a particular tool in the clinical setting and consistency in use of the tool are important. Most of the currently available tools are sensitive to measure mucositis/stomatitis and changes over time and have been used across various treatment modalities, including radiation and chemotherapy. Oral and mucositis assessment begins with a thorough oral examination with a good light source and should include an assessment of objective changes, subjective concerns or experiences (pain, dryness), and functional assessment (communication, swallowing, and nutrition). The frequency of assessment may vary depending on the clinical area. For example, daily assessment should be recorded for patients receiving care on inpatient units, whereas weekly assessments may be carried out in a weekly radiation review clinic, plus additional assessments based on patient needs or when changes are anticipated based on the phase of treatment.

Multiple specific mucositis assessment scales exist, including the OAG (Eilers et al., 1988), the OMAS (Sonis et al., 1999), the OMI-20 (McGuire et al., 1993), the WHO grading scale for mucositis (Miller, Hoogstraten, Staquet, & Winkler, 1981), the WCCNR staging system (Olson et al., 2004), and the MacDibbs Mouth Assessment (Dibble, Shiba, MacPhail, & Dodd, 1996). The OAG, the MacDibbs Mouth Assessment, and the WCCNR scale (Olson et al., 2004) have routinely been used in patients with cancer. The OMI-20 has been used mostly with patients who are undergoing bone marrow transplantation or experiencing graft-versus-host disease as a result of the transplant. The MacDibbs tool was developed for assessment of patients receiving radiation therapy. The OAG, WHO, and WCCNR scales have undergone psychometric testing with content validity established and showing good-to-high correlation for inter-rater reliability.

For the purposes of this review of mucositis assessment tools, the OMAS, OMI, WHO, WCCNR, and MacDibbs tools will be described in more detail. The OMAS (Sonis et al., 1999) has been used with patients receiving chemotherapy and/or radiation therapy. It includes an eight-item assessment of anatomic locations in the mouth, as well as pain and difficulty swallowing, using a 100 mm visual analog scale (VAS), and a categorical scale for the assessment of subjective outcomes, such as the individual's ability to eat various types of food (Harris, Eilers, Harriman, Cashavelly, & Maxwell, 2008; Jaroneski, 2006). The OMAS is used primarily for research purposes and requires some training to be used appropriately.

The OMI tool was originally developed as a research tool and then shortened for use as a clinical tool. It has been evaluated for reliability and validity and has been shown to have content and construct validity, internal consistency (Cronbach's alpha = 0.90–0.94), and test-retest reliability (r = 0.31–0.73, p < 0.0001) (McGuire et al., 2004; Schubert, Williams, Lloid, Donaldson, & Chapko, 1992). The settings where the OMI tool and the OMI-20, a shortened version, have been used are in the context of bone marrow transplantation in patients with leukemia. The scores for both the OMI and OMAS show good correlation between mucosal changes and mucositis pain scores using a VAS for pain assessment (Sonis et al., 2004). Although the objective assessment of mucosal changes does not always correlate well with the functional impact on the patient, the assessment of pain using a VAS is often a good indication of the impact of mucositis on the patient.

The WHO mucositis grading system was developed following international meetings where researchers and clinicians met to develop a tool that could be used worldwide and has been considered a gold standard for the assessment of mucositis. The tool encompasses a five-point grading scale, from 0 to 4, ranging from no side effects to the inability to eat or drink. An oral examination of the mouth is not included in the tool, only the severity of oral mucositis based on the impact on the patient. The scale is simple to use, which is likely why it has been extensively used in clinical practice as well as in research—38% of the clinical trials have used the WHO scale (Putwatana et al., 2009; Sonis et al., 2004). Despite its use in practice, reliability and validity data have not been reported.

The WCCNR Stomatitis Staging System was developed specifically for the assessment of stomatitis/mucositis and not overall oral health (Olson et al., 2004). Interviews were conducted with physicians, nurses, and dentists to develop a list of descriptors that could be used in the development of an assessment tool. The original tool included eight assessment descriptors (lesions, color, bleeding, moisture, edema, infection, pain, and ability to eat and drink) but was later reduced to three (lesions, color, and bleeding) because they were found to predict the stage of stomatitis 96.4% of the time. The tool has been shown to correlate with the OAG and influenced changes to the OAG tool and the development of a new scoring system for the assessment of mucositis caused by chemotherapy or radiation within clinical trials (Sonis et al., 1999). It has been described as being quick and easy to use, as it only assesses mucositis or stomatitis (Jaroneski, 2006). A limitation of the tool is that while it is quick and easy to use, it does not capture the subjective and functional impact of mucositis on the patient.

The MacDibbs Mouth Assessment tool was developed for use in radiation settings. It is a 14-item tool with four sections focusing on patient information or symptoms experienced by the patient, an observational examination of the mouth, a swab taken for fungal growth, and a culture for herpes simplex virus. It has not been used widely in routine clinical practice but has been used in intervention studies (Dodd et al., 2000; Larson et al., 1998) because it is able to distinguish between mucositis resulting from radiation therapy and infections or other oral health concerns (Olson et al., 2004).

The challenge with all of the tools for mucositis assessment is the variation between scores within and between tools. A score may vary depending on the skill and interpretation of the assessor, and changes may exist in item scores within the tool that may not alter the overall total score. Additionally, several of the tools have multiple items of assessment, which affects the nurse's ability to systematically and consistently use the tool in a busy oncology clinic or other setting. A simple, and easy-to-use tool is desirable, but as with all tools, making a choice about which tool to use and using it consistently is far better than not using a tool at all because no one tool to date will meet all needs of the practitioner and be a reliable and valid tool in practice.

Xerostomia Assessment Tools

All patients with cancer are affected physically, emotionally, and spiritually by a number of distressing treatment-related side effects. For patients with head and neck cancer, the side effects of radiotherapy are among the most devastating, and the disfigurement, progressive loss of function, and oral changes that arise as a result of treatment significantly reduce their overall quality of life (Bjordal et al., 1999). The oral changes associated with radiotherapy occur when the major salivary glands (parotid, submandibular, and sublingual glands) fall within the radiation field and receive high-dose radiation (Gosselin & Pavilonis, 2002; van Rij et al., 2008). Changes in salivary gland output and consistency most commonly lead to xerostomia, the sensation of dry mouth (Schiff et al., 2009). However, patients with head and neck cancer commonly report tenderness, burning or pain in the oral cavity, and difficulty with eating or wearing dentures, speaking, and sleeping (Gosselin & Pavilonis, 2002).

Efforts to maximize radiotherapy treatment outcomes and promote optimal quality of life among patients with head and neck cancer have led to the development or modification of oral tools that assess xerostomia, including the XQ (Eisbruch et al., 2001), the OAG (Eilers et al., 1988; Knöös & Östman, 2010) and the EORTC QLQ-H&N35 (Bjordal et al., 2000).

Eisbruch et al. (2001) developed the patient-reported XQ after an extensive literature search of both xerostomia-specific and general head and neck cancer quality-of-life instruments. The questionnaire consists of eight questions—four that address oral dryness when eating or chewing and four that address oral dryness when not eating and chewing. Patients rate each item on a 0 to 10 scale, and each individual score is added to produce a total score ranging from 0 to 100; the higher the score, the worse the xerostomia. The XQ has undergone psychometric testing and has shown high test-retest correlation coefficients (0.82; $p < 0.01$) for each study participant, as well as high internal consistency (0.86). In addition, the patient-reported scores were higher one month after treatment for both bilateral ($p = 0.01$) and unilateral ($p < 0.01$) radiation treatments, indicating that the XQ could detect a statistically significant increase in oral discomfort (Eisbruch et al., 2001). The validity and reliability of the XQ were strengthened when a Taiwanese version (XQ-T) was developed to assess the impact of xerostomia on the quality of life of Taiwanese patients with head and neck cancer (Lin, Jen, Chang, & Lin, 2008). When experts were asked to rate the tool's relevance, clarity, simplicity, and ambiguity, the content reliability was found to be 0.97, and saliva flow was significantly correlated with XQ-T scores at two, four, six, and eight weeks after radiation treatments (Lin et al., 2008).

Recently, Knöös and Östman (2010) tested the reliability and validity of the OAG (Eilers et al., 1988) for assessing the oral side effects of radiotherapy among patients with head and neck cancer. Inter-rater reliability between nurses and oncologists was high (greater than 71% in all categories and greater than 80% in voice and saliva assessments). Examiners reported that the tool was easy to use and was well accepted among patients. However, only a moderate association between radiation dose and side effects could be established. This is most likely because the domains of the OAG represent the whole oral cavity, making it difficult to identify minor oral changes (Knöös & Östman, 2010). For this tool to be successfully used in daily clinical practice in patients with head and neck cancer, further research and examination is necessary to determine the validity of the OAG when assessing oral health after radiotherapy.

Finally, the EORTC QLQ group has developed and tested a patient-reported assessment tool that addresses xerostomia and health-related quality of life. The EORTC QLQ-H&N35 tool (Bjordal et al., 2000) was to be used along with the QLQ-C30, which is a quality-of-life questionnaire previously developed and tested by EORTC. The EORTC QLQ-H&N35 consists of 30 items scored using a Likert scale from 1 (not at all) to 4 (very much) with an additional five questions that require a yes or no answer. Each of these tools is self-administered by the patient. The scores are transformed to a 0 to 100 scale, with a high score indicating significant symptoms or problems (Bjordal et al., 1999, 2000). The EORTC QLQ-H&N35 has been tested in large clinical trials of patients with head and neck cancer before and after receiving radiotherapy, surgery, and chemotherapy and has yielded high compliance among patients. To date, the EORTC QLQ-H&N35 has been extensively tested in 12 countries and successfully translated into nine languages (Bjordal et al. 1999). It is regarded as the most comprehensive assessment tool for quality-of-life assessments in relation to oral changes for patients with head and neck cancer.

Special Populations and Considerations

A number of tools, including those previously discussed, used to assess broad oral changes as well as specific mucosal changes, such as mucositis and xerostomia, have been created and validated in numerous studies (Tomlinson et al., 2009). Therefore, it is imperative that nurses consider population-specific needs in addition to reliability and validity data when selecting an instrument to evaluate oral changes in clinical and research practice.

All patients have individualized needs; however, pediatric and intubated patients are among the most complex and vulnerable patients in healthcare settings because of their unique developmental, cognitive, and communication abilities. For patients who are intubated, poor oral hygiene can lead to a number of complications, including increased morbidity, the spread of infection leading to ventilator-associated pneumonia, and irreversible damage to the teeth related to the development of dental caries (Blot et al., 2008). Several oral assessment tools have been developed, and many existing tools have been modified to meet the unique needs of orally intubated patients. The modified oral assessment tool used by Barnason et al. (1998) was adapted from the OAG (Eilers et al., 1988). Each of the domains (lips, tongue, saliva, mucous membranes, gingiva, and teeth) included were rated on a three-point scale, with a lower total score indicating a healthier mouth.

Treloar and Stechmiller (1995) developed an oral assessment tool to specifically meet the needs of intubated patients. This tool outlines a detailed assessment of all oral structures and assigns a numeric score to salivary flow, plaque and debris status, and gingiva condition. It is recommended that this tool be used daily to accurately assess and monitor mucosal changes; however, the successful transition of this tool into clinical practice has not been clearly demonstrated (McNeill, 2000).

As with intubated patients, the unique needs of pediatric patients have also prompted the development and modification of oral assessment tools (Tomlinson et al., 2009). Again, the OAG (Eilers et al., 1988) has served as a template to develop an age-appropriate oral assessment tool. The Great Ormond Street Hospital Oral Assessment Guide (GOSH OAG), developed by Gibson et al. (2006), consists of the same eight oral domains and numeric (1–3) grading scale as the OAG tool previously described. However, the method of assessment and the verbal descriptors in each category were modified to include age-appropriate approaches and language. For example, in the voice domain, the method of assessment included talking and listening to the child, and a normal rating of 1 was determined by a normal tone and quality when talking or crying. Content validity in each domain of the GOSH OAG was assessed as high (0.78–1) as established by pediatric clinical experts. With further validation and development, this tool could be appropriate for use in daily clinical practice.

The Children's International Mucositis Evaluation Scale (ChIMES) is another pediatric-specific oral assessment tool (Tomlinson et al., 2009). This tool was developed to specifically evaluate mucositis and was based on the OMAS. The self-report ChIMES for children (or parent proxies) addresses three categories: pain, function, and appearance of the oral cavity. Six cartoon faces ranging from a smiling face (0) to a crying face (5) quantify pain and function. A visual inspection of the oral mucosa is prompted at the end of each self-report. In clinical trials, both children and parents reported that the ChIMES was easy to understand. The questions that caused participants the greatest amount of confusion and were consequently rated as "bad questions" were those that addressed pain medication and the presence of ulcers. Overall, the ChIMES tool addresses the needs of pediatric patients. However, further evaluations are necessary before this tool is integrated into daily practice.

The population-specific oral assessment tools mentioned in this section are only a few of the many oral assessment tools available to clinicians to trial and use in practice when conducting oral assessments. Studies reveal that across all patient populations, only 26% of clinicians use a written assessment tool in daily practice (Jones, Newton, & Bower, 2004). In an effort to encourage and increase the use of oral assessment tools in daily nursing practice, Hayes and Jones (1995) developed the BRUSHED Assessment Model. The model is not an assessment tool but rather a guide that can be used in conjunction with an assessment tool. The model assists nurses with assessments of the oral cavity by outlining particular clinical signs using a simple mnemonic: **B**leeding, **R**edness, **U**lceration, **S**aliva, **H**alitosis, **E**xternal factors/endotracheal tubes, **D**ebris. The BRUSHED Assessment Model can be used to guide global or focused oral assessments and is applicable to all patients.

Consideration for population-specific needs is necessary when conducting any assessment. Therefore, an assessment tool that best reflects the needs of the population will ultimately yield the most accurate and consistent assessment data. Unfortunately, the oral assessment guides designed for intubated and pediatric patients are in their infancy and require further exploration, modification, and evaluation before they can be successfully integrated into daily clinical practice.

Naturopathic, Complementary, and Alternative Medicine

In recent years, a growing acceptance for complementary and alternative medicine (CAM) has led to an increase in the number of adult and pediatric patients with cancer who turn to CAM in addition to conventional therapies to manage common symptoms associated with chemotherapy and radiation treatments (Ladas, Post-White, Hawks, & Taromina, 2006). Overlapping toxicities and interactions between treatments, although rare, have prompted the need for reliable evidence-based CAM practice. Small clinical trials testing two biologic CAM therapies (glutamine and Traumeel S® [Heel Inc.]) have reported positive results when trialed in both pediatric and adult patients with cancer with inflammatory or ulcerative oral changes including mucositis and stomatitis (Anderson, Ramsay, et al., 1998; Anderson, Schroeder, & Skubitz, 1998; Oberbaum et al., 2001). Assessment and data of oral changes (mucositis/stomatitis), pain severity, and ability to swallow and maintain nutrition were collected using a variety of methods. Anderson and colleagues used a patient/parent self-report method in clinical trials designed to determine the effect of glutamine on stomatitis (Anderson, Ramsay, et al., 1998; Anderson, Schroeder, et al., 1998). The questionnaire/calendar (Anderson, Schroeder, et al., 1998) prompted patients or their parents to indicate the presence or absence of a sore mouth each day with a "yes" or "no" followed by a numeric rating to indicate how their eating was affected by the presence or absence of a sore mouth using a 0 (no pain) to 4 (painful mucositis, no oral intake except medications) rating scale. Andersson et al. (1999) collected self-report data by asking patients or parents to indicate the presence or absence of stomatitis (an "N" for no pain and an "M" for sore mouth or sore present) in combination with a numeric rating of its effects on oral intake (0, none; 1, mild; 2, soft foods; 3, liquids only; 4, unable to swallow liquids). In a randomized clinical trial, Oberbaum et al. (2000) used the WHO grading system for mucositis (0 = no change to 4 = alimentation not possible) to determine oral changes in combination with a subjective scoring system that asked patients or parents to judge the degree of oral pain or discomfort, dryness of the mouth or tongue, dysphagia, and ability to swallow when trailing the effectiveness of Traumeel S.

Each of the identified studies reported a positive correlation between CAM and either a reduction in the severity of oral changes or a delay in the onset. As complementary therapies continue to emerge and their use becomes more widespread, it will become increasingly important to ensure that validated and reliable assessment tools are used in clinical and research practice in order to accurately determine the usefulness of CAM interventions and ensure reproducible results. The OAG (Eilers et al., 1988) for broad mucosal changes and the OMAS (Sonis et al., 1999), which focuses on mucous membrane changes, should be strongly considered when selecting a tool to guide the evaluation of CAM interventions because these assessment tools have both shown high reliability and validity rates. In addition, these tools have proven beneficial clinical utility, require minimal training to use correctly, and have been successfully modified to meet language- and population-specific characteristics when evaluating the effectiveness of oral therapies and interventions (Gibson et al., 2006; Tomlinson et al., 2009).

Conclusion

A variety of assessment tools exist for oral care and oral symptoms. Currently, assessments are done infrequently or inconsistently in clinical practice. Systematic assessment is needed before, during, and following cancer therapy. Despite the lack of agreement about the frequency of assessment, studies favor the need for daily assessment based on changes that occur in the mouth over a short period of time (Quinn et al., 2008). In addition, assessments should include not only objective measures but also subjective or patient-reported impact and outcomes, including pain. This may require the use of several assessment tools to capture all of the information. As a result, more work is required to develop or adapt a tool to ensure that it is useful not only in clinical trials but in daily routine clinical practice as well.

The Oncology Nursing Society undertook a Patient Outcomes Survey (Mallory & Thomas, 2004) in which members clearly identified the importance of documenting nursing-sensitive patient outcomes. Members indicated the benefits of patient outcomes measurement, including clinical decision making, patient assessment, and quality of care. Interestingly, when asked about the use of assessment tools to assess, measure, and document outcomes, specific tools such as the OAG were used less than 35% of the time. Numeric pain scores were the most commonly used type of assessment tool, and 83.4% of respondents reported using these. Despite the work that has been undertaken to develop and evaluate clinical assessment tools and their ease of use in the clinical setting, a great deal of work remains to be done to ensure that an oral assessment guide is used in clinical practice. Ongoing, consistent, and standardized education for nurses performing oral assessments is warranted to ensure that the data collected are reliable because clinical decisions are and will be made based on assessment findings.

References

Anderson, P.M., Ramsay, N.K.C., Shu, X.O., Rydholm, N., Rogosheske, J., Nicklow, R., ... Skubitz, K.M. (1998). Effect of low-dose oral glutamine on painful stomatitis during bone marrow transplantation. *Bone Marrow Transplantation, 22*, 339–344. doi:10.1038/sj.bmt.1701317

Anderson, P.M., Schroeder, G., & Skubitz, K.M. (1998). Oral glutamine reduces the duration and severity of stomatitis after cytotoxic cancer chemotherapy. *Cancer, 83*, 1433–1439. doi:10.1002/(SICI)1097-0142(19981001)83:7<1433::AID-CNCR22>3.0.CO;2-4

Andersson, P., Persson, L., Hallberg, I.R., & Renvert, S. (1999). Testing an oral assessment guide during chemotherapy treatment in a Swedish care setting: A pilot study. *Journal of Clinical Nursing, 8*, 150–158. doi:10.1046/j.1365-2702.1999.00237.x

Barnason, S., Graham, J., Wild, M.C., Jensen, L.B., Rasmussen, D., Schulz, P., ... Carder, B. (1998). Comparison of two endotracheal tube securement techniques on unplanned extubation, oral mucosa, and facial skin integrity. *Heart and Lung: The Journal of Acute and Critical Care, 27*, 409–417. doi:10.1016/S0147-9563(98)90087-5

Beck, S. (1979). Impact of a systematic oral care protocol on stomatitis after chemotherapy. *Cancer Nursing, 2*, 185–199.

Bjordal, K., de Graeff, A., Fayers, P.M., Hammerlid, E., van Pottelsberghe, C., Curran, D., ... Kaasa, S. (2000). A 12 country field study of the EORTC QLQ-C30 (version 3.0) and the head and neck cancer specific module (EORTC QLQ-H&N35) in head and neck patients. EORTC Quality of Life Group. *European Journal of Cancer, 36*, 1796–1807.

Bjordal, K., Hammerlid, E., Ahlner-Elmqvist, M., de Graeff, A., Boysen, M., Evensen, J.F., ... Kaasa, S. (1999). Quality of life in head and neck cancer patients: Validation of the European Organization for Research and Treatment of Cancer Quality of Life Questionnaire-H&N35. *Journal of Clinical Oncology, 17,* 1008–1019.

Blot, S., Vandijck, D., & Labeau, S. (2008). Oral care of intubated patients. *Clinical Pulmonary Medicine, 15,* 153–160. doi:10.1097/CPM.0b013e3181729250

Catlin-Huth, C., Haas, M., & Pollock, V. (Eds.). (2002). *Radiation therapy patient care record: A tool for documenting nursing care.* Pittsburgh, PA: Oncology Nursing Society.

Cella, D., Pulliam, J., Fuchs, H., Miller, C., Hurd, D., Wingard, J.R., ... Giles, F. (2003). Evaluation of pain associated with oral mucositis during the acute period after administration of high-dose chemotherapy. *Cancer, 98,* 406–412. doi:10.1002/cncr.11505

Chen, C.-F., Wang, R.-H., Cheng, S.-N., & Chang, Y.-C. (2004). Assessment of chemotherapy-induced oral complications in children with cancer. *Journal of Pediatric Oncology Nursing, 21,* 33–39. doi:10.1177/1043454203259947

Chen, H.-M. (2008). Patients' experiences and perceptions of chemotherapy-induced oral mucositis in a day unit. *Cancer Nursing, 31,* 363–369. doi:10.1097/01. NCC.0000305762.89109.29

Chen, Y., Trotti, A., Coleman, C.N., Machtay, M., Mirimanoff, R.O., Hay, J., ... Jeremic, B. (2006). Adverse event reporting and developments in radiation biology after normal tissue injury: International Atomic Energy Agency consultation. *International Journal of Radiation Oncology, Biology, Physics, 64,* 1442–1451. doi:10.1016/j.ijrobp.2005.10.014

Coleman, S. (1995). An overview of the oral complications of adult patients with malignant haematological conditions who have undergone radiotherapy or chemotherapy. *Journal of Advanced Nursing, 22,* 1085–1091. doi:10.1111/j.1365-2648.1995.tb03109.x

Colevas, A.D., & Setser, A. (2004). The NCI Common Terminology Criteria for Adverse Events (CTCAE) v3.0 is the new standard for oncology clinical trials. *Journal of Clinical Oncology, 22*(Suppl. 14), Abstract No. 6098.

Dibble, S.L., Shiba, G., MacPhail, L., & Dodd, M.J. (1996). MacDibbs Mouth Assessment: A new tool to evaluate mucositis in the radiation therapy patient. *Cancer Practice, 4,* 135–140.

Dodd, M.J., Dibble, S.L., Miaskowski, C., MacPhail, L., Greenspan, D., Paul, S.M., ... Larson, P. (2000). Randomized clinical trial of the effectiveness of 3 commonly used mouthwashes to treat chemotherapy-induced mucositis. *Oral Surgery, Oral Medicine, Oral Pathology, Oral Radiology and Endodontics, 90,* 39–47. doi:10.1067/moe.2000.105713

Eilers, J., Berger, A.M., & Petersen, M. (1988). Development, testing, and application of the oral assessment guide. *Oncology Nursing Forum, 15,* 325–330.

Eilers, J., & Epstein, J.B. (2004). Assessment and measurement of oral mucositis. *Seminars in Oncology Nursing, 20,* 22–29. doi:10.1053/j.soncn.2003.10.005

Eisbruch, A., Kim, H.M., Terrell, J.E., Marsh, L.H., Dawson, L.A., & Ship, J.A. (2001). Xerostomia and its predictors following parotid-sparing irradiation of head-and-neck cancer. *International Journal of Radiation Oncology, Biology, Physics, 50,* 695–704. doi:10.1016/ S0360-3016(01)01512-7

Fox, P.C., Busch, K.A., & Baum, B.J. (1987). Subjective reports of xerostomia and objective measures of salivary gland performance. *Journal of the American Dental Association, 115,* 581–584.

Gibson, F., Cargill, J., Allison, J., Begent, J., Cole, S., Stone, J., & Lucas, V. (2006). Establishing content validity of the oral assessment guide in children and young people. *European Journal of Cancer, 42,* 1817–1825. doi:10.1016/j.ejca.2006.02.018

Ginsberg, M.K. (1961). A study of oral hygiene nursing care. *American Journal of Nursing, 61*(10), 67–69.

Gosselin, T.K., & Pavlonis, H. (2002). Head and neck cancer: Managing xerostomia and other treatment induced side effects. *ORL-Head and Neck Nursing, 20*(4), 15–22.

Harris, D.J., Eilers, J., Harriman, A., Cashavelly, B.J., & Maxwell, C. (2008). Putting evidence into practice: Evidence-based interventions for the management of oral mucositis. *Clinical Journal of Oncology Nursing, 12,* 141–148. doi:10.1188/08.CJON.141-152

Harrison, M.B., Légaré, F., Graham, I.D., & Fervers, B. (2010). Adapting clinical practice guidelines to local context and assessing barriers to their use. *Canadian Medical Association Journal, 182,* E78–E84. doi:10.1503/cmaj.081232

Hayes, J., & Jones, C. (1995). A collaborative approach to oral care during critical illness. *Dental Health, 34*(3), 6–10.

Holmes, S., & Mountain, E. (1993). Assessment of oral status: Evaluation of three oral assessment guides. *Journal of Clinical Nursing, 2*(1), 35–40.

Jaroneski, L.A. (2006). The importance of assessment rating scales for chemotherapy-induced oral mucositis. *Oncology Nursing Forum, 33,* 1085–1092. doi:10.1188/06. ONF.1085-1093

Jones, H., Newton, J.T., & Bower, E.J. (2004). A survey of the oral care practices of intensive care nurses. *Intensive and Critical Care Nursing, 20,* 69–70. doi:10.1016/j.iccn.2004.01.004

Keefe, D.M., Schubert, M.M., Elting, L.S., Sonis, S.T., Epstein, J.B., Raber-Durlacher, J.E., … Peterson, D.E. (2007). Updated clinical practice guidelines for the prevention and treatment of mucositis. *Cancer, 109,* 820–831. doi:10.1002/cncr.22484

Knöös, M., & Östman, M. (2010). Oral assessment guide—Test of reliability and validity for patients receiving radiotherapy to the head and neck region. *European Journal of Cancer Care, 19,* 53–60. doi:10.1111/j.1365-2354.2008.00958.x

Ladas, E.J., Post-White, J., Hawks, R., & Taromina, K. (2006). Evidence for symptom management in the child with cancer. *Journal of Pediatric Hematology/Oncology, 28,* 601–615. doi:10.1097/01.mph.0000212989.26317.52

Larson, P.J., Miaskowski, C., MacPhail, L., Dodd, M.J., Greenspan, D., Dibbble, S., … Ignoffo, R. (1998). The PRO-SELF Mouth Aware program: An effective approach for reducing chemotherapy-induced mucositis. *Cancer Nursing, 21,* 263–268.

Lin, S.C., Jen, Y.M., Chang, Y.C., & Lin, C.C. (2008). Assessment of xerostomia and its impact on quality of life in head and neck cancer patients undergoing radiotherapy and validation of the Taiwanese version of the Xerostomia Questionnaire. *Journal of Pain and Symptom Management, 36,* 141–148. doi:10.1016/j.jpainsymman.2007.09.009

Mallory, G., & Thomas, R. (2004). ONS patient outcomes survey 2004. Retrieved from http://www.ons.org/Research/NursingSensitive/Survey

McGuire, D.B., Altomonte, V., Peterson, D.E., Wingard, J.R., Jones, R.J., & Grochow, L.B. (1993). Patterns of mucositis and pain in patients receiving preparative chemotherapy and bone marrow transplantation. *Oncology Nursing Forum, 20,* 1493–1502.

McGuire, D.B., Rubenstein, E.B., & Peterson, D.E. (2004). Evidence-based guidelines for managing mucositis. *Seminars in Oncology Nursing, 20,* 59–66.

McNeill, H.E. (2000). Biting back at poor oral hygiene. *Intensive and Critical Care Nursing, 16,* 367–372. doi:10.1054/iccn.2000.1531

Miller, A.B., Hoogstraten, B., Staquet, M., & Winkler, A. (1981). Reporting results of cancer treatment. *Cancer, 47,* 207–214.

National Cancer Institute Cancer Therapy Evaluation Program. (2009). *Common terminology criteria for adverse events* [v.4.0]. Bethesda, MD: National Cancer Institute.

Oberbaum, M., Yaniv, I., Ben-Gal, Y., Stein, J., Ben-Zvi, N., Freedman, L.S., & Branski, D. (2001). A randomized, controlled clinical trial of the homeopathic medication TRAUMEEL S® in the treatment of chemotherapy-induced stomatitis in children undergoing stem cell transplantation. *Cancer, 92,* 684–690. doi:10.1002/1097-0142(20010801)92:3<684::AID-CNCR1371>3.0.CO;2-#

Olson, K., Hanson, J., Hamilton, J., Stacey, D., Eades, M., Gue, D., … Oliver, C. (2004). Assessing the reliability and validity of the revised WCCNR stomatitis staging system for cancer therapy-induced stomatitis. *Canadian Oncology Nursing Journal, 14,* 168–174.

Parulekar, W., Mackenzie, R., Bjarnason, G., & Jordan, R.C.K. (1998). Scoring oral mucositis. *Oral Oncology, 34,* 63–71.

Passos, J.Y., & Brand, L.M. (1966). Effects of agents used for oral hygiene. *Nursing Research, 15,* 196–202.

Putwatana, P., Sanmanowong, P., Oonprasertpong, L., Junda, T., Pitiporn, S., & Narkwong, L. (2009). Relief of radiation-induced oral mucositis in head and neck cancer. *Cancer Nursing, 32*, 82–87. doi:10.1097/01.NCC.0000343362.68129.ed

Quinn, B., Potting, C.M.J., Stone, R., Blijlevens, N.M.A., Fliedner, M., Margulies, A., & Sharp, L. (2008). Guidelines for the assessment of oral mucositis in adult chemotherapy, radiotherapy and haematopoietic stem cell transplant patients. *European Journal of Cancer, 44*, 61–72. doi:10.1016/j.ejca.2007.09.014

Rosenthal, D.I., Mendoza, T.R., Chambers, M.S., Asper, J.A., Gning, I., Kies, M.S., ... Cleeland, C.S. (2007). Measuring head and neck cancer symptom burden: The development and validation of the M. D. Anderson symptom inventory, head and neck module. *Head and Neck, 29*, 923–931. doi:10.1002/hed.20602

Russo, G., Haddad, R., Posner, M., & Machtay, M. (2008). Radiation treatment breaks and ulcerative mucositis in head and neck cancer. *Oncologist, 13*, 886–898. doi:10.1634/theoncologist.2008-0024

Rutledge, D.N., & Grant, M. (2002). Introduction. *Seminars in Oncology Nursing, 18*, 1–2. doi:10.1053/sonu.2002.30035

Schiff, E., Mogilner, J.G., Sella, E., Doweck, I., Hershko, O., Ben-Arye, E., & Yarom, N. (2009). Hypnosis for postradiation xerostomia in head and neck cancer patients: A pilot study. *Journal of Pain and Symptom Management, 37*, 1086–1092. doi:10.1016/j.jpainsymman.2008.07.005

Schubert, M.M., Williams, B.E., Lloid, M.E., Donaldson, G., & Chapko, M.K. (1992). Clinical assessment scale for the rating of oral mucosal changes associated with bone marrow transplantation. Development of an oral mucositis index. *Cancer, 69*, 2469–2477.

Sonis, S.T., Eilers, J.P., Epstein, J.B., LeVeque, F.G., Liggett, W.H., Jr., Mulagha, M.T., ... Wittes, J.P. (1999). Validation of a new scoring system for the assessment of clinical trial research of oral mucositis induced by radiation or chemotherapy. Mucositis Study Group. *Cancer, 85*, 2103–2113. doi:10.1002/(SICI)1097-0142(19990515)85:10<2103::AID-CNCR2>3.0.CO;2-0

Sonis, S.T., Elting, L.S., Keefe, D., Peterson, D.E., Schubert, M., Hauer-Jensen, M., ... Rubenstein, E.B. (2004). Perspectives on cancer therapy-induced mucosal injury: Pathogenesis, measurement, epidemiology, and consequences for patients. *Cancer, 100*(Suppl. 9), 1995–2025. doi:10.1002/cncr.20162

Stone, R., Potting, C.M.J., Clare, S., Uhlenhopp, M., Davies, M., Mank, A., & Quinn, B. (2007). Management of oral mucositis at European transplantation centres. *European Journal of Oncology Nursing, 11*(Suppl. 1), S3–S9. doi:10.1016/S1462-3889(07)70002-9

Tomlinson, D., Gibson, F., Treister, N., Baggott, C., Judd, P., Hendershot, E., ... Sung, L. (2009). Understandability, content validity, and overall acceptability of the Children's International Mucositis Evaluation Scale (ChIMES): Child and parent reporting. *Journal of Pediatric Hematology/Oncology, 31*, 416–423. doi:10.1097/MPH.0b013e31819c21ab

Treloar, D.M., & Stechmiller, J.K. (1995). Use of a clinical assessment tool for orally intubated patients. *American Journal of Critical Care, 4*, 355–360.

Trotti, A., Bellm, L.A., Epstein, J.B., Frame, D., Fuchs, H.J., Gwede, C.K., ... Zilberberg, M.D. (2003). Mucositis incidence, severity and associated outcomes in patients with head and neck cancer receiving radiotherapy with or without chemotherapy: A systematic literature review. *Radiotherapy and Oncology, 66*, 253–262. doi:10.1016/S0167-8140(02)00404-8

Trotti, A., Colevas, A.D., Setser, A., Rusch, V., Jacques, D., Budach, V., ... Rubin, P. (2003). CTCAE v3.0: Development of a comprehensive grading system for the adverse effects of cancer treatment. *Seminars in Radiation Oncology, 13*, 176–181.

van Rij, C.M., Oughlane-Heemsbergen, W.D., Ackerstaff, A.H., Lamers, E.A., Balm, A.J.M., & Rasch, C.R.N. (2008). Parotid gland sparing IMRT for head and neck cancer improves xerostomia related quality of life. *Radiation Oncology, 3*, 41. doi:10.1186/1748-717X-3-41

Watt, R.G. (2005). Strategies and approaches in oral disease prevention and health promotion. *Bulletin of the World Health Organization, 83*, 711–718.

Williams, J., Chen, Y., Rubin, P., Finkelstein, J., & Okunieff, P. (2003). The biological basis of a comprehensive grading system for the adverse effects of cancer treatment. *Seminars in Radiation Oncology, 13,* 182–188. doi:10.1016/S1053-4296(03)00045-6

CHAPTER 5

Nutrition Management Strategies for Oral Effects of Cancer Treatment

Maria Q.B. Petzel, RD, CSO, LD, CNSC

Introduction

Cancer itself and the treatments for cancer often lead to changes in nutrition status. Not only does treatment have the potential to alter nutrient needs, but it also may lead to alterations in the ability to meet those needs with usual oral intake (Hurst & Gallagher, 2006). Many patients will seek out information about food choices and symptom management to help improve their tolerance of treatment, quality of life, and healing after treatment.

Basic nutrient requirements for all individuals are based on age, sex, anthropometrics, and physical activity. In patients with cancer, their nutrition status at the time of diagnosis, the type or location of cancer, and the type of treatment also affect nutrient requirements (Hurst & Gallagher, 2006). Nutrition screening is important for all patients undergoing treatment for cancer. Screening and assessment tools and processes should comply with current standards and elements of performance established by the Joint Commission (2010). Prior to starting treatment, patients who have a high potential for treatment-related alterations in nutrition status should, if at all possible, meet with a registered dietitian with experience in oncology (Hayward & Shea, 2009). If feasible, patients should meet with a dietitian who is certified as a specialist in oncology nutrition by the Commission on Dietetic Registration.

Malnutrition is reported to occur in 40%–80% of patients with cancer (Bruera, 1997; National Cancer Institute, 2010). Inadequate nutrient intake may lead to decreases in performance status and quality of life, as well as response to and tolerance of treatment. It also may increase treatment complications, morbidity and mortality, and healthcare costs (Keefe, Rassias, O'Neil, & Gibson, 2007). Patients with poor nutrition are less able to tolerate their prescribed dose and schedule of cancer treatments and therefore may have less favorable results from treatment (Petree, 2005).

This chapter will present suggestions for the management of the nutrition-related oral effects of therapy. Although evidence is available regarding the effect of poor nutrition on cancer treatments, very little exists in the literature regarding evidence-based practices for nutrition treatment of symptoms. Many of the tips provided in this chapter are largely practice based. It is important to recognize and to educate patients that nutrition strategies are an adjunct to other medical interventions that may have a greater impact. Therefore, the nutrition strategies discussed should be implemented in combination with medical therapies for side effect management. Nutrition tips are especially useful for patients who seek an active role in their relief of symptoms and recovery from treatment. The overall goals are to prevent or reverse poor nutrition, support immune function, manage side effects, and aid with successful completion of therapy (Kagan & Sweeney-Cordes, 2005).

Mucositis

Mucositis, as discussed earlier in this book, is an inflammation of the lining of the mouth. Thick mucus or decreased saliva production may accompany mucositis (Kagan & Sweeney-Cordes, 2005); these will be discussed more in the section about xerostomia. Mucositis occurs as a result of stomatotoxic chemotherapy or radiation therapy to the oral mucosa (Shih, Miaskowski, Dodd, Stotts, & MacPhail, 2002). Authors report occurrences of oral mucositis in 40%–90% of patients depending on the type and intensity of treatment (Berendt & D'Agostino, 2005; Cheng, 2007; Elting et al., 2007). Chemotherapy-induced mucositis generally lasts 3–12 days, whereas radiation-induced mucositis may last 3–12 weeks. Concurrent chemotherapy and radiation therapy leads to an earlier onset of more severe mucositis that lasts for an extended duration (Lalla, Sonis, & Peterson, 2008; Rosenthal & Trotti, 2009).

Oral mucositis can affect nutrition intake and quality of life (Duncan et al., 2005). The pain and changes in taste associated with severe mucositis can lessen nutrition intake (Cheng, 2007; Lalla et al., 2008; Raber-Durlacher et al., 2004). Elting et al. (2007) reported that patients with oral mucositis due to radiation treatment are significantly more likely to have a weight loss of more than 5%. Poor nutrition status can also interfere with mucosal regeneration (Cheng, 2007).

In addition to medical treatments including pain control and good mouth care, nutrition techniques can help increase intake of food and fluid as well. Medication regimens should take into account the timing of meals to maximize pain control at the time of oral intake. See Table 5-1 for nutrition tips and techniques for coping with mucositis. Medical nutrition therapy for mucositis should include a soft diet and medical food supplement drinks (see Figure 5-1 and Table 5-2). In cases of severe mucositis, nutrition support may be beneficial (Kagan & Sweeney-Cordes, 2005).

Often, mucositis impairs eating to such a degree that necessitates the use of tube feeding or parenteral nutrition (nutrition support) (Lalla et al., 2008). Per

Table 5-1. Nutrition Interventions for Oral Effects of Treatment	
Symptom	**Intervention**
Dysphagia (difficult or painful swallowing)	Chew and swallow food carefully. Make sure to drink enough fluid. Thicken fluids as directed by the doctor or speech-language pathologist. Use commercially available food thickeners. Use medical nutrition supplement drinks. Choose foods that are high in protein and calories. Continue swallowing as much as possible throughout treatment. Try small, frequent meals of soft, moist, or pureed foods. Avoid bread, cakes, and crackers unless moistened with liquid. If prescribed, follow appropriate dysphagia diet and swallow techniques.
Mucositis (sore mouth and throat)	Eat soft foods that are easy to chew and swallow (see Table 5-2). Avoid foods that irritate the mouth. Avoid citrus fruits and juices. Avoid acidic, tomato-based, or pickled (vinegar) foods. Avoid spicy or salty foods. Avoid rough, coarse, or dry foods. Cook foods until soft and tender. Cut foods into small pieces. Use a straw to drink liquids to bypass mouth sores. Eat foods cold or at room temperature; hot and warm foods can irritate a tender mouth. Increase the fluid content of foods by adding gravy, broth, or sauces. Supplement meals with high-calorie, high-protein drinks. Numb the mouth with ice chips or flavored ice pops. Use a small spoon. Avoid alcohol and carbonated beverages. Avoid tobacco products.
Taste changes	Eat small, frequent meals and healthy snacks throughout the day. Be flexible. Eat meals when hungry rather than at set mealtimes. Use plastic utensils and do not drink directly from metal containers if foods taste metallic. Try favorite foods, if not nauseated. Plan to eat with family and friends. Have others prepare the meal. Try new foods when feeling best. Substitute poultry, fish, eggs, and cheese for red meat. A vegetarian, Indian, or Chinese cookbook can provide useful meatless, high-protein recipes.

(Continued on next page)

Table 5-1. Nutrition Interventions for Oral Effects of Treatment *(Continued)*

Symptom	Intervention
Taste changes *(Cont.)*	Use sugar-free lemon drops, gum, or mints when experiencing a metallic or bitter taste in the mouth. Add spices and sauces to foods. Eat meat with something sweet, such as cranberry sauce, jelly, or applesauce. Choose foods that look and smell appealing. Marinate foods. Try tart foods and drinks. Make foods sweeter. If tastes are dull but not unpleasant, chew food longer to allow more contact with taste receptors.
Thick saliva	Drink plenty of fluids. Use tart drinks to stimulate saliva. Use fresh papaya or pineapple juice (or fruit) to help dissolve thick mucus. Moisten foods.
Xerostomia	Keep water handy at all times to moisten the mouth. Drink plenty of fluids. Avoid rinses containing alcohol. Consume tart foods and beverages to help stimulate saliva. Drink fruit nectar instead of juice. Use a straw to drink liquids. Sip water throughout the day. Eat easy-to-swallow foods (see Table 5-2). Moisten foods by adding gravy, broth, or sauces. Avoid drinking beer, wine, or any other type of alcohol. Avoid tobacco products. Use artificial saliva and oral moisturizers as desired. Use a cool mist humidifier during sleep.

Note. Based on information from Eldridge & Hamilton, 2004; National Cancer Institute, 2010.

Figure 5-1. Medical Food Supplement Drinks

Standard (per can: 250 calories, 9–11 g protein)
- Boost® (Nestlé HealthCare Nutrition)
- Ensure® (Abbott Nutrition)
- Carnation® Instant Breakfast® Lactose Free (Nestlé HealthCare Nutrition)

High-calorie, high-protein (per can: 350 calories, 13–15 g protein)
- Boost Plus® (Nestlé HealthCare Nutrition)
- Ensure Plus® (Abbott Nutrition)
- Carnation® Instant Breakfast® Lactose Free Plus (Nestlé HealthCare Nutrition)

Carbohydrate-controlled (per can: 350 calories, 10–14 g protein)
- Boost Glucose Control® (Nestlé HealthCare Nutrition)
- Glucerna® (Abbott Nutrition)

Note. All of the above are lactose free.

Table 5-2. Soft Foods: Easy to Chew and Swallow	
Food Group	Specific Foods and Suggested Use
Fruit and vegetables	Bananas, applesauce, fruit nectars, canned fruits, pureed or mashed vegetables, avocados
Protein foods	Cottage cheese, yogurt, eggs, custard, pudding, beans, pureed or ground meats, milkshakes, smoothies. Add protein powders to liquid foods and smoothies.
Starches	Cooked cereal, oatmeal, rice or pasta in sauce or oil, potatoes without skin

the National Cancer Institute Cancer Therapy Evaluation Program's (2010) Common Terminology Criteria for Adverse Events scale, grade 3 mucositis is defined as interfering with oral intake and grade 4 as life-threatening, thus requiring nutrition support for either grade (Berendt & D'Agostino, 2005). In patients who are expected to develop severe mucositis, such as those receiving head and neck radiation, a gastrostomy feeding tube may be placed prophylactically (Lalla et al., 2008). Placement of a gastrostomy tube prior to beginning radiation treatment has been successful at preventing weight loss, treatment interruptions, and dehydration in patients (Kagan & Sweeney-Cordes, 2005).

Evidence is emerging regarding the use of certain nutritional supplements or therapies to help decrease the severity, duration, or onset of mucositis. A Cochrane review of interventions for mucositis found no significant differences between glutamine and placebo for prevention of mucositis (Worthington, Clarkson, & Eden, 2007). However, a review by Crowther, Avenell, and Culligan (2009) was completed in the Cochrane style and reviewed an additional two studies of oral glutamine (in patients having undergone stem cell transplantation) and found that glutamine may reduce mucositis in post-transplantation patients. At this time, evidence is not conclusive enough to make glutamine supplementation standard (Hayward & Shea, 2009), but it may be appropriate in individualized cases. The Cochrane review also identified topical use of honey and supplementation with zinc sulfate as promising and suggested additional studies to research the potential benefits and harms of these nutrition therapies for prevention of mucositis (Worthington et al., 2007).

Xerostomia

Xerostomia is often a late effect of treatment for head and neck cancer but can occur during treatment and may exacerbate mucositis (Hayward & Shea, 2009). It can be transient or permanent. Recovery may take up to 12 months after completion of treatment, unless mucositis is permanent (Silverman, 1999). It is characterized by decreased saliva production and can cause food to stick to the teeth or roof of the mouth and make swallowing difficult (Kisak & Klein, 2005).

Thick saliva and copious secretions may accompany xerostomia and may contribute to nausea, gagging, and sometimes vomiting (Hayward & Shea, 2009). Rosenthal and Trotti (2009) reported that xerostomia can be the most vexing symptom for some patients. In addition to mouth care and medication management, implementing some nutrition strategies may be helpful. Table 5-1 provides medical nutrition therapy tips for coping with thick saliva as well as xerostomia.

Dysgeusia and Hypogeusia

Taste changes may be an actual or perceived change in taste sensation (dysgeusia) or decreased sensitivity to taste (hypogeusia) (Berendt & D'Agostino, 2005). Dysgeusia and hypogeusia can happen with chemotherapy, radiotherapy, or other supportive medications. Taste changes are reported to occur in 15%–100% of patients receiving cancer therapy (Hayward & Shea, 2009; Ravasco, 2005). In patients receiving radiation therapy, decreased taste sensitivity typically begins during the first or second week of treatment (Hayward & Shea, 2009).

Taste changes may lead to food aversions or anorexia. Often the altered taste sensation results in a lack of desire for animal proteins such as fish, poultry, or red meat (Berendt & D'Agostino, 2005). Taste dysfunction can result in patients avoiding foods, a behavior that can lead to weight loss and malnutrition. After treatment is finished, the sense of taste may return partially or completely. The cells that make up the taste buds will regenerate within four months of completion of treatment. However, it may take a year before tastes are normal if impairment is not long term (National Cancer Institute, 2010; Silverman, 1999). Table 5-1 gives strategies for coping with taste changes, whether short or long term.

Research is controversial regarding the use of high-dose supplemental zinc to prevent or treat taste changes associated with cancer therapies. In uncontrolled studies, improvement in taste after zinc supplementation in patients receiving radiation therapy showed promising results (Halyard, 2009). A randomized controlled trial by Ripamonti et al. (1998) investigated the recovery of taste acuity following radiation therapy for head and neck cancer. Patients were given 45 mg elemental zinc or placebo three times per day. The study found that patients receiving zinc had a faster recovery of taste than those in the placebo group (Ripamonti et al., 1998). However, Halyard et al. (2007) reported more recent findings of a multicenter double-blinded, placebo-controlled trial where supplementation with zinc sulfate did not show benefit in the amount of time it took for taste to recover. Given these findings, zinc supplementation should not be used routinely to prevent taste changes or speed recovery from treatment-related taste changes.

Dysphagia

For the purposes of this chapter, *dysphagia* will refer to both difficult and painful swallowing; management of these in the short term will be discussed. Long-term (persistent) dysphagia is discussed in Chapter 3. Up to one-half of patients with head and neck cancer may experience dysphagia (Hayward & Shea, 2009). Most acute effects of cancer therapy resolve by about three months following completion of treatment, and swallowing function begins to return. A dysphagia assessment by a qualified speech-language pathologist is recommended at that time (Murphy & Gilbert, 2009).

It is important to be familiar with the common terminology for modified consistency diets. If patients are evaluated by a speech-language pathologist, a specific diet recommendation may be made. In 2002, the American Dietetic Association announced its effort to establish a "National Dysphagia Diet." The goal was to provide standardized language to describe the components of this modified consistency diet. Terminology is used to refer to two components of the diet: the food texture and consistency, and the liquid consistency. Foods and beverages are selected based on texture, cohesiveness, density, viscosity, temperature, and seasonings. The different levels of the diet are termed National Dysphagia Diet Levels 1, 2, and 3 or "Dysphagia Pureed," "Dysphagia Mechanically Altered," or "Dysphagia Advanced." The following terms are recommended for liquid consistencies: spoon-thick, honey-like, nectar-like, and thin liquids, although the actual viscosity of these fluids remains controversial and is still being studied (National Dysphagia Diet Task Force & American Dietetic Association, 2002).

Dysphagia often is associated with weight loss, anorexia, nausea, dehydration, protein-calorie malnutrition, cachexia, and muscle wasting (Berendt & D'Agostino, 2005). Dysphagia can affect quality of life through its impact on social interactions (Hayward & Shea, 2009). Nutrition goals are to modify the diet to ensure safe and adequate oral intake during treatment and recovery (Murphy & Gilbert, 2009). Table 5-1 presents strategies for the management of difficult or painful swallowing (see also the tips for mucositis). If oral intake of food and fluids is inadequate, tube feeding is most appropriate (Kagan & Sweeney-Cordes, 2005).

Other Oral Effects of Treatment

Oral Candidiasis

Oral candidiasis can be mistaken for mucositis (Silverman, 1999). It commonly causes changes in taste. The symptoms may be similar to mucositis, causing sore mouth or throat and leading to decreased intake. Strategies outlined in Table 5-1 for mucositis and taste changes can be used in addition to management with medications. Although studies in patients with cancer have not been done, a double-blind, placebo-controlled study of older adult subjects found that consumption of probiotic-containing cheese decreased the salivary yeast count by 32% in the experimental group (Hatakka et al., 2007). This study shows promise that if patients with cancer consume foods containing probiotics ("good bacteria"), it may reduce their risk of developing oral thrush.

Dental Caries, Trismus, and Osteoradionecrosis

Dental caries, trismus, and osteoradionecrosis can certainly affect nutrition, as they can make eating difficult. Additionally, nutrition can affect these, as malnutrition can intensify the severity of oral infections (Moynihan & Petersen, 2004). Nutrition strategies for coping with these issues should include ongoing good oral care. Food textures should be modified as needed. In patients with trismus or osteoradionecrosis, tube feeding may be necessary to provide adequate nutrition (Kogut & Luthringer, 2005).

Nutrition Support

If the patient's intake of food and fluid is not adequate, the diet may be supplemented with medical food supplement drinks. These are a convenient source of calories, protein, and fluid. Figure 5-1 lists some brands and their characteristics. Ravasco (2005) suggested introducing supplement drinks when patients are experiencing the least symptoms rather than when side effects are at their worst. This will improve the likelihood that the supplement will be acceptable to the patient (Ravasco, 2005).

The oral effects of cancer treatments can limit functional ability to take in adequate food and fluids, both short and long term, even with the modifications described throughout this book. Tube feeding should be considered when oral intake is inadequate because of either a mechanical obstruction from the tumor or severe side effects (Luthringer, 2006). Unless the gastrointestinal tract is impaired, enteral nutrition infusion should be used. The benefits of enteral nutrition over parenteral nutrition are that it stimulates bile flow and prevents cholestasis, may reduce risk of bacterial translocation, and carries a lower risk of infections than parenteral nutrition (Robinson, 2006). Although prophylactic placement of feeding tubes has been found to reduce weight loss, hospitalization, and treatment interruptions in patients receiving treatment for head and neck cancer, prophylactic placement is not standard among practitioners (Hayward & Shea, 2009; Rosenthal & Trotti, 2009). About 10% of patients with head and neck cancer who have feeding tubes placed during treatment will need them long term (Hayward & Shea, 2009).

Conclusion

Good nutrition can improve patients' quality of life and ability to complete the prescribed treatment. Nutrition is a tool that patients can use to play an active role in their treatment and recovery. The healthcare team, including nurses and dietitians, can help empower patients and families by providing practical and sound nutrition advice.

References

Berendt, M., & D'Agostino, S. (2005). Alterations in nutrition. In J.K. Itano & K.N. Taoka (Eds.), *Core curriculum for oncology nursing* (4th ed., pp. 277–317). St. Louis, MO: Elsevier Saunders.

Bruera, E. (1997). ABC of palliative care. Anorexia, cachexia, and nutrition. *BMJ, 315,* 1219–1222.

Cheng, K.K.-F. (2007). Oral mucositis, dysfunction, and distress in patients undergoing cancer therapy. *Journal of Clinical Nursing, 16,* 2114–2121. doi:10.1111/j.1365-2702.2006.01618.x

Crowther, M., Avenell, A., & Culligan, D.J. (2009). Systematic review and meta-analyses of studies of glutamine supplementation in haematopoietic stem cell transplantation. *Bone Marrow Transplantation, 44,* 413–425. doi:10.1038/bmt.2009.41

Duncan, G.G., Epstein, J.B., Tu, D., El Sayed, S., Bezjak, A., Ottaway, J., & Pater, J. (2005). Quality of life, mucositis, and xerostomia from radiotherapy for head and neck cancers: A report from the NCIC CTG HN2 randomized trial of an antimicrobial lozenge to prevent mucositis. *Head and Neck, 27,* 421–428. doi:10.1002/hed.20162

Eldridge, B., & Hamilton, K.H. (2004). *Management of nutrition impact symptoms in cancer and educational handouts* (2nd ed.). Chicago, IL: American Dietetic Association.

Elting, L.S., Shih, Y.-C.T., Stiff, P.J., Bensinger, W., Cantor, S.B., Cooksley, C., … Emmanoulides, C. (2007). Economic impact of palifermin on the costs of hospitalization for autologous hematopoietic stem-cell transplant: Analysis of phase 3 trial results. *Biology of Blood and Marrow Transplantation, 13,* 806–813. doi:10.1016/j.bbmt.2007.03.004

Halyard, M.Y. (2009). Taste and smell alterations in cancer patients—Real problems with few solutions. *Journal of Supportive Oncology, 7,* 68–69.

Halyard, M.Y., Jatoi, A., Sloan, J.A., Bearden, J.D., III, Vora, S.A., Atherton, P.J., … Loprinzi, C.L. (2007). Does zinc sulfate prevent therapy-induced taste alterations in head and neck cancer patients? Results of phase III double-blind, placebo-controlled trial from the North Central Cancer Treatment Group (N01C4). *International Journal of Radiation Oncology, Biology, Physics, 67,* 1318–1322. doi:10.1016/j.ijrobp.2006.10.046

Hatakka, K., Ahola, A.J., Yli-Knuuttila, H., Richardson, M., Poussa, T., Meurman, J.H., & Korpela, R. (2007). Probiotics reduce the prevalence of oral candida in the elderly—A randomized controlled trial. *Journal of Dental Research, 86,* 125–130. doi:10.1177/154405910700860204

Hayward, M.C., & Shea, A.M. (2009). Nutritional needs of patients with malignancies of the head and neck. *Seminars in Oncology Nursing, 25,* 203–211. doi:10.1016/j.soncn.2009.05.003

Hurst, J.D., & Gallagher, A.L. (2006). Energy, macronutrient, micronutrient, and fluid requirements. In L. Elliott, L.L. Molseed, & P.D. McCallum (Eds.), *The clinical guide to oncology nutrition* (2nd ed., pp. 54–71). Chicago, IL: American Dietetic Association.

Joint Commission. (2010). *CAMH: Comprehensive accreditation manual for hospitals: The official handbook.* Retrieved from http://e-dition.jcrinc.com/Frame.aspx

Kagan, S.H., & Sweeney-Cordes, E. (2005). Head and neck cancers. In V.J. Kogut & S.L. Luthringer (Eds.), *Nutritional issues in cancer care* (pp. 103–116). Pittsburgh, PA: Oncology Nursing Society.

Keefe, D.M., Rassias, G., O'Neil, L., & Gibson, R J. (2007). Severe mucositis: How can nutrition help? *Current Opinion in Clinical Nutrition and Metabolic Care, 10,* 627–631. doi:10.1097/MCO.0b013e3282bf90d6

Kisak, A.Z., & Klein, L.B. (2005). Lung cancer. In V J. Kogut & S.L. Luthringer (Eds.), *Nutritional issues in cancer care* (pp. 127–138). Pittsburgh, PA: Oncology Nursing Society.

Kogut, V.J., & Luthringer, S.L. (2005). Appendix D: Nutrition sequelae of radiation therapy and suggested nutritional interventions. In V.J. Kogut & S.L. Luthringer (Eds.), *Nutritional issues in cancer care* (pp. 350–351). Pittsburgh, PA: Oncology Nursing Society.

Lalla, R.V., Sonis, S.T., & Peterson, D.E. (2008). Management of oral mucositis in patients who have cancer. *Dental Clinics of North America, 52,* 61–77. doi:10.1016/j.cden.2007.10.002

Luthringer, S.L. (2006). Nutritional implications of radiation therapy. In L. Elliott, L.L. Molseed, & P.D. McCallum (Eds.), *The clinical guide to oncology nutrition* (2nd ed., pp. 88–93). Chicago, IL: American Dietetic Association.

Moynihan, P., & Petersen, P.E. (2004). Diet, nutrition and the prevention of dental diseases. *Public Health Nutrition, 7,* 201–226. doi:10.1079/PHN2003589

Murphy, B A., & Gilbert, J. (2009). Dysphagia in head and neck cancer patients treated with radiation: Assessment, sequelae, and rehabilitation. *Seminars in Radiation Oncology, 19,* 35–42. doi:10.1016/j.semradonc.2008.09.007

National Cancer Institute. (2010). Nutrition in cancer care (PDQ®) [Health professional version]. Retrieved from http://www.cancer.gov/cancertopics/pdq/supportivecare/nutrition/HealthProfessional

National Cancer Institute Cancer Therapy Evaluation Program. (2010, June 14). *Common terminology criteria for adverse events* [v.4.3]. Retrieved from http://evs.nci.nih.gov/ftp1/CTCAE/CTCAE_4.03_2010-06-14_QuickReference_8.5x11.pdf

National Dysphagia Diet Task Force & American Dietetic Association. (2002). *National dysphagia diet: Standardization for optimal care.* Chicago, IL: American Dietetic Association.

Petree, J.M. (2005). Supportive care: Support therapies and procedures. In J.K. Itano & K.N. Taoka (Eds.), *Core curriculum for oncology nursing* (4th ed., pp. 137–160). St. Louis, MO: Elsevier Saunders.

Raber-Durlacher, J.E., Barasch, A., Peterson, D.E., Lalla, R.V., Schubert, M.M., & Fibbe, W.E. (2004). Oral complications and management considerations in patients treated with high-dose chemotherapy. *Supportive Cancer Therapy, 1,* 219–229. doi:10.3816/SCT.2004.n.014

Ravasco, P. (2005). Aspects of taste and compliance in patients with cancer. *European Journal of Oncology Nursing, 9*(Suppl. 2), S84–S91. doi:10.1016/j.ejon.2005.09.003

Ripamonti, C., Zecca, E., Brunelli, C., Fulfaro, F., Villa, S., Balzarini, A., … De Conno, F. (1998). A randomized, controlled clinical trial to evaluate the effects of zinc sulfate on cancer patients with taste alterations caused by head and neck irradiation. *Cancer, 82,* 1938–1945. doi:10.1002/(SICI)1097-0142(19980515)82:10<1938::AID-CNCR18>3.0.CO;2-U

Robinson, C.A. (2006). Enteral nutrition in adult oncology. In L. Elliott, L.L. Molseed, & P.D. McCallum (Eds.), *The clinical guide to oncology nutrition* (2nd ed., pp. 138–155). Chicago, IL: American Dietetic Association.

Rosenthal, D.I., & Trotti, A. (2009). Strategies for managing radiation-induced mucositis in head and neck cancer. *Seminars in Radiation Oncology, 19,* 29–34. doi:10.1016/j.semradonc.2008.09.006

Shih, A., Miaskowski, C., Dodd, M.J., Stotts, N.A., & MacPhail, L. (2002). A research review of the current treatments for radiation-induced oral mucositis in patients with head and neck cancer. *Oncology Nursing Forum, 29,* 1063–1080. doi:10.1188/02.ONF.1063-1080

Silverman, S., Jr. (1999). Oral cancer: Complications of therapy. *Oral Surgery, Oral Medicine, Oral Pathology, Oral Radiology, and Endodontics, 88,* 122–126.

Worthington, H.V., Clarkson, J.E., & Eden, T.O.B. (2007). Interventions for preventing oral mucositis for patients with cancer receiving treatment. *Cochrane Database of Systematic Reviews* 2007, Issue 4. Art. No.: CD000978. doi:10.1002/14651858.CD000978.pub3

CHAPTER 6

Xerostomia and Cytoprotection

Carrie F. Daly, RN, MS, AOCN®

Introduction

Xerostomia is the medical term for the subjective complaint of dry mouth due to lack of saliva. Xerostomia is not a disease but rather a symptom of certain diseases, or the result of medications or cancer treatments including chemotherapy, radiation, and surgery. Cytoprotection is the use of a chemical (or chemicals) to minimize the damage to normal tissue in the oral cavity that can be caused specifically by radiation therapy. Chemotherapy and surgery, as well as specific diseases, may cause similar damage. Oral cavity tissue includes the salivary glands that produce saliva for the normal processes of eating and speaking and the natural protection of tooth enamel.

The purpose of this chapter is to define xerostomia and present current approved and investigational approaches used to protect cells in the mouth from the adverse effects of radiation therapy, chemotherapy, medications, and disease. The cytoprotectant amifostine (Ethyol®, MedImmune, LLC) and other methods of treating xerostomia, including salivary stimulants such as pilocarpine and the surgical transfer of submandibular salivary glands, will be discussed.

Xerostomia is a debilitating problem that primarily affects middle-age and older adults. Although not life-threatening, xerostomia can affect one's quality of life and can be a life-long problem. However, permanent xerostomia can compromise nutrition and speech and accelerate dental decay (Bhide, Miah, Harrington, Newbold, & Nutting, 2009; Eisbruch et al., 2001). The protective effect of saliva's remineralizing the enamel is no longer present with xerostomia, which can make the mucosa and periodontal tissue of the mouth more vulnerable to infections, as well.

The most common causes of xerostomia include medications, cancer treatments, Sjögren syndrome, dehydration, diabetes, and nerve damage from trauma to the head and neck region. All of these causes of xerostomia are the result of damage to the parotid glands. At least a hundred current medications cause extreme dry mouth. These medication groupings include antihypertensives, antidepressants, analgesics, tranquilizers, diuretics, and antihistamines. Chemotherapy medications can change the flow and the composition of saliva.

Radiation therapy is an effective treatment for patients with oral cancer, showing a high success rate in early-stage disease. However, permanent xerostomia is a common complication leading to dental caries and tooth loss one year after treatment. Xerostomia results from bilateral irradiation of the major salivary-producing glands, mainly the parotids, and the minor salivary glands, which significantly contribute to mucinous secretion (Jensen, Hansen, Jørgensen, & Bastholt, 1994). Advances in radiation therapy techniques, such as intensity-modulated radiation therapy (IMRT), have enabled increased delivery of therapeutic doses of radiation to tumors while limiting exposure to normal tissue, thereby reducing the incidence, duration, and severity of xerostomia in patients with oral cancers. However, xerostomia is a risk when treating the oral cavity. An effective treatment does not yet exist for this late complication once it has occurred, thereby reducing the patient's quality of life (Cerezo, Martín, López, Marín, & Gómez, 2009). Sjögren syndrome is an autoimmune disease that causes xerostomia and dry eyes. Other diseases that cause xerostomia include endocrine disorders (i.e., diabetes), stress, anxiety, depression, and nutritional deficiencies.

Because xerostomia can be a common problem with multiple causes for numerous people, an individual may present to various clinicians for treatment, such as a primary care physician, dentist, otolaryngologist, oral surgeon, speech or swallow therapist, radiation oncologist, or medical oncologist. Because of the aging population, the number of prescribed medications, and the number of patients going through cancer therapy, dentists and other clinicians can expect an increasing number of patients to present with xerostomia in the coming years. To treat xerostomia, the condition and the cause need to be identified. If it is medication induced, the medications can be reduced or discontinued if possible. Clinicians need to be aware of the groupings/classifications of medications that result in dry mouth. The current published evidence-based literature shows little correlation between patient symptoms and objective tests of salivary flow. Therefore, clinical management should be based on patient symptoms (Visvanathan & Nix, 2010).

A thorough intraoral and extraoral clinical examination is important for the diagnosis of xerostomia (Cassolato & Turnbull, 2003). Treatment involves finding any correctable causes and fixing them when possible. In many cases, it may not be possible to correct the xerostomia itself; therefore, the treatment focuses on reducing or relieving the symptoms, preventing cavities, and preventing infections. Palliative treatments would include a prescription for a salivary stimulant such as pilocarpine (Salagen® [Eisai Inc.] 5 mg four times a day); blended and moist foods that are easier to swallow; over-the-counter artificial saliva substitutes; sipping water throughout the day; alcohol-free oral products (i.e., Biotene® [Glaxo-SmithKline] mouth care products); and humidified air. For radiation-induced xerostomia, significant evidence exists supporting the use of a cytoprotective agent approved by the U.S. Food and Drug Administration (FDA) such as amifostine (Ethyol). Amifostine was created by the U.S. Army in Nuclear Warfare Project (WR-2721). Amifostine is a prodrug that is dephosphorylated by alkaline phosphate in tissues to a pharmacologically active free thiol metabolite. The active free metabolite is believed to be responsible for the reduction of the toxic effects of radiation on normal tissue (Wasserman et al., 2000).

Another possibility to reduce radiation-induced xerostomia is the surgical transfer of submandibular salivary glands. Researchers hypothesized that surgical transfer of a submandibular salivary gland to the submental space outside of the proposed radiation field, before starting radiation treatments, would prevent xerostomia (Al-Qahtani, Hier, Sultanum, & Black, 2006). They conducted a prospective clinical trial in which the surgical transfer was performed before chemoradiation therapy in eight patients. These patients were clinically followed with salivary flow studies, salivary gland scans, and the University of Washington quality-of-life questionnaire. All of the transferred salivary glands were positioned outside of the proposed radiation field, were partially shielded from radiation, and were functional. All of the patients completed their chemotherapy and radiation therapy. Four of the eight (50%) patients did not have xerostomia, three (37.5%) had only minor symptoms, and no surgical complications occurred. Therefore, surgical transfer of a submandibular salivary gland to the submental space (outside the radiation field) showed promise in preserving its function and minimizing the development of radiation-induced xerostomia, but this surgery has not been embraced by physicians and patients (Al-Qahtani et al., 2006).

Dentists need to be particularly involved with patients who experience dry mouth caused by medication, disease, surgery, or cancer-related therapies. Current evidence indicates that many patients who undergo radiation therapy do not receive adequate oral or dental care and are frequently lost in follow-up (Brosky, 2007). Additionally, patient compliance with oral care recommendations is frequently poor (Brosky, 2007). Because a marked increase in dental caries is a common occurrence in patients with xerostomia, it is important that the xerostomia be controlled. Patient appointments with a dentist must be scheduled to monitor dental caries. Infections of the mouth should be aggressively treated. Daily fluoride treatments are recommended, as well as frequent cleaning of the teeth by a dentist—every three months (Brosky, 2007). Careful observation of the color, texture, and location of dental caries is necessary to prevent loss of teeth. Good oral hygiene will reduce infections and patient discomfort.

Sjögren Syndrome of the Oral Cavity

Sjögren syndrome is one of the most frequently seen autoimmune diseases. It is a chronic and systemic disorder predominantly found in women and is characterized by the appearance of a lymphocytic inflammatory syndrome with dryness of the oral cavity and eyes secondary to involvement of the salivary and lacrimal glands (Margaix-Muñoz, Bagán, Poveda, Jiménez, & Sarrión, 2009). This syndrome is not clearly understood, but an autoimmune response is known to be triggered, with the accumulation of immune complexes in the gland acini that interfere with the gland's function. In the oral cavity, xerostomia is the most disabling manifestation for patients and is accompanied by rapidly progressing caries, candidiasis, and worsening oral health. Patients typically present with difficulties speaking, chewing, and swallowing; dry mouth sensation reported to be like a burning sensation; taste alterations such as a salty, bitter, or metallic taste; and pain in the salivary glands associated with eating and swallowing (Soto-Rojas & Kraus, 2002). A reduction in estrogen levels could explain the predominance of Sjögren syndrome in females and the development of the disease after menopause (Nakamura, Kawakami, & Eguchi, 2006).

A number of hypotheses have been proposed to account for dry mouth in Sjögren syndrome, such as destruction of the duct and acinar cells of the salivary glands, and neural degeneration or inhibition of nerve transmission. Because almost half of the gland acini remains intact in a large proportion of patients, a defect or alteration in nerve transmission could be a possible cause; however, the most decisive factor appears to be the progressive infiltration of mononuclear cells and the consolidation of autoimmune disease (Soto-Rojas & Kraus, 2002). Sjögren syndrome is the main cause of noniatrogenic xerostomia, whereas the iatrogenic presentation of dry mouth fundamentally corresponds to polymedication and radiation therapy targeted to the oral cavity and head and neck region. Bilateral parotid swelling is often seen as a result of ductal obstruction induced by the lymphocyte inflammatory infiltrate; swelling is usually recurrent.

The most serious complication of Sjögren syndrome is the appearance of parotid gland lymphomas. People with this syndrome have a 44-fold increased risk of developing non-Hodgkin lymphoma compared with the general population (Margaix-Muñoz et al., 2009). Unfortunately, no cure exists for Sjögren syndrome, and treatment is symptomatic and empirical and involves the use of saliva secretion stimulators and saliva substitutes.

In the oral cavity, saliva substitutes are based on solutions of carboxymethylcellulose, mucin, and polyacrylic acid, which offer limited and transient effects. Many commercial brands are available, such as Mouth Kote® (Parnell Pharmaceuticals, Inc.), and Biotene Oral Balance® (GlaxoSmithKline) and other Biotene products. Saliva substitutes have minimal acceptance among patients. The best known and most widely used saliva stimulant is the cholinergic agent pilocarpine (Salagen), which acts upon all the muscarinic receptors. Salagen is recommended at 5 mg orally four times daily. The adverse effects include confusion, rubor, perspiration, diarrhea, and increased micturition (Venables, 2006). If the patient shows no response to treatment after two to three months, the medication is stopped. Another more novel approach is cevimeline 30 mg orally three times daily, which has specific activity on M1 and M3 muscarinic receptors. Other treatments are targeted to the B cells of the glandular lymphocytic infiltrate. The use of agents against CD20 (a B lymphocyte surface antigen), such as rituximab, has been proposed because of the hyperreactivity that characterizes these cells. Rituximab deletes circulating B lymphocytes and is used safely in the treatment of non-Hodgkin lymphomas (Pijpe et al., 2005).

Dental treatment and prophylaxis aim to improve and prevent the consequences of chronic xerostomia and rampant dental caries in these patients. Topical fluoride rinses or gels can help a little. Patients need close professional dental monitoring. For control of the bacterial flora, daily 0.12% chlorhexidine rinses are recommended, as well as brushing and dental flossing after eating and at bedtime (Selwitz, Ismail, & Pitts, 2007).

Review of Oral Cancers

Patients with oral cavity cancers can be the most challenging to treat and care for in the oncology setting because of the acute and chronic effects that can occur from cancer treatments. Treatment of oral cancers is ideally a multidisciplinary approach involving the efforts of surgeons, radiation oncologists, medical oncologists, dentists, nutritionists, and rehabilitation and restorative specialists. Oral cancers are particularly dangerous because in their early stages they may not be noticed by the patient, as they can frequently grow without producing pain or symptoms that might be readily recognized. These tumors have a high risk of producing a second primary tumor (Schwartz et al., 1998). Several types of oral cancers exist, but around 90% are squamous cell carcinomas that line the aerodigestive tract (Schwartz et al., 1998). Other histologies include adenocarcinoma, lymphoepithelioma, adenoid cystic, mucoepidermoid spindle cell, verrucous, undifferentiated, and lymphoma tumors (American Cancer Society [ACS], 2010). Patients are also diagnosed with metastatic squamous cell cancer of the head and neck with unknown primary and present with positive lymph nodes of the neck with no evidence of organ-specific cancer. Those who smoke and drink alcohol have a 15-times greater risk of developing oral cancers than those who do not drink and smoke (ACS, 2010). Signs and symptoms of oral cancers include a sore or lesion in the mouth that does not heal within two weeks; a lump or thickening in the cheek; a white or red patch on the gums, tongue, tonsil, or lining of the mouth; a sore throat or a feeling that something is caught in the throat; difficulty moving the jaw or tongue; swelling of the jaw that causes dentures to fit poorly or become uncomfortable; and numbness of the tongue or the other areas of the mouth (ACS, 2010).

ACS estimated that more than 51,000 new cases of new head and neck cancer will be diagnosed in 2010. The majority of the cancers are expected to be of the oral cavity or pharyngeal cancers (36,540 cases). An estimated 7,880 deaths from oral cavity and pharynx cancers were expected in 2010 (ACS, 2010). The next common are laryngeal and hypopharynx cancers, and the least common are nasal cavity, paranasal sinus, and nasopharyngeal cancers. Squamous cell carcinoma continues to be the most common type of head and neck cancer. Men older than the age of 50 are at greatest risk, particularly men who use tobacco or consume excessive amounts of alcohol. Incidence rates continue to be twice as high in men as in women (ACS, 2010).

The oral symptoms experienced by patients with oral cancer correspond to the function of the area or tissue affected by the treatment or the cancer. It is known that treatment to the oral cavity affects swallowing, articulation, and taste. Treatment to the oropharynx affects swallowing, emesis, articulation, coughing, and yawning. Treatment to the nasal cavity affects olfactory humidification, temperature control, filtration, and smell, and treatment to the larynx affects speech and breathing. Treatment to the salivary glands affects the production of saliva. Negative outcomes associated with oral cancers include significant morbidity, increased mortality, and altered quality of life (Samuels, 2004).

Human papillomavirus (HPV)-associated squamous cell cancer of the head and neck occurs in 26% of all head and neck cancer (Gillison et al., 2009). HPV-16 is predominant viral isolate. Oropharyngeal, lingual, and palatine tonsil cancers occur in greater than 50% of HPV-related cancers in the United States. HPV-related head and neck cancers usually show a poorly differentiated basaloid pathology and occur in nonsmokers, nondrinkers, and younger patients. Patients with advanced forms of a cancer in the upper portion of their throat have a better outcome if their tumors are positive for HPV, according to the new data from a phase III clinical trial presented at the 2009 annual meeting of the American Society of Clinical Oncology (Gillison et al., 2009). Although other studies have suggested a link between HPV status and outcome in patients who have oropharyngeal cancer, these new data provide the most definitive evidence. Oropharyngeal cancers may now be divided into two groups: those linked to prolonged use of tobacco and alcohol and those linked to HPV. Determining HPV status may now be part of routine clinical care because of its prognostic implications in these patients (Gillison et al., 2009). The findings come from a correlative study in the Radiation Therapy Oncology Group (RTOG) 0129 clinical trial, a phase III trial in which patients with stage III or IV oropharyngeal cancer were randomly assigned to receive different regimens of radiation and chemotherapy (cisplatin). Tumor HPV status was evaluable for 73% (317/433) of oropharyngeal cases, and nearly two-thirds of the tumors tested were HPV positive. In this study, 88% of the HPV-positive patients were alive two years after treatment compared with 66% of the HPV-negative patients (Gillison et al., 2009). The absolute difference in survival increased over time. Because of the dramatic differences in treatment response, RTOG and the Eastern Cooperative Oncology Group will stratify all their clinical trials by HPV status. The clinical trials will be designed specifically for HPV-positive or HPV-negative patients.

Oral HPV infection seems to be the main risk factor for carcinogenesis of HPV-positive oropharyngeal cancer, and HPV-16 is found in the majority of cases of HPV-positive oral cancers (Kreimer, Clifford, Boyle, & Franceschi, 2005). For this reason, it might be possible to prevent or even treat these cancers by means of vaccines designed to elicit appropriate virus-specific immune responses. The impact of current HPV vaccines on the incidences of persistent oral HPV infection remains to be identified (Mannarini et al., 2009). All vaccine trials reported to date have been designed to investigate the ability of the vaccines to generate protection against the consequences of anogenital HPV infection in women. However, there is a reason to be optimistic that the existing vaccines may be protective against other HPV infections and therefore potentially effective in preventing vaccine-type HPV-associated head and neck cancer in both men and women (Mannarini et al., 2009).

Treatment for Oral Cancers

Radiation therapy, surgery, chemotherapy, and targeted therapy can be used alone or in combination for the treatment of oral cavity cancers. Radiation therapy and surgery separately or in combination are common treatments. In advanced disease, chemotherapy is added to surgery and/or radiation. Targeted therapy with cetuximab may be combined with radiation in initial treatment or used alone to treat recurrent cancer.

Radiation therapy is the local treatment that is site specific, which leads to significant damage to normal tissue when it is exposed in the treatment field (Köstler, Hejna, Wenzel, & Zielinski, 2001). Adverse effects of radiation therapy to the oral cavity region include xerostomia, mucositis, esophagitis, candidiasis, skin reactions, and osteoradionecrosis. These adverse effects from radiation to the oral cavity region can lead to significant weight loss, taste alterations, pain, dental complications, extreme fatigue, and dehydration, which can lead to treatment interruptions, dose reduction, discontinuation of treatments, hospitalizations, and ultimately poor outcomes (Vissink, Jansma, Spijkervet, Burlage, & Coppes, 2003; Wendt et al., 1998). An increasing body of evidence suggests that chemotherapy combined with radiation yields a survival advantage over radiation alone, but with increased toxicities (Calais et al., 1999; Rosenthal & Trotti, 2009; Wendt et al., 1998). Both radiation therapy and chemotherapy can lead to both acute and chronic toxicities.

With the use of the targeted therapy such as cetuximab, patients with head and neck cancer receiving radiation may experience increased skin reaction toxicities in the treatment field. Cetuximab is a monoclonal antibody that blocks the epidermal growth factor receptor and is a potentially less toxic targeted therapy. Early studies suggest that treatment with cetuximab might boost the effectiveness of radiation therapy in patients with advanced cancer (Koukourakis et al., 2010). Patients treated with cetuximab develop a temporary acneform skin reaction (rash) on the face and body that usually disappears after treatment. The presence and intensity of the rash have been associated with better survival in several cancers (Koukourakis et al., 2010).

Acute complications are defined as early adverse effects that occur within the first two weeks of radiation therapy and persist for some weeks or months after the completion of treatment. The effects of external radiation therapy are cumulative, and patients may not begin to experience any significant adverse effects until a specific threshold dose for normal tissue damage is reached during radiation therapy. These adverse effects include changes to the skin and soft tissue, mucosal changes, alterations in taste, and alterations in quality, quantity, and consistency of saliva.

The feeling of oral dryness and saliva-related complaints were reported in a study of patients with breast cancer who received cyclophosphamide, epirubicin, methotrexate, and 5-fluorouracil (Jensen, Mouridsen, Reibel, Brünner, & Nauntofte, 2008). Findings suggested that chemotherapy acutely affected salivary gland function when compared to a control group of patients with breast cancer who did not receive chemotherapy (Jensen et al., 2008). Flow rates and composition of unstimulated and stimulated whole saliva, as well as stimulated parotid saliva, were measured. Xerostomia scores were elevated during chemotherapy and stayed elevated for up to one year after completion of chemotherapy (Jensen et al., 2008).

Late complications of radiation therapy are those that occur months to years after the completion of therapy and tend to be chronic in nature. Some late complications can be the result of persistence or progression of some of the acute complications of radiation. These chronic effects include prolonged xerostomia, dental caries, skin and soft tissue fibrosis, and damage to bone, teeth, and tongue mobility, which all affect eating, oral hygiene, and articulation.

Davies, Broadley, and Beighton (2001) investigated features of xerostomia in 120 patients with advanced cancer. The protocol involved completion of the Memorial Symptom Assessment Scale and measurement of the unstimulated and stimulated whole salivary flow rates. Xerostomia was the fourth most common symptom (78%) of the patients, and there was an association with poor performance status (p = 0.01) (Eisbruch et al., 2003; Epstein et al., 1999). The usual cause of xerostomia was drug treatment, and the median number of xerostomia-producing drugs prescribed was four. Study participants ranked xerostomia as the third most distressing chronic symptom, which was correlated with oral discomfort, dysphagia, dysphoria, and anorexia (Eisbruch et al., 2003; Epstein et al., 1999).

Advances in Radiation Therapy

The extent of the damage caused by radiation therapy to the oral cavity region depends on both the volume of the tissue being irradiated and on the dose of radiation delivered. Prevention of radiation-induced xerostomia is a goal. In the mid-1990s, IMRT became available, which facilitated a higher degree of dose conformality and offered opportunities for additional clinical gains. Preserving salivary gland function while maintaining locoregional control is essential. IMRT involves the use of radiation fields for which intensity varies across the field depending on the thickness of the target and the existence of critical organs or critical noninvolved tissue in its path. Treating the targets with multiple beams of varying intensity allows a relatively uniform dose in an irregularly shaped target while avoiding delivering a high dose to the surrounding structures. Techniques in clinical practice have made it possible to spare a portion of the parotid gland by the implementation of three-dimensional (3-D) conformal radiation therapy and IMRT. A high dose is administered to a small part of the parotid gland and is positioned close to the tumor, while the rest of the gland receives a low dose or no dose. This parotid-sparing protocol prevents permanent xerostomia (Dirix, Nuyts, & Van den Bogaert, 2006).

The ability of 3-D conformal radiation therapy and IMRT to produce dose distributions that allow preservation of parotid gland tissue and reduction of xerostomia has been demonstrated abundantly. Evidence has also shown that reduction of xerostomia results in improved quality of life (Lin et al., 2003). A mean gland dose of less than or equal to 28 Gy was initially proposed as a planning objective for substantial sparing of parotid gland function by Eisbruch, Ten Haken, Kim, Marsh, and Ship (1999). Researchers from Washington University reported very similar results, finding that a mean parotid dose of greater than or equal to 25.8 Gy was likely to reduce salivary flow to 25% of its pretreatment value (Blanco et al., 2005). Gradually, consensus was formed that using a mean parotid dose of less than 26 Gy to 30 Gy can achieve a significant reduction of xerostomia.

Image-guided radiotherapy provides the opportunity for better precision of patient setup and for tracking tumor regression and anatomic changes in noninvolved tissue during the course of radiation. This relates to patient and tumor imaging using electronic portal imaging devices or computed tomography before each fraction or every few fractions of therapy to ensure tracking of the tumor by the treatment beams. Tracking these anatomic changes may facilitate future replanning during the course of radiation therapy to address them and reduce tissue toxicities (Eisbruch, Foote, O'Sullivan, Beitler, & Vikram, 2002; Eisbruch et al., 1999). In cancer of the oral cavity or head and neck region, where breathing-related motion is nonconsequential, image-guided radiotherapy has two main goals: minimizing setup uncertainties and enabling the specific tumor margins, and assessing anatomic changes in the tumor and critical tissue during the course of radiation therapy (Eisbruch, 2009; Eisbruch et al., 1999, 2002).

The anatomy of the neck and oral cavity is very complex with many critical and radiation-sensitive organs in close proximity to the targets. Doses are tight around the target, which limits the dose to noninvolved tissues. IMRT is used for this reason—to spare or limit the radiation dose or toxicity to noninvolved tissue. Noninvolved tissue sparing may offer tangible gains for the major salivary glands, the minor salivary glands dispersed within the oral cavity, the mandible, and the pharyngeal musculature (Eisbruch et al., 2002; Kam et al., 2007). The inner and middle ears, temporomandibular joints, temporal brain lobes, and optic pathways can be partly spared with IMRT to the nasopharyngeal and paranasal sinus cavity. Growing evidence in the literature supports that patients with early-stage oropharyngeal and oral cavity cancers have a low incidence of contralateral node involvement; hence, radiation therapy can be limited to the ipsilateral neck without compromising locoregional control (Eisbruch, 2009; Eisbruch et al., 2002; Kam et al., 2007). However, bilateral neck irradiation continues to be the standard approach for most patients, especially those with ipsilateral clinical node-positive presentation. One argument for the continued bilateral approach is that morbidity is low using IMRT because parotid sparing can be easily achieved with this technique, but mucositis may be greater (Samuels, 2004). However, IMRT may not be universally available.

IMRT eliminates the need for posterior neck electron fields commonly used in conventional radiation therapy and their associated deficiencies. When using IMRT in patients with oral cancer, multiple factors need to be taken into account, such as patient setup uncertainties, swallowing-related organ movements, and changes in target and organ positions related to tumor shrinkage and patient weight loss during radiation treatment. IMRT is work intensive and lengthens treatment time.

Patients who would benefit the most from IMRT are those with oropharyngeal sinus cancer where the targets are near the optic pathway; patients with pharyngeal or nasopharyngeal cancer in whom standard radiation therapy would encompass the majority of the salivary glands; and patients in whom standard radiation therapy techniques would require a compromise in the tumor doses because of the proximity of the tumor to the spinal cord or brain stem (Eisbruch et al., 2002). IMRT may not be of benefit to all patients, such as those with laryngeal cancer and clinically noninvolved neck cancers. The main advantage to IMRT is that it spares normal structures, such as the parotid gland or larynx, while still delivering a sufficient dose of radiation to areas of gross or clinical disease.

The only pitfall or concern with IMRT is that by increasing the precision of the radiation, some clinical treatment areas at risk could be excluded (Eisbruch et al., 1999). When treating mucosal sites, care must be taken to include all mucosal surfaces of anatomic areas included in the clinical treatment volume so as not to underdose and undertreat potential target areas.

Most studies assessing clinical reduction of the salivary glands in the treatment field using IMRT have concentrated on reduced xerostomia through the sparing of the parotid salivary glands (Kam et al., 2007; Lin et al., 2003). The large majority of the glands receiving a mean dose of greater than 26 Gy did not produce measurable saliva and did not recover, whereas glands receiving lower mean doses produced variable salivary output that increased over time (Chambers et al., 2005). One year after radiotherapy, parotid glands receiving a moderate dose (mean dose of 17–26 Gy) recovered, on average, to the pretreatment salivary production levels. The common finding in all the data is that a relationship seems to exist between the mean doses to the glands and their residual salivary output. These findings motivate reducing the dose to the salivary glands to the lowest levels possible.

Regardless of the dose threshold, it is now apparent that spared glands not only partially retain the salivary output but also that the output increased over time through at least two years after radiotherapy. This is compared with generally no improvement over time following standard radiotherapy, in which most of the parotid glands received full radiotherapy doses. Once preservation of the salivary output is achieved, there is improvement in patients' reported xerostomia symptoms.

The correlation between the salivary output from the major salivary glands and xerostomia symptoms is significant but not very high. The problem is that the minor salivary glands are scattered throughout the oral cavity, notably on the surface of the palate, and produce much of the saliva (salivary mucin). It has been found that the dose delivered to the oral cavity affects both the major and the minor salivary glands (Chao et al., 2001; Eisbruch et al., 2003).

An optimal practice is to add the sparing of the oral cavity as an objective in radiotherapy, in addition to the sparing of the parotid glands. Researchers at the University of Michigan validated a patient-reported xerostomia questionnaire, which demonstrated that xerostomia improved significantly over time in tandem with the increase in saliva production (Kam et al., 2007). Two years following radiation therapy, xerostomia reported by patients receiving parotid-sparing bilateral neck radiation was only slightly worse than in patients receiving unilateral neck radiotherapy. Kam et al. (2007) showed the advantage of IMRT in terms of improvement of the salivary flow rates, but not in xerostomia symptoms. Other studies demonstrated significant improvement of both salivary flow rates and xerostomia-related quality of life in patients with nasopharyngeal cancer randomized to IMRT compared with those randomized to conventional radiation therapy (Hassan & Weymuller, 1993; Lin et al., 2003). It is apparent that partial sparing of the salivary glands, made possible by IMRT, achieves gains in both the retention of saliva production and the symptoms of xerostomia. Additional potential functional gains from IMRT compared with conventional radiation include reduced long-term dysphagia and aspiration, suggesting that sparing pharyngeal constrictors, the glottis, and the supraglottic larynx may be of benefit.

Compared with conventional radiation, IMRT caused less grade 2 and 3 xerostomia, but even with IMRT, about 30% of patients suffer permanent significant dry mouth symptoms (Samuels, 2004; Thorstad, Chao, & Haughey, 2004;

Vissink et al., 2003). In addition, grade 2–4 mucositis was more common with IMRT than with conventional radiation because IMRT brings beams in from many directions and exposes more of the oral mucosa to a significant radiation dose (Samuels, 2004).

Cytoprotection

A major dose-limiting effect of radiation therapy and chemotherapy is damage to normal tissue, thereby compromising the efficiency of treatment. Protection of normal tissues against adverse effects from radiation therapy and chemotherapy may permit dose escalation, increased patient survival, and better quality of life for patients requiring cancer treatments (Samuels, 2004; Wasserman et al., 2000). Cytoprotection, also referred as radioprotection, is defined as chemical modifiers designed to minimize normal tissue damage resulting from radiation therapy without compromising local tumor control (Capizzi, 1999; Kemp et al., 1996). The goals of cytoprotection are to reduce early and late toxicities of treatment, thereby improving a patient's quality of life. Also, the use of cytoprotection can enhance the antineoplastic activity of radiation and chemotherapy and avoid unnecessary delays in radiation therapy treatments. Therefore, cytoprotective agents need to be considered even with the advantages of IMRT; consideration should be given to combining amifostine and IMRT in an attempt to decrease the acute and chronic toxicity of radiation therapy (Thorstad et al., 2004). With conventional radiation, xerostomia causing hyposalivation, which may be reversible, has been seen with doses of 30–50 Gy, while higher doses generally produce irreversible destruction of the salivary gland and permanent dryness (Anand et al., 2008; Carr, 2005; Vissink et al., 2003). Radioprotective agents or cytoprotective agents being investigated include intratumor injection of manganese superoxide dismutase plasmid, liposome (SOD2-PL), transforming growth factor-beta, keratinocyte growth factor, glutamine interleukin-15, melatonin, and omega-3 fatty acids (Jatoi & Thomas, 2002). It is difficult to find information on clinical data for any of these therapies in use as a radioprotective agent at this time.

The only FDA-approved agent for cytoprotection used in patients undergoing radiation therapy is amifostine. Amifostine is FDA-approved as a radioprotector to reduce the incidence of moderate to severe xerostomia in patients undergoing postoperative radiation for head and neck cancer where the radiation field includes the parotid gland (Capizzi, 1999; Kouvaris, Kouloulias, & Vlahos, 2007). Based on extensive data, additions were made to the compendia listing of amifostine for the off-label use of amifostine for mucosal protection in radiation therapy or radiation therapy combined with chemotherapy according to the U.S. Pharmacopeia drug information database June 2002 update (U.S. Pharmacopeia, 2002).

Amifostine is a supportive therapy used to reduce adverse effects, both acute and chronic, from radiation and chemotherapy. Amifostine is a prodrug that is dephosphorylated by alkaline phosphatase in tissues to pharmacologically active free thiol metabolite. The active free metabolite is believed to be responsible for the reduction of the toxic effects of radiation on normal tissue (Capizzi, 1999). The free thiol metabolite is much more readily absorbed by normal tissue. The higher concentrations of free thiol protect normal tissue such as bone marrow, the kidneys, and the heart (Calais et al., 1999; MedImmune, LLC, 2009).

The use of amifostine has not been embraced as fully as other strategies to reduce the toxic effects of radiation and chemotherapy. Many radiation oncologists remain hesitant to adopt cytoprotective therapies because of their limited use of and experience with injectable medications, and lack of appreciation of symptom burden (i.e., nausea/vomiting, hypotension, rash) (Rosenthal & Trotti, 2009; Samuels, 2004). Also, many radiation and medical oncologists have questions about the risk-benefit profiles of cytoprotective agents, including the potential for tumor protection and the belief that IMRT eliminates the need for cytoprotectant agents (Rosenthal, 2006; Samuels, 2004). Published trials and guidelines from the American Society of Clinical Oncology for the use of protectants for chemotherapy and radiotherapy note that there is no evidence that amifostine leads to tumor protection (Hensley et al., 1999).

In a phase III randomized trial with amifostine as a radioprotector in squamous cell cancer of the head and neck, amifostine reduced acute and chronic xerostomia while preserving antitumor efficacy and reducing the overall evidence of grade 2 or higher xerostomia from 78% to 51% (p < 0.0001) (Brizel et al., 2000). The median time to onset of grade 2 or higher acute xerostomia was longer in the amifostine and radiation group at 45 days compared to the control group at 30 days (p = 0.0001). Patients in the amifostine group were able to tolerate a higher dose of radiation at 60 Gy compared to the radiation-alone group at 42 Gy. The radiation dose necessary to cause grade 2 or higher acute xerostomia was 40% higher in the amifostine and radiation group. In an 18–24-month follow-up, it was confirmed that amifostine did not compromise antitumor efficacy of radiation therapy (Brizel et al., 2000). An eight-item, validated Patient Benefit Questionnaire (PBQ) was done during and up to 11 months after completion of radiation therapy to measure the clinical benefit of amifostine. Amifostine-treated patients reported better PBQ scores at week 4 of radiation. This was indicative of improved oral toxicity-related outcomes and improved clinical benefits (Wasserman et al., 2000).

Antonadou, Pepelassi, Synodinou, Puglisi, and Throuvalas (2000) administered amifostine 300 mg/m^2 IV push to patients with head and neck cancer 15 minutes before daily radiation therapy. These patients were also receiving weekly carboplatin. It was found that acute mucositis was almost nonexistent in the amifostine group versus the control group. Similarly, late-phase toxicity of xerostomia was similarly diminished in the amifostine group in the three-month follow-up: only 27% of the amifostine group had grade 2 xerostomia, compared to 74% in the control group (Antonadou et al., 2002).

Dosing and Administration of Amifostine for Radioprotection

The recommended dose of amifostine to protect against xerostomia from radiation therapy to the head and neck area is 200 mg/m^2 once daily administered IV push 15–30 minutes before radiation (Boccia, 2002). However, IV push amifostine given in a rapid one-minute push has demonstrated reduction in hypertension and nausea and vomiting and improved the tolerability of the drug (Boccia, 2002).

The subcutaneous (SC) injection of amifostine is not FDA-approved but has shown some advantage and comfort in giving the drug SC versus IV (Anné & Curran, 2002; Bardet et al., 2002; Koukourakis et al., 2000). Less nausea and vomiting and hypotension was discovered when the medication was given SC versus IV. When giving the medication subcutaneously, there is a reduction in time and staff required to administer amifostine. Koukourakis et al. (2000) tested the feasibility of amifostine administered by SC injection in patients undergoing radiation therapy for head and neck and other tumors. Patients were given a 500 mg dose diluted in 2.5 ml of normal saline administered SC 20 minutes before radiation therapy daily. The results demonstrated that amifostine administered SC was well tolerated, and patients experienced less nausea and vomiting and less hypotension than with IV administration (Koukourakis et al., 2000). SC amifostine at 500 mg in 2.5 ml of normal saline is a convenient dosing option in trials of patients with head and neck cancer receiving radiation with and without chemotherapy (Koukourakis et al., 2000). SC administration of amifostine may lessen the risk of adverse events compared to IV administration, but it does not eliminate the need for hydration and recommended antiemetics. Proper techniques for SC injections are recommended, and site rotation is necessary.

Adverse Effects of Amifostine

Common adverse effects are associated with both IV and SC amifostine in patients with oral cavity cancer receiving radiation therapy with or without chemotherapy to reduce acute and chronic xerostomia and possibly mucositis. These adverse effects include nausea and vomiting, transient hypotension, local injection-site reaction, and generalized rash. Other reported adverse effects include hypocalcemia, sneezing, fatigue, dizziness, flushing, hiccups, fever, and chills. Fevers can be a precursor to a systemic rash. Although rare, allergic reactions can also occur with amifostine. Some have speculated that sulfa allergies may possibly be correlated with allergic reaction to amifostine. An increase of adverse effects has occurred when amifostine is used as a chemoprotectant IV at 740 mg/m^2 or 910 mg/m^2 (as done per package insert) compared to the radioprotector dose of 200 mg/m^2 or 500 mg flat dose given IV or SC (Boccia, 2002; MedImmune, LLC, 2009).

Increased nausea and vomiting may result when the patient is also receiving chemotherapy with radiation therapy, leading to uncertainty as to the cause of the nausea and vomiting. Amifostine is typically not given when patients are receiving targeted therapy such as cetuximab because of the acute skin reaction (rash) that patients develop when receiving targeted therapy (Koukourakis et al., 2010). It would be hard to distinguish the cause of a cetuximab skin reaction or generalized rash with amifostine.

Hydration is key for patients tolerating this medication. To minimize hypotension, the patient receiving amifostine should be well hydrated before amifostine administration. Patients are encouraged to drink two to three 8 oz glasses of water or sports drink before receiving amifostine. If the patient has a gastrostomy or percutaneous endoscopic gastrostomy tube, extra water or other liquids can be added through the tube. Before administering amifostine, a baseline blood pressure should be performed daily and every 5–15 minutes or until stable or as clinically indicated (Daly, Holloway, & Ameen, 2003). Amifostine should be held if the patient becomes dehydrated or hypotensive. Symptoms of dehydration are dizziness, light-headedness, hypotension, tachycardia, and concentrated urine. Lowered blood pressure during amifostine administration is usually transient and easily reversible with IV or oral fluids.

Amifostine has the potential to be an emetogenic medication, with the incidence being at 53% in patients receiving amifostine (MedImmune, LLC, 2009). Risk factors for nausea and vomiting include highly emetogenic chemotherapy; emesis with previous chemotherapy and/or amifostine; younger patients; poorly hydrated patients; women prone to nausea and vomiting during pregnancy; and patients with a history of motion sickness (Daly et al., 2003). To minimize nausea and vomiting, antiemetic medication should be administered 90–120 minutes before daily amifostine. Common oral antiemetics are prochlorperazine 10 mg, ondansetron 8 mg, and lorazepam 1 mg. Prochlorperazine 10 mg orally is tried first for the low-risk patients. High-risk patients may need a 5-HT$_3$ antagonist (such as ondansetron). Other effective medications used to reduce nausea and vomiting are dexamethasone and metoclopramide. These medications can be used alone or in combination.

Pilocarpine

Pilocarpine is an FDA-approved drug for relieving radiation-induced xerostomia. Pilocarpine stimulates the activity of the salivary glands and allows patients to get symptomatic relief when radiation has caused damage to the parotid glands. To have an effect, pilocarpine therapy requires that some functioning parotid acinar tissue remain. On a theoretical basis, one would expect that pilocarpine therapy would be most effective clinically in patients who have benefited from some degree of salivary tissue protection from physical techniques, such as IMRT, and from cytoprotection, such as amifostine. In a double-blind randomized placebo-controlled study, pilocarpine 5 mg orally four times daily given during radiotherapy for protection against radiation-induced xerostomia was investigated (Burlage et al., 2008). Overall, no statistically significant differences were noted between the pilocarpine group and the placebo group. However, the study results suggest that the beneficial effect of pilocarpine depends on the radiation dose distribution in the parotid glands, indicating that when the mean parotid dose exceeds 40 Gy, pilocarpine significantly spares parotid flow and reduces patient-rated xerostomia, particularly after 12 months (Burlage et al., 2008). Pilocarpine can be given to patients in whom even advanced radiation techniques fail to sufficiently spare the parotid gland, and it should be considered for patients treated at institutions in which advanced techniques (IMRT) for radiation delivery are not available. Pilocarpine is used more to stimulate salivary production than to protect the salivary glands.

Quality of Life

Quality-of-life considerations are important in deciding treatment modalities in patients with oral cancer. The acute and chronic effects of treatment can be devastating to patients. *Quality of life* is defined as the value a person places on health status and function. Social isolation may occur as a result of physical appearance or inability to speak, interact, taste, or eat normally (Hassan & Weymuller, 1993; List, Ritter-Sterr, & Lansky, 1990). Also, tooth decay can occur after radiation therapy to the head and neck area because of lack of saliva, which will affect one's quality of life and body image.

Quality-of-life research has matured with the development of assessment tools that have been validated in research studies. The University of Washington Quality of Life Scale is perhaps the most commonly used quality-of-life assessment tool (Rogers, Lowe, Brown, & Vaughan, 1999). This tool is a questionnaire covering quality-of-life issues that patients with oral cavity cancer experience during cancer therapies. These issues include pain, appearance, activity, recreation, swallowing, chewing, speech, shoulder problems, taste, saliva, mood, and anxiety. Another common assessment tool is the Functional Assessment of Cancer Therapy–Head and Neck scale. Other factors that affect quality of life in these patients that need to be considered are age, sex, tumor site, tumor size, stage of disease, marital status, and income (List et al., 1990).

Conclusion

Nurses need to understand what xerostomia is and how devastating it can be as an acute and chronic problem for patients who are polymedicated, have underlying diseases that cause xerostomia such as Sjögren syndrome, or are receiving cancer therapies. Nurses have a significant impact on patient outcomes through diligent assessment and ongoing education regarding symptom management. A definite need exists for research on the management of xerostomia and quality-of-life issues for all of these groups of patients. A multidisciplinary team is essential in providing the best practices for patients experiencing xerostomia, which would include a nurse; a primary care physician; a dentist; an oral surgeon or ear, nose, and throat physician; a speech and swallow therapist; a medical oncologist; and a radiation oncologist.

It is important for oncology nurses to understand the complications—both acute and chronic—of radiation therapy and chemotherapy for patients with oral cancer. Xerostomia can significantly negatively affect one's quality of life, which includes problems in eating, swallowing, chewing, speaking, and sleeping; acceleration of dental caries and loss of teeth; and other factors. Proper patient management and assessment are critical and significant to improve and reduce acute and chronic complications from radiation therapy. This can be accomplished by using IMRT to spare the parotid glands, cytoprotection such as amifostine to protect the parotid glands, artificial saliva, close monitoring of oral hygiene and dental care, and follow-up. Both IMRT and cytoprotection can reduce treatment-related toxicities, both acute and chronic problems of the oral cavity; decrease treatment breaks; and possibly improve quality of life and overall survival. Certainly more evidence-based practices are necessary to improve on the practices that are already being implemented to reduce xerostomia, both acute and long term.

References

Al-Qahtani, K., Hier, M.P., Sultanum, K., & Black, M.J. (2006). The role of submandibular salivary gland transfer in preventing xerostomia in the chemoradiotherapy patient. *Oral Surgery, Oral Medicine, Oral Pathology, Oral Radiology, and Endodontics, 101,* 753–756. doi:10.1016/j.tripleo.2005.12.017

American Cancer Society. (2010). *Cancer facts and figures, 2010.* Atlanta, GA: Author.

Anand, A.K, Chaudhoory, A.R, Shukla, A., Negi, P.S, Sinha, S.N, Babu, A.A., … Vaid, A.K. (2008). Favourable impact of intensity-modulated radiation therapy on chronic dysphagia in patients with head and neck cancer. *British Journal of Radiology, 81,* 865–871. doi:10.1259/bjr/31334499

Anné, P.R., & Curran, W.J., Jr. (2002). A phase II trial of subcutaneous amifostine and radiation therapy in patients with head and neck cancer. *Seminars in Radiation Oncology, 12*(1, Suppl. 1), 18–19.

Antonadou, D., Pepelassi, M., Synodinou, M., Puglisi, M., & Throuvalas, N. (2002). Prophylactic use of amifostine to prevent radiochemotherapy-induced mucositis and xerostomia in head-and-neck cancer. *International Journal of Radiation Oncology, Biology, Physics, 52,* 739–747.

Bardet, E., Martin, L., Calais, G., Tuchais, C., Bourhis, J., Rhein, B., … Alphonsi, M. (2002). Preliminary data of the GORTEC 2000-02 phase III trial comparing intravenous and subcutaneous administration of amifostine for head and neck tumors treated by external radiotherapy. *Seminars in Oncology, 29*(6, Suppl. 19), 57–60. doi:10.1053/sonc.2002.37348

Bhide, S.A., Miah, A.B., Harrington, K.J., Newbold, K.L., & Nutting, C.M. (2009). Radiation-induced xerostomia: Pathophysiology, prevention and treatment. *Clinical Oncology, 21,* 737–744. doi:10.1016/j.clon.2009.09.002

Blanco, A.I., Chao, K.S., El Naqa, I., Franklin, G.E., Zakarian, K., Vicic, M., & Deasy, J.O. (2005). Dose-volume modeling of salivary function in patients with head-and-neck cancer receiving radiotherapy. *International Journal of Radiation Oncology, Biology, Physics, 62*, 1055–1069. doi:10.1016/j.ijrobp.2004.12.076

Boccia, R.V. (2002). Improved tolerability of amifostine with rapid infusion and optimal patient preparation. *Seminars in Oncology, 29*(6, Suppl. 19), 9–13. doi:10.1053/sonc.2002.37358

Brizel, D.M., Wasserman, T.H., Henke, M., Strnad, V., Rudat, V., Monnier, A., ... Sauer, R. (2000). Phase III randomized trial of amifostine as a radioprotector in head and neck cancer. *Journal of Clinical Oncology, 18*, 3339–3345.

Brosky, M.E. (2007). The role of saliva in oral health: Strategies for prevention and management of xerostomia. *Journal of Supportive Oncology, 5*, 215–225.

Burlage, F.R., Roesink, J.M., Kampinga, H.H., Coppes, R.P., Terhaard, C., Langendijk, J.A., ... Vissink, A. (2008). Protection of salivary function by concomitant pilocarpine during radiotherapy: A double-blind, randomized, placebo-controlled study. *International Journal of Radiation Oncology, Biology, Physics, 70*, 14–2. doi:10.1016/j.ijrobp.2007.06.016

Calais, G., Alfonsi, M., Bardet, E., Sire, C., Germain, T., Bergerot, P., ... Bertrand, P. (1999). Randomized trial of radiation therapy versus concomitant chemotherapy and radiation therapy for advanced-stage oropharynx carcinoma. *Journal of the National Cancer Institute, 91*, 2081–2086. doi:10.1093/jnci/91.24.2081

Capizzi, R.L. (1999). The preclinical basis for broad-spectrum selective cytoprotection of normal tissues from cytotoxic therapies by amifostine. *Seminars in Oncology, 26*(2, Suppl. 7), 3–21.

Carr, E. (2005). Head and neck malignancies. In C.H. Yarbro, M.H. Frogge, & M. Goodman (Eds.), *Cancer nursing: Principles and practice* (6th ed., pp. 1295–1324). Sudbury, MA: Jones and Bartlett.

Cassolato, S.F., & Turnbull, R.S. (2003). Xerostomia: Clinical aspects and treatment. *Gerodontology, 20*, 64–77. doi:10.1111/j.1741-2358.2003.00064.x

Cerezo, L., Martín, M., López, M., Marín, A., & Gómez, A. (2009). Ipsilateral irradiation for well lateralized carcinomas of the oral cavity and oropharynx: Results on tumor control and xerostomia. *Radiation Oncology, 4*, 33. doi:10.1186/1748-717X-4-33

Chambers, M.S., Garden, A.S., Rosenthal, D., Ahamad, A., Schwartz, D.L., Blanco, A.I., ... Weber, R.S. (2005). Intensity-modulated radiotherapy: Is xerostomia still prevalent? *Current Oncology Reports, 7*, 131–136.

Chao, K.S., Deasy, J.O., Markman, J., Haynie, J., Perez, C.A., Purdy, J.A., & Low, D.A. (2001). A prospective study of salivary function sparing in patients with head-and-neck cancers receiving intensity-modulated or three-dimensional radiation therapy: Initial results. *International Journal of Radiation Oncology, Biology, Physics, 49*, 907–916. doi:10.1016/S0360-3016(00)01441-3

Daly, C., Holloway, N., & Ameen, D. (2003). Subcutaneous administration of amifostine during radiotherapy: A clinical perspective. *Proceedings of the American Society of Clinical Oncology, 22*, Abstract No. 3154.

Davies, A.N., Broadley, K., & Beighton, D. (2001). Xerostomia in patients with advanced cancer. *Journal of Pain and Symptom Management, 22*, 820–825. doi:10.1016/S0885-3924(01)00318-9

Dirix, P., Nuyts, S., & Van den Bogaert, W. (2006). Radiation-induced xerostomia in patients with head and neck cancer: A literature review. *Cancer, 107*, 2525–2534. doi:10.1002/cncr.22302

Eisbruch, A. (2009). Novel radiation therapy techniques in the management of head and neck cancer. In L.B. Harrison, R.B. Sessions, & W.K. Hong (Eds.), *Head and neck cancer: A multidisciplinary approach* (3rd ed., pp. 98–112). Philadelphia, PA: Lippincott Williams & Wilkins.

Eisbruch, A., Foote, R.L., O'Sullivan, B., Beitler, J.J., & Vikram, B. (2002). Intensity-modulated radiation therapy for head and neck cancer: Emphasis on the selection and delineation of the targets. *Seminars in Radiation Oncology, 12*, 238–249. doi:10.1053/srao.2002.32435

Eisbruch, A., Kim, H.M., Terrell, J.E., Marsh, L.H., Dawson, L.A., & Ship, J.A. (2001). Xero-stomia and its predictors following parotid-sparing irradiation of head and neck cancer. *International Journal of Radiation Oncology, Biology, Physics, 50,* 695–704. doi:10.1016/S0360-3016(01)01512-7

Eisbruch, A., Rhodus, N., Rosenthal, D., Murphy, B., Rusch, C., Sonis, S., … Brizel, D. (2003). The prevention and treatment of radiotherapy-induced xerostomia. *Seminars in Radiation Oncology, 13,* 302–308. doi:10.1016/S1053-4296(03)00027-4

Eisbruch, A., Ten Haken, R.K., Kim, H.M., Marsh, L.H., & Ship, J.A. (1999). Dose, volume, and function relationships in parotid salivary glands following conformal and intensity-modulated irradiation of head and neck cancer. *International Journal of Radiation Oncology, Biology, Physics, 45,* 577–587. doi:10.1016/S0360-3016(99)00247-3

Epstein, J.B., Emerton, S., Kolbinson, D.A., Le, N.D., Phillips, N., Stevenson-Moore, P., & Osoba, D. (1999). Quality of life and oral function following radiotherapy for head and neck cancer. *Head and Neck, 21,* 1–11. doi:10.1002/(SICI)1097-0347(199901)21:1<1::AID-HED1>3.0.CO;2-4

Gillison, M.L., Harris, J., Westra, W., Chung, C., Jordan, R., Rosenthal, D., … Ang, K. (2009). Survival outcomes by tumor human papillomavirus (HPV) status in stage III–IV oropharyngeal cancer (OPC) in RTOG 0129. *Journal of Clinical Oncology, 27*(Suppl. 15), Abstract No. 6003.

Hassan, S.J., & Weymuller, E.A., Jr. (1993). Assessment of quality of life in head and neck cancer patients. *Head and Neck, 15,* 485–496.

Hensley, M.L., Schuchter, L.M., Lindley, C., Meropol, N.J., Cohen, G.I., Broder, G., … Pfister, D.G. (1999). American Society of Clinical Oncology clinical practice guidelines for the use of chemotherapy and radiotherapy protectants. *Journal of Clinical Oncology, 17,* 3333–3355.

Jatoi, A., & Thomas, C.R., Jr. (2002). Esophageal cancer and the esophagus: Challenges and potential strategies for selective cytoprotection of the tumor-bearing organ during cancer treatment. *Seminars in Radiation Oncology, 12*(1, Suppl. 1), 62–67.

Jensen, A.B., Hansen, O., Jørgensen, K., & Bastholt, L. (1994). Influence of late side-effects upon daily life after radiotherapy for laryngeal and pharyngeal cancer. *Acta Oncologica, 33,* 487–491.

Jensen, S.B., Mouridsen, H.T., Reibel, J., Brünner, N., & Nauntofte, B. (2008). Adjuvant chemotherapy in breast cancer patients induces temporary salivary gland hypofunction. *Oral Oncology, 44,* 162–173. doi:10.1016/j.oraloncology.2007.01.015

Kam, M.K., Leung, S.F., Zee, B., Chau, R.M., Suen, J.J., Mo, F., … Chan, A.T. (2007). Prospective randomized study of intensity-modulated radiotherapy on salivary gland function in early-stage nasopharyngeal carcinoma patients. *Journal of Clinical Oncology, 25,* 4873–4879. doi:10.1200/JCO.2007.11.5501

Kemp, G., Rose, P., Lurain, J., Berman, M., Manetta, A., Roullet, B., … Glick, J. (1996). Amifostine pretreatment for protection against cyclophosphamide-induced and cisplatin-induced toxicities: Results of a randomized control trial in patients with advanced ovarian cancer. *Journal of Clinical Oncology, 14,* 2101–2112.

Köstler, W.J., Hejna, M., Wenzel, C., & Zielinski, C.C. (2001). Oral mucositis complicating chemotherapy and/or radiotherapy: Options for prevention and treatment. *CA: A Cancer Journal for Clinicians, 51,* 290–315. doi:10.3322/canjclin.51.5.290

Koukourakis, M.I., Kyrias, G., Kakolyris, S., Kouroussis, C., Frangiadaki, C., Giatromanolaki, A., … Georgoulias, V. (2000). Subcutaneous administration of amifostine during fraction-ated radiotherapy: A randomized phase II study. *Journal of Clinical Oncology, 18,* 2226–2233.

Koukourakis, M.I., Tsoutsou, P.G., Karpouzis, A., Tsiarkatsi, M., Karapantzos, I., Daniilidis, V., & Kouskoukis, C. (2010). Radiochemotherapy with cetuximab, cisplatin, and amifostine for locally advanced head and neck cancer: A feasibility study. *International Journal of Radiation Oncology, Biology, Physics, 77,* 9–15. doi:10.1016/j.ijrobp.2009.04.060

Kouvaris, J.R., Kouloulias, V.E., & Vlahos, L.J. (2007). Amifostine: The first selective-target and broad-spectrum radioprotector. *Oncologist, 12,* 738–747. doi:10.1634/theoncologist.12-6-73

Kreimer, A.R., Clifford, G.M., Boyle, P., & Franceschi, S. (2005). Human papillomavirus types in head and neck squamous cell carcinomas worldwide: A systematic review. *Cancer Epidemiology, Biomarkers and Prevention, 14*, 467–475. doi:10.1158/1055-9965.EPI-04-0551

Lin, A., Kim, H.M., Terrell, J.E., Dawson, L.A., Ship, J.A., & Eisbruch, A. (2003). Quality of life after parotid-sparing IMRT for head-and-neck cancer: A prospective longitudinal study. *International Journal of Radiation Oncology, Biology, Physics, 57*, 61–70. doi:10.1016/S0360-3016(03)00361-4

List, M.A., Ritter-Sterr, C., & Lansky, S.B. (1990). A performance status scale for head and neck cancer patients. *Cancer, 66*, 564–569.

Mannarini, L., Kratochvil, V., Calabrese, L., Silva, L.G., Morbini, P., Betka, J., & Benazzo, M. (2009). Human papilloma virus (HPV) in head and neck region: Review of literature. *Acta Otorhinolaryngologica Italica, 29*, 119–126.

Margaix-Muñoz, M., Bagán, J.V., Poveda, R., Jiménez, Y., & Sarrión, G. (2009). Sjögren's syndrome of the oral cavity. Review and update. *Medicina Oral Patología Oral y Cirugía Bucal, 14*, E325–E330.

MedImmune, LLC. (2009, January). *Ethyol®* [Package insert]. Retrieved from http://www.ethyol.com/resources/pdf/Ethyol-PI.pdf

Nakamura, H., Kawakami, A., & Eguchi, K. (2006). Mechanisms of autoantibody production and the relationship between autoantibodies and the clinical manifestations in Sjögren's syndrome. *Translational Research, 148*, 281–288. doi:10.1016/j.trsl.2006.07.003

Pijpe, J., van Imhoff, G.W., Spijkervet, F.K., Roodenburg, J.L., Wolbink, G.J., Mansour, K., ... Bootsma, H. (2005). Rituximab treatment in patients with primary Sjögren's syndrome: An open-label phase II study. *Arthritis and Rheumatism, 52*, 2740–2750. doi:10.1002/art.21260

Rogers, S.N., Lowe, D., Brown, J.S., & Vaughan, E.D. (1999). The University of Washington head and neck cancer measure as a predictor of outcome following primary surgery for oral cancer. *Head and Neck, 21*, 394–401. doi:10.1002/(SICI)1097-0347(199908)21:5<394::AID-HED3>3.0.CO;2-Q

Rosenthal, D. (2006). Established and emerging uses of cytoprotection in head and neck cancer [Editorial]. *Archives of Otolaryngology—Head and Neck Surgery, 132*, 129–130.

Rosenthal, D.I., & Trotti, A. (2009). Strategies for managing radiation-induced mucositis in head and neck cancer. *Seminars in Radiation Oncology, 19*, 29–34. doi:10.1016/j.semradonc.2008.09.006

Samuels, M.A. (2004). Cytoprotection in head and neck cancer: Issues in oral care. *Journal of Supportive Oncology, 2*(6, Suppl. 3), 9–12.

Schwartz, S.M., Daling, J.R., Doody, D.R., Wipf, G.C., Carter, J.J., Madeleine, M.M., ... Galloway, D.A. (1998). Oral cancer risk in relation to sexual history and evidence of human papillomavirus infection. *Journal of the National Cancer Institute, 90*, 1626–1636.

Selwitz, R.H., Ismail, A.I., & Pitts, N.B. (2007). Dental caries. *Lancet, 369*, 51–59. doi:10.1016/S0140-6736(07)60031-2

Soto-Rojas, A.E., & Kraus, A. (2002). The oral side of Sjögren syndrome. Diagnosis and treatment. A review. *Archives of Medical Research, 33*, 95–106. doi:10.1016/S0188-4409(01)00371-X

Thorstad, W.L., Chao, K.S., & Haughey, B. (2004). Toxicity and compliance of subcutaneous amifostine in patients undergoing postoperative intensity-modulated radiation therapy for head and neck cancer. *Seminars in Oncology, 31*(6, Suppl. 18), 8–12. doi:10.1053/j.seminoncol.2004.12.005

U.S. Pharmacopeia. (2002). *Amifostine, finalized drug information.* Rockville, MD: Author.

Venables, P.J. (2006). Management of patients presenting with Sjogren's syndrome. *Best Practice and Research Clinical Rheumatology, 20*, 791–807. doi:10.1016/j.berh.2006.05.003

Vissink, A., Jansma, J., Spijkervet, F.K.L., Burlage, F.R., & Coppes, R.P. (2003). Oral sequelae of head and neck radiotherapy. *Critical Reviews in Oral Biology and Medicine, 14*, 199–212. doi:10.1177/154411130301400305

Visvanathan, V., & Nix, P. (2010). Managing the patient presenting with xerostomia: A review. *International Journal of Clinical Practice, 64,* 404–407. doi:10.1111/j.1742-1241.2009.02132.x

Wasserman, T., Mackowiak, J.I., Brizel, D.M., Oster, W., Zhang, J., Peeples, P.J., & Sauer, R. (2000). Effect of amifostine on patient assessed clinical benefit in irradiated head and neck cancer. *International Journal of Radiation Oncology, Biology, Physics, 48,* 1035–1038. doi:10.1016/S0360-3016(00)00735-5

Wendt, T.G., Grabenbauer, G.G., Rödel, C.M., Thiel, H.J., Aydin, H., Rohloff, R., ... Schalhorn, A. (1998). Simultaneous radiochemotherapy versus radiotherapy alone in advanced head and neck cancer: A randomized multicenter study. *Journal of Clinical Oncology, 16,* 1318–1324.

CHAPTER 7

Pain Management

Ingrid Bowser, MS, APRN-BC, AOCNP®, ADM-BC

Introduction

The reasons that pain management should be included as a fifth vital sign (Jacox et al., 1994) in any nursing assessment are numerous. Pain has a negative impact on daily activities, interaction with family and friends, motivation, quality of life, and, potentially, overall disease survival (von Gunten & Cole, 2009). Pain affects nutrition status, oral hygiene, and the quality of life of patients with cancer. If not dealt with adequately and in a timely manner, unresolved pain leads to anxiety, depression, hopelessness, and fear of disease progression or recurrent disease. Pain management has been studied over many years, and there is an assertion that it should be considered a fundamental human right (Brennan, Carr, & Cousins, 2007). An unreasonable attempt (such as poor assessment and evaluation) to treat pain adequately is thought by some to be malpractice (Brennan et al., 2007). It is estimated that pain occurs in approximately 50%–60% of patients with cancer that are actively undergoing treatment and often occurs in 80%–90% of patients in the advanced stage of disease (Caraceni & Portenoy, 1999; Chiu, Hu, & Chen, 2000; Potter, Hami, Bryan, & Quigley, 2003). The prevalence of pain in head and neck cancer is rated among the highest, at 67%–91% of patients (von Gunten & Cole, 2009). Most pain can be managed by fairly simple means; however, pain associated with cancer often is undertreated. An organized approach to assess and treat the symptoms of patients with advanced disease is frequently necessary (Vogel & Rosiak, 2009).

Causes of Oral Pain

Chemotherapy, radiation therapy, and surgical procedures can lead to oral pain. Bone metastasis and invasive tumors can lead to nerve compression and destruction of the bones and soft tissues of the oral cavity in the head and neck. Pain in the oral cavity may be considered acute or chronic. Acute pain may be the result of mucositis, infection, ulceration, or hemorrhage. Chronic discomfort may result from trismus and soft tissue or bone destruction (Carr, 2005).

Chemotherapy and radiation treatments, on occasion, can lead to mucositis, osteonecrosis, or osteoradionecrosis, along with chronic discomfort. Tissue injury categorized as nociceptive pain is the primary symptom of oral mucositis (Bruner, Haas, & Gosselin-Acomb, 2005). For many years, it was widely believed that mucositis was the result of an interruption in the normal sequence of a renewing epithelium. However, recent studies have indicated that mucosal injury occurs as a result of a five-stage sequence: initiation, primary damage with response, signal amplification, ulceration, and healing. The ulceration phase is the most symptomatic of the phases and is the stage in which pain management needs to take place (Treister & Sonis, 2007). The most common chemotherapy agents associated with mucositis include methotrexate, fluorouracil, cisplatin, cytarabine, etoposide, cyclophosphamide, vinblastine, vincristine, hydroxyurea, and procarbazine. Oral mucositis occurs in approximately 40% of patients receiving standard chemotherapy and can be as high as 70% of patients who are receiving higher doses of chemotherapy (Borbasi et al., 2002). Radiation therapy can lead to mucositis but is dose and site dependent (Berendt & D'Agostino, 2005).

Other treatment-related causes of oral pain include osteonecrosis and osteoradionecrosis. Osteonecrosis of the jaw (ONJ) is associated with bisphosphonate treatment for osteoporosis or bone metastasis. The incidence of ONJ is estimated to be 1%–11% of patients receiving bisphosphonates (Levy, Chwistek, & Mehta, 2008). Osteoradionecrosis is seen most commonly in patients who have received radiation therapy of 60 Gy or more to the jaw. The incidence of osteoradionecrosis of the jaw is estimated at 3% (Blanchaert & Harris, 2008). Osteoradionecrosis of the jaw following radiation therapy is an effect that can manifest months to years after receiving radiation therapy and can be a significant source of pain (Levy et al., 2008).

Surgical procedures such as radical neck dissection can lead to tightness due to lymphedema or burning or shock-like pain (Jacox et al., 1994). Radical neck dissection can cause pain associated with direct injury to the cervical plexus, which can result in neuropathic pain at the surgical site. However, it is more common for chronic pain to be associated with tissue damage to the muscles and nerve fibers, which may result in scarring and fibrosis (Levy et al., 2008). Dressing changes and care after the surgical procedure also can produce acute or chronic episodes of pain that should be addressed in advance of the event.

Tumor-related pain can be caused by local extension into the surrounding tissues, which then leads to nociceptive or neuropathic pain. Nociceptive pain arises from direct injury to the mucosa of the oral cavity, in contradistinction to neuropathic pain, which is secondary to nerve injury and may radiate to the ear. Cranial neuropathies may occur as a result of tumor progression in head and neck cancer, trigeminal neuralgia, or herpetic neuralgia, which then leads to facial pain (Shaiova, 2006).

Limited or nonuse of the jaw frequently leads to trismus, which describes a tonic contraction of the jaw muscle at the temporomandibular joint. The sequelae of trismus are dysphagia, compromised oral hygiene, odynophagia, dysphasia, dysphonia, and pain. Pain management is essential during rehabilitation of the jaw muscle. Inadequate pain management can lead to muscle guarding and, in turn, decreased compliance and effectiveness of therapy (Oral Cancer Foundation, 2001–2010).

Assessment

Assessment of oral pain is necessary to help determine the etiology of the patient's pain and allow the initiation of appropriate interventions. One of the most important keys when assessing pain in patients with cancer is to remember that pain is a subjective symptom. Therefore, it should be accepted that the patient's pain is whatever the patient or family says it is (McCaffery, 1968).

It is important to regularly question the patient about pain. Several tools are available that can assist the patient with pain descriptors to allow for objectivity. This objectivity allows the pain to be assessed and understood by multiple healthcare providers. When selecting a pain assessment tool, the amount of patient and healthcare provider burden should be considered (Eaton, 2009). The most commonly used pain scale is the Brief Pain Inventory. This tool includes a numeric scale (1–10), picture scales, verbal rating cues, or visual analog scales. It is recommended that nurses assess the pain intensity currently, at its worst, at its best, and the average over a specified period of time. It is also important to document how the pain interferes with activities of daily living. The Brief Pain Inventory is a reliable and valid assessment tool that has been used widely in cancer research and several studies of pain (Passik, Kirsh, Donaghy, & Portenoy, 2006).

Acute pain is defined as lasting less than six months. The etiology of pain is usually known, and objective pain behaviors often are exhibited. Objective pain behaviors are evident in the process of assessment. Objective behaviors can include grimacing, tachypnea, tachycardia, hypertension, pallor, and diaphoresis. Chronic pain is characterized as lasting longer than three months, having unknown etiology, and usually not including evidence of objective behaviors (Brant, 2005). However, patients may report insomnia, fatigue, depression, decreased appetite, decreased libido, constipation, and social withdrawal (Vogel & Rosiak, 2009). Breakthrough pain produces sudden, severe flares in pain that are transient (Hwang, Chang & Kasimis, 2003; Mercadente et al., 2002). It is estimated that 65% of patients with cancer experience breakthrough pain at some time even though the pain is well controlled with long-acting medications (Fromer, 2007). Breakthrough pain can bring on anxiety, particularly in patients who have been living fairly pain-free, because they are encountering discomfort for no apparent reason or identifiable cause.

Assessing the patient's pain status provides a good opportunity for education. Teach the patient and caregivers why the medication was chosen and what relief should be achieved with the medication. Discuss why short- and long-acting medications were prescribed and when to use them. Encourage the patient and family to actively participate in the management of pain symptoms, and teach them to use pain assessment tools in their homes. Reassure patients that many pain management options are available, and encourage those who are reluctant to report pain that their fears will be addressed and discussed.

Pain assessment should occur at regular intervals before and during treatment. The goals of the initial assessment should include determining the pathophysiology of the pain along with the intensity and impact on quality of life. To meet the goals of the initial assessment, the following are essential components: detailed history, physical examination, psychosocial assessment, and diagnostic evaluation. Ongoing pain assessment should include descriptive words about the level of pain, the location, changes in the pattern of pain or development of new pain, pain intensity, characteristics, aggravating or relieving factors, cognitive response to pain, cognitive impairment related to the pain or medications, and, finally, the patient and family's goals for pain control (National Cancer Institute [NCI], 2010).

Interventions for Oral Pain

In 1990, the World Health Organization (WHO) developed an analgesic ladder model that emphasized a three-step approach to pain management. Step one of the ladder incorporates strategies to alleviate mild pain. The recommendations include nonopioid analgesics such as nonsteroidal anti-inflammatory drugs (NSAIDs). If step one does not adequately relieve discomfort or the patient is having moderate pain, step two suggests adding a weak opioid such as codeine or tramadol. If pain is still unrelieved or is described as moderate to severe, step three recommends replacement of the weak opioid with a strong opioid such as morphine, oxycodone, or fentanyl (WHO, 2008). Because patients with head and neck cancer are among the highest in reporting moderate to severe pain (von Gunten & Cole, 2009), it would be appropriate to start with a stage two or three analgesic at presentation (NCI, 2010). The WHO analgesic ladder incorporates a starting point for pain management and guidelines for advancement of pain medication. There is still a need to customize pain medication to be patient-specific. Important and equally essential factors need to be taken into account when deciding on pain medication regimens, including the cause of pain, patient compliance, route of administration, and the patient's financial capability to purchase the medication. Timing of the administration of the medication is just as important as the medication being chosen. "Analgesics should be given by mouth, by the clock, by the ladder, and for the individual" (NCI, 2010). Regular scheduling of pain medications, in addition to as-needed dosing, is required to help maintain good pain control. The oral route is the preferred route of administration but should always be customized for the individual (NCI, 2010).

Nonsteroidal Anti-Inflammatory Drugs

NSAIDs are suggested for mild to moderate pain (see Table 7-1). They can also be combined with opioids for a drug-sparing effect that can reduce some

Table 7-1. Acetaminophen and Nonsteroidal Anti-Inflammatory Drugs (NSAIDs)			
Drug	Usual Starting Adult Dose	Indications	Common Side Effects
Over-the-Counter NSAIDs			
Acetamino-phen	650 mg every 4 hours 975 mg every 6 hours	Mild to moderate pain: Acetaminophen inhibits prostaglandin in the central nervous system and not peripherally; other NSAIDs inhibit peripherally as well.	Jaundice, allergic skin eruptions, hypoglycemia
Ibuprofen	400–600 mg every 6 hours		Gastrointestinal disturbances
Naproxen	250–275 mg every 6–8 hours		
Naproxen sodium	275 mg every 6–8 hours		
Prescription NSAIDs			
Etodolac	200–400 mg every 6–8 hours	Anti-inflammatory; used for mild to moderate pain	Gastrointestinal disturbances, heartburn, nausea/vomiting
Fenoprofen calcium	300–600 mg every 6 hours		
Ketoprofen	25–60 mg every 6–8 hours		
Parenteral NSAIDs			
Ketorolac tromethamine	60 mg initially, then 30 mg every 6 hours; IV administration not to exceed 5 days	Anti-inflammatory; use is limited to short-term acute pain, usually in postoperative setting.	Gastrointestinal ulceration, perforation, bleeding

Note. Based on information from Drugs.com, 2010; *Monthly Prescribing Reference*, 2010; National Cancer Institute, 2010.

of the associated side effects of narcotics. Several options for over-the-counter NSAIDs are aspirin, ibuprofen, naproxen, and magnesium salicylate. Prescription NSAIDs include drugs such as etodolac, ketoprofen, ketorolac tromethamine, and celecoxib (NCI, 2010). Acetaminophen is not used very often clinically because of its lack of peripheral anti-inflammatory activity; however, it is most often used as an antipyretic or an analgesic for mild pain. Acetaminophen lacks antiplatelet effect and has only mild action on the gastrointestinal system (Aiello-Laws, Ameringer, Delzer, Peterson, & Reynolds, 2009).

Dosages for NSAIDs are based on patient response and on the maximum tolerated dose recommendations. If the pain has not been relieved by one drug in this group, it is important to try a different medication before abandoning this important therapy. Multiple routes of administration can be used. Tablets, capsules, and liquids are available orally and suppositories are available when nausea and vomiting are present. However, ketorolac tromethamine is the only NSAID available for parenteral use (NCI, 2010).

The side effects of NSAIDs can range from mild gastrointestinal problems to more severe gastrointestinal ulceration and hepatic dysfunction. Renal insufficiency can occur and may be due to the prolonged use of some of these drugs. In addition, it has been found that NSAIDs such as diclofenac can lead to myocardial infarction (JAMA and Archives Journals, 2006). Renal and hepatic function needs to be carefully monitored when patients are taking these medications. Drug-drug interactions can occur with other medications that follow the same pharmacologic pathway and are highly protein bound. The drugs that most commonly have interactions with NSAIDs are warfarin, methotrexate, cyclosporine, oral antidiabetic medications, and sulfonamide-containing drugs (NCI, 2010). NSAIDs will remain a popular choice for analgesia because they do not produce any physiologic or psychological dependency (Aiello-Laws et al., 2009).

Opioids

Opioids are the drugs of choice for moderate to severe acute and chronic pain (see Table 7-2 and Figure 7-1). They are very effective, easily titrated, and have a low risk-to-benefit ratio. Step one of the analgesic ladder should not be abandoned when adding an opioid. Opioids are classified as full morphine-like agonists, partial agonists, or mixed agonist-antagonists depending on which pain receptor they bind to and the activity within these receptors. Full agonists include morphine, hydromorphone, codeine, oxycodone, hydrocodone, methadone, levorphanol, and fentanyl and are classified as such because their effectiveness with dose increases is not limited by a ceiling. Partial agonists include buprenorphine. They have less effect than full agonists and are subject to ceiling doses. Mixed agonist-antagonists include pentazocine, butorphanol tartrate, dezocine, and nalbuphine hydrochloride, which block or are neutral at one type of opioid receptor while being effective on other opioid receptors. Mixed agonist-antagonists are contraindicated for use in patients receiving full agonists because they may induce withdrawal symptoms and cause an increase in pain. Their effectiveness is limited by a dose-related ceiling (NCI, 2010).

Opioid analgesics produce pain relief "by binding to the opioid receptors within and outside the central nervous system" (Miaskowski, 2010, p. 394). The

Table 7-2. Opioids			
Drug	Usual Starting Adult Dose	Indications	Common Side Effects
Atypical Opioid			
Tramadol	50 mg PO 1–2 times/day; gradual titration up to 400 mg PO daily	Weak opioid; inhibits reuptake of norepinephrine and serotonin	Drowsiness, constipation, dizziness, nausea, orthostatic hypotension Use with caution in patients taking SSRIs and SNRIs.
Full Agonist Opioids • Short-acting agonists: Analgesic effect in 30 minutes • Controlled-release agonists: Analgesic effect in 1 hour, peak 2–3 hours			
Morphine	15–30 mg every 4 hours	Moderate to severe pain	Common side effects for all opioids: Constipation, nausea and vomiting, cognitive and neurotoxicity, respiratory depression, reduced libido Less common side effects: Dry mouth, urinary retention, pruritus, dysphoria, euphoria, sleep disturbances, inappropriate secretion of antidiuretic hormone
Hydromorphone	2–4 mg every 4–6 hours		
Codeine plus acetaminophen	30/300–60/300 every 4 hours		
Oxycodone	5 mg every 6 hours		
Fentanyl Available as transdermal, transmucosal/ buccal, or parenteral	For use in opioid-tolerant patients who are converting from a previous narcotic	Provides relief for 72 hours in transdermal patch. Buccal doses are used for breakthrough pain.	
Hydrocodone	5/500 every 4–6 hours	Moderate to severe pain	
Oxymorphone	5 mg every 6 hours		

PO—by mouth; SSRI—selective serotonin reuptake inhibitor; SNRI—serotonin norepinephrine reuptake inhibitor

Note. Based on information from Drugs.com, 2010; *Monthly Prescribing Reference*, 2010; National Cancer Institute, 2010.

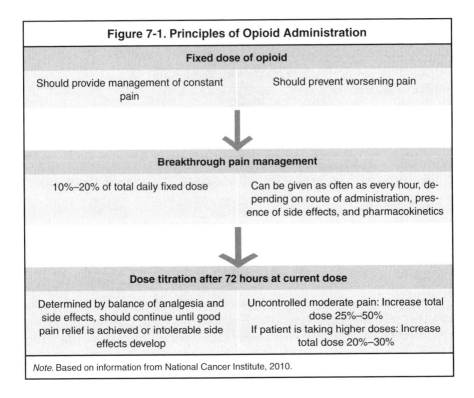

Figure 7-1. Principles of Opioid Administration

Fixed dose of opioid

Should provide management of constant pain	Should prevent worsening pain

Breakthrough pain management

10%–20% of total daily fixed dose	Can be given as often as every hour, depending on route of administration, presence of side effects, and pharmacokinetics

Dose titration after 72 hours at current dose

Determined by balance of analgesia and side effects, should continue until good pain relief is achieved or intolerable side effects develop	Uncontrolled moderate pain: Increase total dose 25%–50% If patient is taking higher doses: Increase total dose 20%–30%

Note. Based on information from National Cancer Institute, 2010.

receptors are present in many areas of the body, including the central nervous system and gastrointestinal tract (Miaskowski, 2010). Some of the consequences associated with long-term opioid use include tolerance and physical dependence. Patients and healthcare providers should discern the difference and discuss this issue with the patient. A lack of understanding of these two concepts can easily lead to ineffective prescribing, administering, or dispensing of opioids, which in turn can lead to the undertreatment of pain (NCI, 2010).

Two common opioids prescribed for oral pain are morphine and methadone. Morphine is the most commonly used opioid in patients with cancer; however, when appropriate levels of pain management are not maintained, hydromorphone, oxycodone, methadone, and fentanyl may be initiated. Morphine is readily available in many forms, including immediate release and sustained release. The administration methods of morphine are numerous, so it lends itself well to be customized to the patient's needs and abilities. Methadone has received more interest recently for use in oncology pain management. Methadone is a synthetic opioid agonist that is distinct and continues to have controversy. The benefits of methadone are excellent oral and rectal absorption, no known active metabolites, prolonged duration of action, and affordability. The controversy surrounding methadone is related to its unpredictable half-life and prolongation of the QT interval, which may lead to torsades de pointes and ventricular arrhythmia (NCI, 2010). Methadone should only be prescribed by healthcare providers who understand its complex pharmacology (Miaskowski, 2010).

One drug that is not used in cancer pain management is meperidine because of its short duration of action and neurotoxic effects. Accumulation of the normeperidine metabolite may lead to delirium or seizures. Multifocal myoclonus seizures usually precede seizures initiated by the meperidine metabolite and may be a useful warning sign if recognized early (NCI, 2010).

Most opioids have similar side effects. The most common side effects include nausea, somnolence, and constipation. Nausea and somnolence tend to decrease over the first 72 hours after initiation and escalation of opioid doses. Constipation will be an ongoing issue that needs to be continually monitored and treated. Patient education is essential, and an anticonstipation bowel regimen should be initiated at the same time as the opioid. Other opioid side effects that may occur include dry mouth, urinary retention, pruritus, dysphoria, euphoria, and sleep disturbances (NCI, 2010).

Topical Medications

Topical analgesics frequently are used to treat acute mucositis. A variety of formulations of topical analgesics are used to numb the mucous membranes. However, most of them contain some form of a numbing agent, such as diphenhydramine, kaolin, milk of magnesia, or sucralfate, and are swished and swallowed. The oral mucosa contains opioid receptors. Topical morphine has been studied to determine the effectiveness of its use on mucositis; however, it is unknown whether the effects are due to local or systemic pathways. Therefore, systemic management of pain with morphine and other opioid pain medications is considered the standard of care for oral pain management (Treister & Sonis, 2007).

Several mucosal adhesive agents are available, or are in the development process, that help relieve pain simply by coating the oral cavity, thereby decreasing the irritation felt by the patient. The currently available products include Caphosol® (EUSA Pharma), which has shown effectiveness in decreasing symptoms of pain and xerostomia. Gelclair® (EKR Therapeutics, Inc.) and Mucotrol® (CURA Pharmaceutical Co., Inc.) are used to coat and adhere to the oral cavity and provide a physical barrier to the exposed nerve endings in the ulcerated membranes (Treister & Sonis, 2007). These agents provide some relief; however, systemic pain therapy is usually additionally required to provide adequate pain relief.

Neuropathic Pain Management

Neuropathic pain management can be clinically challenging. However, several medications are available to help alleviate the discomfort that these patients feel and improve their quality of life. The signs of neuropathic pain include dysesthesias, hyperesthesia, allodynia, hyperalgesia, and hyperpathia, and the pain may follow a neural pathway (Vogel & Rosiak, 2009). The effectiveness of the analgesic is variable, and the onset of pain relief may be delayed. First-line treatment medications include tricyclic antidepressants as well as serotonin norepinephrine reuptake inhibitors, calcium channel ligands, and topical lidocaine. Opioid analgesics and tramadol should be considered first line if the patient is experiencing moderate to severe pain or if the pain is refractory to the other first-line medications. Second-line medications for neuropathic pain include other anticonvulsant and antidepressant medications, as well as cannabinoids, mexiletine, N-methyl-D-aspartate receptor antagonists, topical capsaicin (Aiello-Laws et al., 2009), tricyclic antidepressants, and corticosteroids. Antiepileptic medications are used because of their calming effect on neuronal hyperexcitability. Neuropathic pain is more recently being categorized as an increase in sensation caused by the upregulation of Na^+ and Ca^{2+} membrane channels. Therefore, the medications that are more helpful are the calcium channel ligands, such as gabapentin (Shaiova, 2006).

Breakthrough Cancer Pain Management

"Breakthrough pain is an English term, and an equivalent term does not exist in other European languages such as French, Italian, and Spanish" (von Gunten & Cole, 2009, p. 15). Other descriptors that have been used to characterize breakthrough pain across cultures and languages include episodic, flare, transient, transitory, brief, and abrupt pain. Most often, breakthrough pain occurs in the setting of chronic or persistent pain. Breakthrough pain typically will occur over a 3–5-minute period and continue to increase to moderate or severe intensity over 30 minutes or longer if pain management is not initiated. Distinguishing breakthrough pain from a general lack of overall pain management should be a priority. Breakthrough pain generally is defined as four or fewer episodes of pain in a 24-hour period. Several subcategories for breakthrough pain exist, which describe whether the pain is occurring spontaneously or predictably, if it has identifiable triggers, or if there is a relationship to the baseline analgesia dosing (von Gunten & Cole, 2009).

The goal of pain management for oral breakthrough pain should be to reduce the intensity, severity, and impact of every episode. Once the pain is determined to be a true transitory pain that is occurring and not related to an end-dose failure of long-acting pain analgesia, the characteristics of the pain should be clearly identified. The goal of identifying the characteristics associated with the pain is to determine the pathophysiology and etiology of the pain in order to appropriately remove or modify the trigger or alleviate the pain more effectively. The most common pharmacologic treatment for breakthrough medication is supplemental analgesics already being used to control pain for the patient. However, immediate-release opioids are considered the drug of choice in breakthrough pain because of the multiple choices of route and the relatively rapid onset of several drugs (von Gunten & Cole, 2009).

Breakthrough doses of opioids should be calculated to 10%–20% of the total dose in the fixed-dose schedule (NCI, 2010).

Other Treatments

Some pain syndromes can be related to bone metastasis and inflammation in which corticosteroids would be beneficial (Miaskowski, 2010) (see Table 7-3). Corticosteroids have several uses as adjuvants in the treatment of oral pain. They often provide an increase in energy and feeling of well-being, stimulate appetite, provide an anti-inflammatory effect, and lower hypercalcemia (NYU Langone Medical Center, 2004). Although corticosteroids are frequently useful, they are not recommended for long-term use (Miaskowski, 2010).

"In most cases, pain can be controlled by straightforward methods; however, some patients have more resistant pain. Other options such as nerve blocks,

Table 7-3. Adjuvant Drugs			
Drug	**Usual Adult Dose**	**Indications**	**Common Side Effects**
Antidepressants			
Amitriptyline	10–25 mg daily	Neuropathic pain, depression	Tricyclic antidepressants: constipation, dry mouth, blurred vision, cognitive changes, tachycardia, urinary retention
Nortriptyline	10–100 mg daily		
Desipramine	10–150 mg daily		
Duloxetine	20–30 mg BID		Nausea, dry mouth, constipation, somnolence, hyperhidrosis, decreased appetite, dizziness, decreased libido
Venlafaxine	37.5–225 mg daily		
Anticonvulsants			
Carbamazepine	100–400 mg TID	Limited because of bone marrow suppression; used for neuropathic pain	Leukopenia, nystagmus, dizziness, diplopia, cognitive impairment, mood and sleep disturbances
Valproate	500–1,000 mg TID	Neuropathic pain, seizures	Nausea, vomiting, increased liver enzymes, hallucinations, headache
			(Continued on next page)

Table 7-3. Adjuvant Drugs *(Continued)*			
Drug	**Usual Adult Dose**	**Indications**	**Common Side Effects**
Anticonvulsants *(Cont.)*			
Clonazepam	0.5–4 mg BID	Used for sharp, stabbing pain and paroxysmal neuropathic pain	Drowsiness, cognitive impairment
Phenytoin	100 mg TID, increase weekly to maximum dose of 200 mg TID	Neuropathic pain, seizures	Nystagmus, ataxia, slurred speech, decreased coordination, dizziness, GI upset
Gabapentin	100–1,000 mg TID	Neuropathic pain not relieved with opioids alone	Somnolence, dizziness, ataxia, fatigue
Pregabalin	150 mg divided into 2–3 doses; increase to 300 mg starting at day 3–7; if needed, increase to 600 mg 7 days later		
Local Anesthetics			
Mexiletine	100 mg BID to 300 mg TID	Chronic neuropathic pain	Nausea, dizziness, may alter blood vessel constriction, cardiac evaluation may be required with patients with history of cardiac disease
Lidocaine patch	5% patch contains 700 mg; one patch, 12 hours on, 12 hours off		
Corticosteroids			
Dexamethasone	1–10 mg BID	Cancer pain of bone, visceral pain, and pain of neuropathic origin	Neuropsychiatric syndromes, GI disturbances, proximal myopathy, hyperglycemia, aseptic necrosis, capillary fragility, immunosuppression Adverse reactions increase with increased duration of use.
Prednisone	5–10 mg BID		

(Continued on next page)

Table 7-3. Adjuvant Drugs *(Continued)*			
Drug	**Usual Adult Dose**	**Indications**	**Common Side Effects**
Bisphosphonates			
Pamidronate	60–90 mg IV every 3–4 weeks	Bone pain, metastatic disease to bone	Osteonecrosis, possibility of severe bone, joint and/or muscle pain
Zoledronic acid	4–8 mg IV every 3–4 weeks		
Miscellaneous			
Baclofen	5–20 mg TID	Spasticity, neuropathic pain	Drowsiness, dizziness, ataxia, confusion, nausea and vomiting
Calcitonin	100–200 IU SC or intranasally	Bone and neuropathic pain	Nasal: Rhinitis, respiratory symptoms, back pain, GI upset Injection: Local inflammation, flushing, rash, antibody formation, hypersensitivity
Clonidine	0.1–0.3 mg BID, can be given PO, epidural, and transdermally	Neuropathic pain	Dry mouth, dizziness, hypotension, sedation, constipation
Methylphenidate	2.5–20 mg BID	May enhance analgesic effects of opioids, reduce opioid induced sedation	Insomnia, nervousness, CNS overstimulation, anorexia, abdominal pain, dizziness, headache, tachycardia

BID—twice a day; CNS—central nervous system; GI—gastrointestinal; PO—by mouth; SC—subcutaneous; TID—three times a day

Note. Based on information from Drugs.com, 2010; Monthly Prescribing Reference, 2010; National Cancer Institute, 2010.

subcutaneous or spinal infusions, palliative radiation, or chemotherapy and even palliative surgery can offer optimum quality of life" (Fromer, 2007, p. 10). The use of a single IV injection of a beta particle–emitting agent, such as iodine-131, phosphorus-32, strontium, or samarium, may relieve bone metastasis pain. Radiofrequency ablation is also used to relieve painful osteolytic bone lesions. Surgical procedures to reduce the bulk of the tumor may reduce pain and relieve pain symptoms directly related to compression. Nerve blocks can help control intractable pain by use of local anesthetic or neurolytic agents (NCI, 2010).

A dentist should always be involved in the care of patients at risk for oral pain. He or she can assist in evaluation of denture fit and general dental health. Patients should be encouraged to visit their dentist before any intervention that may result in a change in their oral health. They should also continue to follow up with their dentist at regular intervals after they have received chemotherapy, radiation therapy, or a surgical procedure that may have altered the integrity of their oral cavity.

Nonpharmacologic Interventions

The National Comprehensive Cancer Network has published guidelines associated with nonpharmacologic strategies to reduce pain in patients with cancer that include massage, acupuncture/acupressure, guided imagery, relaxation training, and cognitive-behavioral training in conjunction with pharmacologic therapy for consistently elevated pain scores based on the Brief Pain Inventory (Tsai, Chen, Lai, Lee, & Lin, 2007). Nonpharmacologic and self-care measures can be used concurrently with medications to manage oral pain. The effectiveness of nonpharmacologic interventions generally depends on the patient's participation and communication of which methods alleviate the pain most effectively (NCI, 2010).

Physical Modalities

The physical modalities most often used to help relieve pain associated with weakness, deconditioning, and musculoskeletal pain include application of heat or cold, massage, pressure, vibration, exercise, repositioning, immobilization, stimulation techniques, and acupuncture. Some of these modalities work well for patients with oral pain, whereas others do not have a role. However, it is important to explore the different options and attempt to apply the appropriate modality for the patient.

Application of heat or cold can help alleviate discomfort in the muscles surrounding the oral cavity. It is important to instruct the patient to use a timer to prevent burns, and the time should not exceed 15 minutes at a time. The use of heat sources is contraindicated on recently irradiated tissues. Cold sources should be used with caution. Cold treatments help reduce swelling and may provide longer-lasting pain relief than the use of heat (NCI, 2010).

Massage, pressure, and vibration are physical stimulation techniques that can enhance relaxation when gently applied. Studies have suggested that massage has an immediate benefit on pain and mood, but the effects are not long-lasting (Kutner et al., 2008). Precautions associated with massage include avoiding direct massage to open wounds, hematomas, or areas with skin breakdown, tumors that are visible at the skin surface, and known acute deep venous thrombosis (NCI, 2010).

Exercise, repositioning, and immobilization can be used to help relieve discomfort, especially in patients with trismus because of the benefit of mobilization of stiff muscles and strengthening of weak muscles. Speech therapists are important to involve in this process because they can teach the patient proper techniques to increase range of motion. Speech therapists also may be able to assist patients in finding appropriate positions to help relieve discomfort. Immobilization of the jaw may be necessary when a fracture has occurred or if the patient is battling osteonecrosis or osteoradionecrosis. Avoidance of prolonged immobilization is recommended because it can lead to a decrease in function (NCI, 2010).

Acupuncture has been used more widely for pain management in recent years. It involves the insertion of small, solid needles into the skin with or without an electrical current. The exact mechanism for pain relief is still uncertain; however, theories indicate that pain relief is due to the release of endorphins and immune cells or to alteration of the brain chemistry by affecting the release of neurotransmitters and neurohormones (Passik et al., 2006). Needle placement follows the Eastern theory of vital energy flow (NCI, 2010).

Transcutaneous electrical nerve stimulation (TENS) is gaining popularity for pain relief. Several current theories, related to neuromodulation, exist related to the nature of pain relief from this device. The TENS unit may provide presynaptic inhibition in the spinal cord, encourage the body to increase endorphin production, inhibit abnormally excited nerves, or restore afferent input. The TENS unit generally consists of one or more electrical generators, a battery, and a set of electrodes. The unit is programmable to be patient specific and delivers variable current strengths, pulse rates, and pulse widths. When using a TENS unit for oral pain, it is important to avoid the anterior neck because of the risk for laryngospasms. It is also important to avoid areas that have impaired skin integrity, such as breaks, thinning, burns, or inflamed areas (Kaye & Brandstater, 2008).

Cognitive-Behavioral Interventions

Relaxation techniques were the second most commonly reported methodology used as alternative therapy by adults in the general population and by patients diagnosed with cancer and undergoing treatment (Eisenberg et al., 1998). A study by Tsai et al. (2007) "demonstrated the first evidence that relaxation-breathing training with visual and auditory electromyography biofeedback signals is both feasible and effective in reducing cancer-related pain in advanced cancer patients" (p. 351). Further information obtained from the study indicated that the improvement in pain status was most likely related to a break in the pain-anxiety-muscle tension cycle. With adequate training, most patients were able to learn how to induce the relaxation response and increase the success rate of pain management (Tsai et al., 2007). Other behavioral therapies that can be initiated include distraction, humor therapy, hypnosis, imagery and visualization, meditation, music therapy, psychotherapy, counseling, spirituality, and prayer.

Barriers to Pain Management

It is imperative to fully explore patients' beliefs and perceptions about pain management because many myths and misconceptions are associated with pain that can affect pain management. Patients may hold fatalistic views about cancer pain and believe that pain is a part of cancer that cannot be changed. Some falsely believe that they have to accept the fact that very little can be done to relieve pain. There is also a misconception that pain is indicative of advancing disease, and that misconception leads to fear. Some patients falsely conclude that the use of pain medication early on will lead to ineffective pain control as the need for medication increases. It is important to teach patients that there is no upper limit to the dose of opioids. Patients may be reluctant to report pain because they are fearful that the pain they are experiencing will become a distraction to the provider and place the cancer treatment in a secondary role. Gunnarsdottir, Donovan, Serlin, Voge, and Ward (2002) concluded that some patients indicated that they felt there is an exchange between curing cancer and treating pain. Patients and families have concerns of side effects such as constipation, nausea, vomiting, and decreased mental alertness. There is a belief among some patients that in order to be a good patient they should not report pain because healthcare providers do not want to hear about it and will become annoyed if they bring up the subject (Paice, Toy, & Shott, 1998). It is necessary for healthcare providers to be cognizant of how each person views the experience of pain in order to dispel any counterintuitive views (Cohen et al., 2008).

Because of a basic misunderstanding of psychological addiction and physical dependence among those undergoing treatment for pain control, patients frequently have a fear of developing a tolerance of or an addiction to the medication. It is important for healthcare providers to stress the difference between the two situations. People who are addicted to drugs are taking them to escape from their life and "get high." Patients who are taking narcotics for pain are trying to get back in their life; when their pain is relieved, they no longer look for more pain medication (Fromer, 2007).

Provider barriers to pain management include inadequate knowledge of pain management, poor assessment of pain, concern about regulation of controlled substances, fear of patient addiction, concern about side effects of analgesics, and concern about patients becoming tolerant to analgesics. Healthcare system barriers to pain management include low priority given to cancer pain treatment, inadequate reimbursement for pain assessment and treatment, most appropriate treatment may not be reimbursed or may be too costly for patients, restrictive regulations of controlled substances, problems of availability of treatment or access to it, opioids are unavailable in the patient's pharmacy, and unaffordable medications (NCI, 2010; Vogel & Rosiak, 2009).

Ethnicity

Nursing staff often encounter diverse ethnic populations who generally express differences in pain behavior. Each person offers a unique perception of pain and reactions with individual emotions and behaviors. "Lack of cultural competence can result in cultural conflicts, miscommunication, misdiagnosis, inappropriate care, and patient discontent" (Al-Atiyyat, 2009, p. 155). People learn appropriate conduct and reactions by observing others in the group with whom they closely associate. Therefore, pain and perceptions of discomfort will be demonstrated differently among social groups. Some cultures, such as the Pokot people of Kenya, view stoic reactions to pain as very honorable and, in turn, view the expression of pain as shameful.

Several variables related to culture and pain have been identified (Al-Atiyyat, 2009), including

- The personal meaning of pain
- Sex and age
- Living and working environments
- Social class
- Religion
- Language
- Level of assimilation and acculturation.

When a patient describes his or her pain, the personal definition of the experience needs to be explored. For example, some patients may perceive an increase in pain as a sign that they are dying or have progressive disease and may not want to face that possibility; thus, it is easier for them to ignore the symptom. Most cultures train men to be more stoic in response to painful stimuli. Findings suggest that older individuals practice ethnic traditions more so than their younger counterparts (Al-Atiyyat, 2009). Social class and living and working environments correlate with the fact that people who are used to harsh living and working conditions become insensitive to painful stimuli and do not report pain symptoms as frequently as those of higher social classes. Religion gives meaning to life and offers coping strategies. However, some religious groups, such as Christians and Muslims, view pain and suffering as a test of faith, while Buddhists believe the pain should be endured with patience. Language can become a barrier in pain description because some languages offer many words to describe pain while other languages offer very few words. Translating pain descriptors also may be difficult because many times there are no equivalent words between languages. Finally, it is important to assess whether a person has become acculturated into the environment. Assessment of verbal and nonverbal expressions of pain becomes easier when the culture of the patient more closely resembles that of the healthcare provider (Al-Atiyyat, 2009).

According to a study performed using the Multicultural Personality Questionnaire, the most frequently reported pain descriptors across all ethnic backgrounds were aching, tiring, and tender pain symptoms (Im et al., 2007). The two leading symptoms reported were pain and lack of energy. The investigators found strong evidence to suggest ethnic differences existed in the pain experience but noted no difference between the reported symptoms that often accompany cancer pain. An important observation showed that Asians feel more comfortable reporting physical symptoms over psychological symptoms.

Older Adults

The probability of developing oral cancer increases with age, with 50% of all oral cancers occurring in people older than 68 years of age (American Cancer Society, 2007). Many older adult patients have multiple comorbidities and are already taking complex medication regimens, which can lead to drug-drug and drug-disease interactions. The relatively low side effect profile of NSAIDs in the younger population may lead to gastric and renal toxicity in the older adult population. Older adults also can have slower drug clearance, which leads to more sensitivity to medications. Clinicians need to assess visual, hearing, motor, and cognitive impairments on an ongoing basis to ensure that the patients understand the action of the medications and are able to take the prescribed route of administration (NCI, 2010).

History of Substance Abuse

Patients with a history of substance abuse often experience inadequate pain management because of their own personal fear or the perception by their healthcare providers that they may be aiding in an addictive disease. A patient with a history of substance abuse requires a higher dose of opioids to achieve adequate pain control. This is due to the higher tolerance of narcotics and a lower pain threshold in this population. Relapse into drug abuse is also a concern because drug and alcohol abusers are more likely to return to their habits when they are experiencing uncontrolled pain (Carlson, 2006).

Passik et al. (2006) identified behaviors that were indicative of addiction among patients in pain. Behaviors less associated with addiction included anxiety or depression over recurrent symptoms, hoarding medications, taking someone else's pain medication, asking healthcare providers for more pain medication, specifically asking for certain medications by name, using more opioids than prescribed, drinking alcohol or smoking cigarettes when in pain, or expression of worry or anxiety over changing pain medications. Behaviors more associated with addiction included buying pain medications from a street dealer, stealing money to buy drugs, trying to get opioids from more than one source or provider, stealing drugs from other people, forging prescriptions, and prostituting oneself or others to obtain drugs. These behaviors are clearly distinct in that illegal activity points to addiction, whereas trying to obtain medications by legal means indicates less probability of addiction.

Conclusion

Pain is a frequent complication of cancer, and with the five-year relative survival rate for all stages of oral cancer approaching 60% (ACS, 2007), many patients will need ongoing symptom management. Pain is among the most commonly reported fears associated with a cancer diagnosis. The treatment of oral pain involves many facets and requires the use of multiple modalities to effectively control the discomfort. Uncontrolled pain inhibits cancer rehabilitation, increases suffering, and leads to diminished quality of life.

Assessment of the type and causes of oral pain helps define the proper treatment. Management of pain should include a multidisciplinary approach that involves individualized plans based on the physical, psychological, cultural, and social facets of the patient. Incorporating all of these facets will lead to greater adherence, communication, and understanding of pain regimens. Ongoing education of patients and healthcare providers will continue to improve pain management quality.

References

Aiello-Laws, L.B., Ameringer, S.W., Delzer, N.A., Peterson, M.E., & Reynolds, J.K. (2009). ONS PEP resource: Pain. In L.H. Eaton & J.M. Tipton (Eds.), *Putting evidence into practice: Improving oncology patient outcomes* (pp. 223–234). Pittsburgh, PA: Oncology Nursing Society.

Al-Atiyyat, N.M.H. (2009). Cultural diversity and cancer pain. *Journal of Hospice and Palliative Nursing, 11,* 154–164. doi:10.1097/NJH.0b013e3181a1aca3

American Cancer Society. (2007). Oral cancer. Retrieved from http://www.cancer.org/docroot/PRO/content/PRO_1_1x_oral_cancer.pdf

Berendt, M., & D'Agostino, S. (2005). Alterations in nutrition. In J.K. Itano & K.N. Taoka (Eds.), *Core curriculum for oncology nursing* (4th ed., pp. 277–317). St. Louis, MO: Elsevier Saunders.

Blanchaert, R.H., Jr., & Harris, M. (2008). Osteoradionecrosis of the mandible. Retrieved from http://emedicine.medscape.com/article/851539-overview

Borbasi, S., Cameron, K., Quested, B., Olver, I., To, B., & Evans, D. (2002). More than a sore mouth: Patients' experience of oral mucositis. *Oncology Nursing Forum, 29,* 1051–1057. doi:10.1188/02.ONF.1051-1057

Brant, J.M. (2005). Comfort. In J.K. Itano & K.N. Taoka (Eds.), *Core curriculum for oncology nursing* (4th ed., pp. 3–28). St. Louis, MO: Elsevier Saunders.

Brennan, F., Carr, D.B., & Cousins, M. (2007). Pain management: A fundamental human right. *International Anesthesia Research Society, 105,* 205–221. doi:10.1213/01.ane.0000268145.52345.55

Bruner, D.W., Haas, M.L., & Gosselin-Acomb, T.K. (Eds.). (2005). *Manual for radiation oncology nursing practice and education* (pp. 52–54). Pittsburgh, PA: Oncology Nursing Society.

Caraceni, A., & Portenoy, R.K. (1999). An international study of cancer pain characteristics and syndromes. IASP Task Force on Cancer Pain. International Association for the Study of Pain. *Pain, 82,* 263–274. doi:10.1016/S0304-3959(99)00073-1

Carlson, R.H. (2006). A forgotten group: Helping cancer patients who are drug addicts receive adequate pain management. *Oncology Times, 28*(14), 44, 45. doi:10.1097/01.COT.0000303168.96079.1f

Carr, E. (2005). Nursing care of the client with head and neck cancer. In J.K. Itano & K.N. Taoka (Eds.), *Core curriculum for oncology nursing* (4th ed., pp. 624–655). St. Louis, MO: Elsevier Saunders.

Chiu, T.Y., Hu, W.Y., & Chen, C.Y. (2000). Prevalence and severity of symptoms in terminal cancer patients: A study in Taiwan. *Supportive Care in Cancer, 8,* 311–313. doi:10.1007/s005209900112

Cohen, E., Botti, M., Hanna, B., Leach, S., Boyd, S., & Robbins, J. (2008). Pain beliefs and pain management of oncology patients. *Cancer Nursing, 31*(2), E1–E8. doi:10.1097/01. NCC.0000305693.67131.7d

Drugs.com. (2010). Drug information online. Retrieved from http://www.drugs.com

Eaton, L. (2009). Pain. In L.H. Eaton & J.M. Tipton (Eds.), *Putting evidence into practice: Improving oncology patient outcomes* (pp. 215–221). Pittsburgh, PA: Oncology Nursing Society.

Eisenberg, D.M., Davis, R.B., Ettner, S.L., Appel, S., Wilkey, S., Van Rompay, M., & Kessler, R.C. (1998). Trends in alternative medicine use in the United States, 1990–1997: Results of a follow-up national survey. *JAMA, 280,* 1569–1575.

Fromer, M.J. (2007). Minimizing cancer pain: Update on new drugs and treatments. *Oncology Times, 29*(11), 9–11. doi:10.1097/01.COT.0000282533.48028.98

Gunnarsdottir, S., Donovan, H.S., Serlin, R.C., Voge, C., & Ward, S. (2002). Patient-related barriers to pain management: The Barriers Questionnaire II (BQ-II). *Pain, 99,* 385–396. doi:10.1016/S0304-3959(02)00243-9

Hwang, S.S., Chang, V.T., & Kasimis, B. (2003). Cancer breakthrough pain characteristics and responses to treatment in a VA medical center. *Pain, 101,* 55–64. doi:10.1016/S0304-3959(02)00293-2

Im, E.O., Chee, W., Guevara, E., Liu, Y., Lim, H.J., Tsai, H.M., ... Shin, H. (2007). Gender and ethnic differences in cancer pain experience. *Nursing Research, 56,* 296–306. doi:10.1097/01.NNR.0000289502.45284.b5

Jacox, A., Carr, D.B., Payne, R., Berde, C.B., Brietbart, W., Cain, J.M., ... Weissman, D.E. (1994). *Management of cancer pain, clinical practice guideline number 9* (AHCPR Publication No. 94-0592). Rockville, MD: Agency for Health Care Policy and Research, U.S. Department of Health and Human Services, Public Health Service.

JAMA and Archives Journals. (2006, September 18). New evidence on risks associated with Cox-2 inhibitors and NSAIDs. *ScienceDaily.* Retrieved from http://www.sciencedaily.com/releases/2006/09/060915203524.htm

Kaye, V., & Brandstater, M.E. (2008). Transcutaneous electrical nerve stimulation. Retrieved from http://emedicine.medscape.com/article/325107-overview

Kutner, J.S., Smith, M.C., Corbin, L., Hemphill, L., Benton, K., Mellis, B.K., ... Fairclough, D.L. (2008). Massage therapy versus simple touch to improve pain and mood in patients with advanced cancer: A randomized trial. *Annals of Internal Medicine, 149,* 369–379.

Levy, M.H., Chwistek, M., & Mehta, R.S. (2008). Management of chronic pain in cancer survivors. *Cancer Journal, 14,* 401–409. doi:10.1097/PPO.0b013e31818f5aa7

McCaffery, M. (1968). *Nursing practice theories related to cognition, bodily pain, and man-environment interactions.* Los Angeles, CA: Student Store.

Mercadente, S., Radbruch, L., Caraceni, A., Cherny, N., Kaasa, S., Nauck, F., ... De Conno, F. (2002). Episodic (breakthrough) pain: Consensus conference of an expert working group of the European Association for Palliative Care. *Cancer, 94,* 832–839. doi:10.1002/cncr.10249

Miaskowski, C.A. (2010). Cancer pain. In C.G. Brown (Ed.), *A guide to oncology symptom management* (pp. 389–403). Pittsburgh, PA: Oncology Nursing Society.

Monthly Prescribing Reference. (2010, April). New York, NY: Haymarket Media Publications.

National Cancer Institute. (2010, April 20). Pain (PDQ®) [Health professional version]. Retrieved from http://www.cancer.gov/cancertopics/pdq/supportivecare/pain/health professional/allpages/print

NYU Langone Medical Center. (2004). Head and neck cancer pain. Retrieved from http://www.med.nyu.edu/PainManagement/patients/neckpain.html

Oral Cancer Foundation. (2001–2010). What is trismus? Retrieved from http://www.oral cancerfoundation.org/dental/trismus.htm

Paice, J.A., Toy, C., & Shott, S. (1998). Barriers to cancer pain relief: Fear of tolerance and addiction. *Journal of Pain and Symptom Management, 16,* 1–9. doi:10.1016/S0885-3924(98)00025-6

Passik, S.D., Kirsh, K.L., Donaghy, K.B., & Portenoy, R.K. (2006). Pain and aberrant drug-related behaviors in medically ill patients with and without histories of substance abuse. *Clinical Journal of Pain, 22,* 173–181.

Potter, J., Hami, F., Bryan, T., & Quigley, C. (2003). Symptoms in 400 patients referred to palliative care services: Prevalence and patterns. *Palliative Medicine, 17,* 310–314.

Shaiova, L. (2006). Difficult pain syndromes: Bone pain, visceral pain, and neuropathic pain. *Cancer Journal, 12,* 330–340.

Treister, N., & Sonis, S. (2007). Mucositis: Biology and management. *Current Opinion in Otolaryngology and Head and Neck Surgery, 15,* 123–129. doi:10.1097/MOO.0b013e3280523ad6

Tsai, P.S., Chen, P.L., Lai, Y.L., Lee, M.B., & Lin, C.C. (2007). Effects of electromyography biofeedback-assisted relaxation on pain in patients with advanced cancer in a palliative care unit. *Cancer Nursing, 30,* 347–401. doi:10.1097/01.NCC.0000290805.38335.7b

Vogel, W.H., & Rosiak, J.M. (2009). Pain, fatigue, and cognitive dysfunction. In B.H. Gobel, S. Triest-Robertson, & W.H. Vogel (Eds.), *Advanced oncology nursing certification review and resource manual* (pp. 357–403). Pittsburgh, PA: Oncology Nursing Society.

von Gunten, C.F., & Cole, B.E. (2009). *Clinical management of breakthrough cancer pain.* Somerset, NJ: Meda Pharmaceuticals.

World Health Organization. (2008). Analgesia ladder. Retrieved from http://www.who.int/cancer/palliative/painladder/en

CHAPTER 8

Speech, Voice, and Swallowing Problems: The Speech Pathologist's Role

Mary J. Bacon, MA, CCC-SLP, BRS-S

Introduction

It is well known that surgery for head and neck cancers can have adverse effects on speech, voice, and swallowing (Hirano et al., 1992; Olson & Shedd, 1978). Organ-sparing treatments, it was hoped, would conserve function. However, it now is clear that organ preservation does not necessarily result in preservation of function. Swallowing and communication deficits can occur when organ preservation protocols are employed (Fung et al., 2001; Goguen et al., 2006; Langerman et al., 2007). Regardless of the method of treatment used, the speech pathologist is a valuable member of the team of healthcare providers assisting patients after a diagnosis of head and neck cancer.

The speech pathologist evaluates and treats impairments of speech, voice/resonance, and swallowing that arise from head and neck cancer or the treatment of that cancer. The speech pathologist is best utilized when patients are seen before, during, and after treatment. The goal of the speech pathologist's care is to return the patient to the most adequate speech, voice, and swallowing function possible in the shortest amount of time and to assist the patient in maintaining that function.

This chapter will focus on the patient with oral or oropharyngeal cancer treated with radiation therapy and/or chemotherapy. However, the speech pathologist has a central role in the evaluation and treatment of patients requiring surgical treatment for oral, pharyngeal, and laryngeal cancers as well.

Common Speech, Voice, and Swallowing Problems Related to Radiation Therapy and Chemotherapy for Oral and Oropharyngeal Cancers

Impairments can relate to effects of the original tumor, additional procedures required before or during treatment such as tracheostomy, pain from mucositis during treatment, xerostomia related to treatment, auto-amputation of structures as treatment progresses, and fibrosis due to radiation treatment. Some of these impairments can develop even before treatment begins; some are most troublesome during and immediately after treatment; and some can persist and even worsen for many years following treatment.

Speech impairments caused by chemotherapy and radiation therapy typically are mild to moderate in severity and relate to minor effects of treatment on the lips, tongue, teeth, or palate. Patients may have difficulty articulating quickly when the mouth is extremely dry. Speech may become temporarily difficult when significant pain is present because of mucositis.

Voice impairments can range from mild to moderately severe. The patient's voice may become strained, harsh, or breathy. Persistent edema in the larynx, impairment of vocal fold mobility, changes in compliance of the vocal folds, and changes to the vibrating edge of the vocal folds can affect voice quality. Patients suffering from xerostomia may notice voice changes resulting from dryness of laryngeal mucosa. Changes in palatal function or edema in the oropharynx can alter resonance.

Swallowing impairments are common after radiation therapy with or without chemotherapy for head and neck tumors. Dysphagia can range from mild to severe. Difficulties may include inability to masticate because of removal of teeth or because of the inability to move food on and off the chewing surfaces of the teeth, loss of material from the lips, loss of material from the tongue surface to the floor of the mouth, long oral transit time, premature spillage of material into the pharynx, nasal regurgitation, stasis of material in the pharynx, and aspiration of food or liquid. Swallowing safety, swallowing efficiency, or both may be affected by treatment for oral or oropharyngeal cancer (Lazarus et al., 1996). Many of the patients who aspirate may do so "silently," that is, without coughing or choking (Langerman et al., 2007). Special mention should be made of the possible long-term effects of radiation on swallowing function. It is not uncommon for patients to appear with complaints of significant dysphagia many years after radiation therapy. The long-term effects of tissue fibrosis ultimately may produce a degree of dysfunction for which the patient cannot compensate (Eisele, Koch, Tarazi, & Jones, 1991).

Pretreatment Involvement of Speech Pathology

The speech pathologist will use a pretreatment session to gather baseline information about a patient's speech, voice/resonance, and swallowing. It can be very helpful to the team to have a record of pretreatment function, especially when evaluating quality of life and functional outcomes of treatment.

Education will naturally accompany the pretreatment evaluation. The speech pathologist will discuss likely short- and long-term changes to speech, voice, and swallowing that a patient may expect. In addition, the speech pathologist can assure the patient that assistance will be available when and if changes in speech, voice, or swallowing are encountered.

Some evidence supports that prophylactic exercises to maintain function of the oral and pharyngeal structures important to speech, voice, and swallowing may be of benefit to patients undergoing treatment for head and neck cancers (Carroll et al., 2008; Kulbersh et al., 2006). Such exercises can be taught at the pretreatment speech pathology session.

Speech Pathology Evaluations

The evaluations performed by the speech pathologist before, during, and after treatment will follow the same general pattern, although evaluation will vary somewhat depending on the anatomic region to be treated and depending on the patient. A patient hoping to return to work as a salesman or broadcaster may require more detailed evaluation of speech and voice, for example. In general, the team can expect the speech pathologist to evaluate the following.

Oral-Motor Function

The speech pathologist should evaluate the strength, range of motion, and coordination of oral structures to determine whether function can support normal speech and swallowing.

General Intelligibility of Speech

The speech pathologist typically will estimate the percentage of words understood during a face-to-face conversation. If more detail is desired, a formal test of articulation may be administered with a notation made as to the patient's method of production for each phoneme (sound) produced. Additional comments will be made regarding rate of speech and other prosodic features if abnormalities are noted.

Voice Quality and Resonance

A rating system can be used that will allow the speech pathologist to judge various perceptual aspects of voice quality such as roughness, breathiness, strain, pitch, and loudness. The Consensus Auditory-Perceptual Evaluation of Voice (CAPE-V) assessment (Kempster, Gerratt, Abbott, Barkmeier-Kraemer, & Hillman, 2009) provides a useful rating system. Additional rating of hyponasality, hypernasality, or altered oropharyngeal resonance will be included when pertinent. If desired, additional acoustic, aerodynamic, or endoscopic/stroboscopic assessments may be conducted. For patients with a tracheostomy, evaluation of voice will be modified to include information related to the artificial airway. The size and type of tracheostomy tube will be noted. The patient's ability to produce a voice with digital occlusion or use of a one-way speaking valve will be assessed. The characteristics of the voice will be rated, and the understandability of the speech produced will be documented.

Oropharyngeal Swallowing

Use of a feeding tube should be noted along with an estimate of the percentage of nutrition/hydration taken via feeding tube versus by mouth, and the route used for medications. A clinical swallowing examination should be conducted to document mastication, oral transit of food and liquid, and signs and symptoms of pharyngeal swallowing problems such as pharyngeal residue or aspiration of food or liquid. Because pharyngeal swallowing cannot be observed directly during a clinical evaluation, pharyngeal impairments must be inferred. Multiple swallows after every bite or sip, wet voice quality, throat clearing, or coughing can indicate the possibility of pharyngeal swallowing impairment. However, some patients with pharyngeal impairment may show few signs during a clinical examination. For example, in one retrospective review of objective (videofluoroscopic) swallowing examinations, more than half of the patients who aspirated failed to exhibit a cough response (Smith, Logemann, Colangelo, Rademaker, & Pauloski, 1999). Patients who aspirate without a cough response may not appear to be dysphagic when examined at the bedside or in the clinic. Objective evaluation of the pharyngeal stage of swallowing requires examination via endoscopy or fluoroscopy. The speech pathologist can treat swallow dysfunction more accurately and more adequately if objective data, such as that obtained via videofluoroscopic evaluation of swallowing, are obtained (Langerman et al., 2007; Logemann et al., 1992).

Hearing

A hearing screening should take place at the first visit with the speech pathologist, with referral for full audiometric evaluation for any patient who fails the screening. Also, any complaint from the patient about changes in hearing, such as speech sounding "muffled," should trigger referral to otolaryngology and audiology. If patients are to receive chemotherapeutic agents that are known to be ototoxic, full audiometric evaluation by the audiologist is preferred to screening. Hodges and Lonsbury-Martin (1999) provide detailed information regarding hearing management for patients with cancer.

Brief Evaluation of Language and Cognition

Most patients with head and neck cancer do not have an aphasia or significant cognitive-communication deficit. However, an initial evaluation should include an informal assessment of the patient's receptive and expressive language ability and cognitive status.

Other

Measurements of interdental distance at the incisors for patients experiencing trismus and ratings or measurements of xerostomia are additional evaluations that the speech pathologist may provide. Because poor dental health and oral hygiene can greatly increase a patient's risk of aspiration pneumonia (Langmore et al., 1998), the speech pathologist is likely to include an observation regarding oral health.

The speech pathologist should provide interpretation of evaluation results, separating impairments due to tumor and treatment from those unrelated to the head and neck cancer. For repeat evaluations, results should be compared to previous evaluations so that improvement or worsening of symptoms is made clear.

Speech Pathology Treatment

Some recent evidence has shown that therapy exercises during treatment may be of benefit (Carroll et al., 2008; Kulbersh et al., 2006). The speech pathologist often provides exercises to maintain or maximize movement of structures involved in speech and swallowing. A regimen of prophylactic exercises should include those to maintain range of motion, strength, and flexibility of structures. Typically, the patient will be instructed to complete exercises to maintain jaw opening, maintain movement and strength of the oral tongue and the tongue base, maintain hyolaryngeal elevation, and maintain pharyngeal contraction. An optimal practice schedule for such exercises has not been studied. A reasonable regimen might consist of 10 of each exercise morning and night each day (or even every other day). Most patients can complete 10 of each exercise in 10–15 minutes.

There is some thought among clinicians caring for patients with head and neck cancer that patients who continue to swallow some food or liquid throughout their treatment have better swallowing outcomes than those who do not. Obviously, this may simply be because patients who are not able to continue to swallow may have more severe dysphagia during (and after) treatment. However, because the act of swallowing activates pharyngeal musculature more adequately than any nonswallowing exercise (Perlman, Luschei, & Du Mond, 1989), there is reason to attempt to find some materials that a patient may continue to swallow safely during treatment. Swallowing, thus, may be considered an exercise at certain points in treatment rather than a means of nutrition or hydration.

During and after treatment, recommendations and therapy provided by the speech pathologist typically target specific impairments. The purpose for each recommendation or exercise should be clear to the patient and to the care team.

Speech Problems

Strategies to improve intelligibility of speech may be taught. For example, a patient may be guided to modify speech rate, especially over the phone when visual cues are not available to the listener. The patient and family may be taught to use either low-tech or high-tech augmentative or alternative communication options. Something as simple as a list of commonly used phrases may be helpful for some. For others, a computer-based communication system may be pursued. The speech pathologist has a range of such options to explore with patients and families. Therapy programs to help a patient regain precise production of specific speech sounds may be required, especially if the patient relies on speech for employment. In some cases, a compensatory sound production may be taught if there are articulatory placements that can no longer be achieved.

Voice Problems

The speech pathologist may provide recommendations for modified voice rest during treatment. Avoidance of bad habits, such as straining the voice, during treatment can ward off long-term voice changes. If treatment has caused a change to the vocal folds, voice therapy can help the patient optimize voice quality.

If a patient has a tracheostomy, the speech pathologist can evaluate the patient for use of a one-way speaking valve and provide training in its use. Alternatively, the patient can be trained to use digital coverage of the tracheostomy for purposes of improved voice and speech.

The use of a nose clip can temporarily modify hypernasality. Communication between the speech pathologist and a prosthedontist will be required, in most cases, for the long-term management of hypernasality.

Swallowing Problems

In order to improve swallowing function, the speech pathologist might teach the patient compensatory postures (such as head turn or chin tuck), compensatory swallowing maneuvers (such as breath hold prior to swallow), compensatory dietary changes (such as use of thickened fluids), or exercises (such as those to maximize tongue base retraction).

Most dysphagia exercises target specific biomechanical aspects of the patient's swallowing that have been affected by tumor or treatment thereof. Some exercises are meant to globally improve the entire swallowing sequence. The speech pathologist's plan should indicate the specific purpose of each compensation or exercise. Swallowing therapy recommendations usually are based on an objective evaluation of swallowing using videofluoroscopy or flexible endoscopy. Martin-Harris, Logemann, McMahon, Schleicher, and Sandidge (2000) illustrated the significant impact that data from videofluoroscopic swallowing studies can have on patient care. Certainly, some treatments may be based on the results of clinical swallowing evaluations; however, because the important pharyngeal stage of swallowing is largely inferred during clinical examination, objective evaluation at intervals is preferred.

Although treatment of pharyngoesophageal segment stricture is not done by the speech pathologist, it is worth noting that such strictures may be suspected when the speech pathologist analyzes the videofluoroscopic swallow studies. Thus, the videofluoroscopic swallow study may facilitate prompt and sufficient dilation of such strictures by the patient's physicians (Goguen et al., 2006).

The speech pathologist should assist the care team with recommendations regarding the need for supplementary hydration and nutrition. The dietitian and speech pathologist customarily cooperate to give the team an assessment of the patient's ability to maintain adequate hydration and nutrition via oral feeding.

Other Problems

Patients with trismus or at risk for trismus may be offered an exercise device to maintain or improve jaw opening. The speech pathologist can teach proper use of the device and determine an appropriate treatment regimen. The speech pathologist may suggest a modified diet as a compensation for dysphagia and may guide a patient toward recipe books, such as the *Easy-to-Swallow, Easy-to-Chew Cookbook* by Weihofen, Robbins, and Sullivan (2002), to help patients find foods with the recommended properties. General reminders regarding oral health and hints for xerostomia relief may be given to patients. Other members of the healthcare team may be consulted for these purposes as well. The dietitian, dentist, nurse, and speech pathologist may all reinforce one another in instructing patients about oral health and diet.

End-of-Life Care

The speech pathologist's goals will be somewhat different for patients receiving palliative care at the end of life. However, the speech pathologist can be a valuable member of the care team when patients are receiving palliative care.

Patients should have every opportunity to communicate to their loved ones and caregivers at the end of life. Speech pathologists can evaluate a patient's abilities to use a wide array of communication options. Possibilities include various options for written or typed communication, use of amplifiers for the patient with a soft or breathy voice, rate control and use of over-articulation to improve speech that is difficult to understand, use of picture boards, and optimal use of yes-no questions by those needing to communicate with the patient.

If the patient approaching the end of life has dysphagia and yet desires some oral intake, the speech pathologist often can help the patient to arrive at a way to swallow with greater ease. Risk of aspiration can be kept to a minimum. A patient who desires water or some oral intake will enjoy the experience more if he or she can ingest the material efficiently without coughing. A speech pathologist may be able to find simple compensations that will allow the patient to successfully swallow what he or she desires.

Conclusion

In patients with oral and oropharyngeal cancer, the speech pathologist can function most effectively if involved before, during, and after treatment. Some patients need little or no speech pathology involvement, others need occasional input, and still others require ongoing therapy for a period of months. A speech pathologist trained to manage patients with head and neck cancer will provide appropriate services. The care team should expect the speech pathologist to evaluate speech, voice/resonance, and swallowing. Swallowing concerns may be seen as primary, but many patients with head and neck cancer have speech and voice impairments as well. After evaluation of a patient, the speech pathologist should be able to give opinions regarding appropriate evidence-based treatment for any communication or swallowing difficulties.

• Will a given patient be likely to experience significant short- or long-term speech or swallowing deficits?
• Will the patient be likely to regain functional speech and functional swallowing?
• Is the patient's speech, voice, or swallowing problem related to the effects of cancer treatment or to some other factor?
• Is speech therapy or swallowing therapy likely to be of benefit?
• Should speech or swallowing therapy be deferred or start right away?
• When might the patient see some improvement?
• Are there things the patient can do to avoid speech or swallowing difficulties later on?
• Can the patient eat efficiently enough to meet his or her caloric and hydration requirements?
• Can the tube-fed patient take *some* foods or liquid by mouth?

These all are questions that come up with some regularity as teams of healthcare professionals assist patients with head and neck cancer; the speech pathologist can provide data to assist the care team in arriving at answers.

Functional speech, voice, and swallowing are important outcomes for patients with head and neck cancer. Optimal long-term outcomes and optimal quality of life can be attained through the provision of appropriate speech pathology services.

References

Carroll, W.R., Locher, J.L., Canon, C.L., Bohannon, I.A., McColloch, N.L., & Magnuson, J.S. (2008). Pretreatment swallowing exercises improve swallow function after chemoradiation. *Laryngoscope, 118,* 39–43. doi:10.1097/MLG.0b013e31815659b0

Eisele, D.W., Koch, D.G., Tarazi, A.E., & Jones, B. (1991). Case report: Aspiration from delayed radiation fibrosis of the neck. *Dysphagia, 6,* 120–122.

Fung, K., Yoo, J., Leeper, H.A., Bogue, B., Hawkins, S., Hammond, J.A., ... Venkatesan, V.M. (2001). Effects of head and neck radiation therapy on vocal function. *Journal of Otolaryngology, 30,* 133–139.

Goguen, L.A., Posner, M.R., Norris, C.M., Tishler, R.B., Wirth, L.J., Annino, D.J., ... Haddad, R.I. (2006). Dysphagia after sequential chemoradiation therapy for advanced head and neck cancer. *Otolaryngology—Head and Neck Surgery, 134,* 916–922. doi:10.1016/j.otohns.2006.02.001

Hirano, M., Kuroiwa, Y., Tanaka, S., Matsuoka, H., Sato, K., & Yoshida, T. (1992). Dysphagia following various degrees of surgical resection for oral cancer. *Annals of Otology, Rhinology, and Laryngology, 101,* 138–141.

Hodges, A., & Lonsbury-Martin, B. (1999). Hearing management. In P.A. Sullivan & A.M. Guilford (Eds.), *Swallowing intervention in oncology* (pp. 269–290). San Diego, CA: Singular.

Kempster, G.B., Gerratt, B.R., Abbott, K.V., Barkmeier-Kraemer, J., & Hillman, R.E. (2009). Consensus auditory-perceptual evaluation of voice: Development of a standardized clinical protocol. *American Journal of Speech-Language Pathology, 18,* 124–132. doi:10.1044/1058-0360(2008/08-0017)

Kulbersh, B.D., Rosenthal, E.L., McGrew, B.M., Duncan, R.D., McColloch, N.L., Carroll, W.R., & Magnuson, J.S. (2006). Pretreatment, preoperative swallowing exercises may improve dysphagia quality of life. *Laryngoscope, 116,* 883–886. doi:10.1097/01.mlg.0000217278.96901.fc

Langerman, A., MacCracken, E., Kasza, K., Haraf, D.J., Vokes, E.E., & Stenson, K.M. (2007). Aspiration in chemoradiated patients with head and neck cancer. *Archives of Otolaryngology—Head and Neck Surgery, 133,* 1289–1295.

Langmore, S.E., Terpenning, M.S., Schork, A., Chen, Y., Murray, J.T., Lopatin, D., & Loesche, W.J. (1998). Predictors of aspiration pneumonia: How important is dysphagia? *Dysphagia, 13,* 69–81.

Lazarus, C.L., Logemann, J.A., Pauloski, B.R., Colangelo, L.A., Kahrilas, P.J., Mittal, B.B., & Pierce, M. (1996). Swallowing disorders in head and neck cancer patients treated with radiotherapy and adjuvant chemotherapy. *Laryngoscope, 106,* 1157–1166.

Logemann, J.A., Pauloski, B.R., Rademaker, A., Cook, B., Graner, D., Milianti, F., ... Lazarus, C. (1992). Impact of the diagnostic procedure on outcome measures of swallowing rehabilitation in head and neck cancer patients. *Dysphagia, 7,* 179–186.

Martin-Harris, B., Logemann, J.A., McMahon, S., Schleicher, M., & Sandidge, J. (2000). Clinical utility of the modified barium swallow. *Dysphagia, 15,* 136–141. doi:10.1007/s004550010015

Olson, M.L., & Shedd, D.P. (1978). Disability and rehabilitation in head and neck cancer patients after treatment. *Head Neck Surgery, 1,* 52–58.

Perlman, A.L., Luschei, E.S., & Du Mond, C.E. (1989). Electrical activity from the superior pharyngeal constrictor during reflexive and nonreflexive tasks. *Journal of Speech and Hearing Research, 32,* 749–754.

Smith, C.H., Logemann, J.A., Colangelo, L.A., Rademaker, A.W., & Pauloski, B.R. (1999). Incidence and patient characteristics associated with silent aspiration in the acute care setting. *Dysphagia, 14,* 1–7.

Weihofen, D.L., Robbins, J., & Sullivan, P.A. (2002). *Easy-to-swallow, easy-to-chew cookbook: Over 150 tasty and nutritious recipes for people who have difficulty swallowing.* New York, NY: Wiley.

CHAPTER 9

Complementary and Alternative Medicine and the Mouth

Katherine Katen Moore, MSN, ANP-C, AOCN®,
and M. Renee Yanke, ARNP, MN, AOCN®

Introduction

The mouth is a primary opening to the human body. It is used for a variety of essential human activities—bestowing affection, eating, drinking, speaking, and frequently, breathing. The mouth is a source of pleasure through taste and the sensation of textures. For these reasons, adverse symptoms of cancer and cancer therapies that occur in the mouth seem to be particularly noxious.

Two distinct groups present with oral symptoms: patients with head and neck (H&N) cancers who experience direct effects of treatment to the mouth (surgery or radiation) and the larger group that experience oral side effects secondary to treatment modalities. The second group includes all those individuals on anthracyclines, pyrimidines, or platins, as well as those receiving radiation to anatomic areas that include the oral cavity or pharynx, such as the cervical spine.

Information and research analysis and synthesis are readily available in the Cochrane Collaboration (Clarkson et al., 2010) regarding the best practices known for the assessment, prevention, and intervention for mucositis. Best practice recommendations and evidence exist for the management of oral mucositis. On the other hand, appropriate assessment, intervention, and care of other adverse oral symptoms such as xerostomia, dysgeusia, dental problems and oral pain continue to need research. Patients with cancer who still experience the complex constellation of oral symptoms will often turn to complementary and alternative medicine (CAM) interventions for relief.

Research has shown that people choose to use CAM therapies because of a lack of effective assessment or intervention to provide relief, distrust in providers' concern for the patient's personal well-being, and a desire to control outcome, among other reasons (Humpel & Jones, 2006; Shen et al., 2008). As a result of the public's interest in CAM, the National Institutes of Health formed the National Center for Complementary and Alternative Medicine (NCCAM) in 1998 for the purpose of providing research support for evidence-based information on CAM therapies. Periodically, NCCAM will commission large surveys to learn about the public's use of CAM therapies, with the most recent completed in 2007. Results of this survey indicated that 4 out of 10, or about 38%, of all adults in the United States used some form of CAM at one time or another.

The numbers of patients with cancer who have used or tried a CAM therapy concurrent with allopathic (conventional) medical treatment in the United States range anywhere from 2% to 84% (Cassileth & Deng, 2004; Tascilar, de Jong, Veweij, & Mathijssen, 2006). A similar study conducted throughout Europe of CAM use in patients undergoing active cancer treatment found that patients with H&N and lung cancers comprised the smallest subsets of those using CAM (Molassiotis et al., 2005). This study used a cross-sectional survey design. Fourteen European member countries of the European Oncology Nursing Society participated in the research and surveyed more than 900 patients. The patient groups with the highest use-prevalence rate were those with pancreatic, liver, bone/spine, and brain cancers. The H&N cancer group was consistently around 20% in the various European countries surveyed. The reasons for these results were not studied, but the researchers theorized that perhaps those diagnosed with H&N cancer perceived high rates of cure with current treatment and therefore were confident in their treatment outcome.

Complementary and alternative treatments are used around the world for a wide variety of problems and continue to grow in popularity. People choose these methods for reasons such as philosophical beliefs of health and well-being, to treat problems and symptoms not otherwise treated, and for cost (Humpel & Jones, 2006; Shen et al., 2008). People may be satisfied with their overall cancer care but unsatisfied with the treatment of the side effects, with mucositis being a perfect example—a symptom that continues to be a struggle to manage. Tascilar et al. (2006) cited a Canadian survey that identified dissatisfaction with symptom and side effect management as a primary reason for use of CAM.

According to NCCAM (2010), the treatments most commonly used were nonvitamin, nonmineral products, such as omega-3, echinacea, and flaxseed oil, and deep breathing. Between 2002 and 2007, significant growth in the use of acupuncture and meditation was also noted (Barnes, Bloom, & Nahin, 2008).

As a result of these surveys confirming high use of CAM, healthcare providers are well advised to heed the importance of recognizing the use of CAM, as reflected in documents such as the Oncology Nursing Society's (2009) position statement on CAM and integrative therapies in cancer care and the Association of Community Cancer Centers' (2009) *Cancer Program Guidelines*, which includes discussion on integrative therapies. Both organizations state the expectation that healthcare providers shall listen to patients and support their choices and autonomy. The Society for Integrative Oncology has made several recommendations for utilizing integrative therapies in safe and effective manners (see www.integrativeonc.org) to help providers support their patients (Cassileth et al., 2007).

Definitions

The terms *complementary, alternative,* and now *integrative* have often been used interchangeably; however, they are, in fact, distinct terms with different definitions (NCCAM, 2010).
- **Complementary:** treatments used concurrently *with* allopathic or conventional treatment; usually focus on symptom management and quality of life; and are noninvasive (e.g., acupuncture to treat pain or nausea and vomiting)
- **Alternative:** treatments used in replacement of allopathic treatment (e.g., chelation therapy to remove heavy metals from a person's blood)
- **Integrative:** treatments that include the body, mind, and soul; are blended with conventional treatments for best effect; and the interventions have evidence supporting their safety and efficacy (e.g., omega-3 fatty acid supplement in addition to a prescription statin medication to reduce cholesterol)

Evidence for Use

The challenge to all healthcare providers, including nurses, in providing sound, evidence-based care using integrative therapies is in the persisting lack of strong evidence for most CAM interventions, regardless of their use. Although research is growing, it is limited because of poor funding, few qualified investigators, and problems with methodology and ethical issues (Cassileth et al., 2007). Smith, Olaku, Michie, and White (2008) assessed the interests of cancer researchers in collaborating with CAM practitioners as well as the researchers' concerns in regard to the barriers to conducting CAM research via a survey. Three hundred twenty-one respondents completed the survey, and 298 had participated in cancer research. Symptom and side effect management was identified as one of the high-priority areas for research. More than 80% of the respondents were willing to collaborate with a CAM practitioner for research. The lack of available funding to support this collaboration was identified as the largest barrier to carrying out the studies.

Interventions for Dysgeusia

Alteration in taste is a disturbing side effect of cancer treatment that is common and distressing. Taste changes can, and often do, lead to taste fatigue, poor oral intake, poor nutrition, and weight loss, all of which have an impact on overall outcome (Ravasco, 2005). Permanent taste changes are highly likely at radiation doses of 6,000 cGy, and at lower doses may take up to a year to even partially recover (Rubira et al., 2007). To date, no CAM interventions have evidence to support their use in mitigating this very irritating side effect. However, anecdotally, lemon juice and citrus flavors have been traditionally recommended to improve taste changes and facilitate eating.

Not effective—zinc sulfate: A large, phase III, double blind, two-arm, placebo controlled, multisite study of zinc sulfate 45 mg (n = 61) or placebo (n = 71) given three times a day to patients receiving more than 2,000 cGy radiation over at least 30% of the oral cavity was conducted. The intervention was given during the therapy and for one month after completion. No effect on preventing taste changes with the zinc supplementation was found (Halyard et al., 2007).

Interventions for Oral Mucositis

Oral mucositis is an inflammatory process that can range from oral irritation to a severe reaction necessitating the disruption of therapy, risking serious effects on disease outcome. Oral mucositis has been estimated to occur in up to 100% of patients receiving high-dose chemotherapy for bone marrow transplantation. It is estimated at 80% incidence with standard chemotherapy doses for patients with H&N cancers, both with and without radiation to the oral cavity, and 50% for other cancers (Chiappelli, 2005; Rubenstein et al., 2004). Risk factors for mucositis include the following (Chiappelli, 2005; Rubenstein et al., 2004).
- Oral mucosa in the radiation field (including upper cervical spine metastatic treatment)
- Chemotherapy
  - Pyrimidines (fluorouracil, capecitabine)
  - Anthracyclines (daunorubicin, doxorubicin, epirubicin, idarubicin, mitoxantrone)
- Poor oral hygiene
- Poor dental health

Research-Based Prevention

Cryotherapy: Cryotherapy has been used for many years and has shown effectiveness the longest. Chewing on ice for 20–30 minutes causes the mouth to cool down and the mucosal tissue to vasoconstrict. This limits the mucosal cells' exposure to the chemotherapy. Cryotherapy has been shown to be effective in the reduction of mucositis incidence and severity when used prior to, during, and after doses of chemotherapy with short half-lives such as bolus-only fluorouracil, high-dose melphalan, and edatrexate (Migliorati, Oberle-Edwards, & Schubert, 2006). It is too difficult to continually chew ice for the full time of continuous fluorouracil infusion (Rubenstein et al., 2004). There were attempts to lengthen the duration of the cryotherapy, hoping for better coverage and efficacy. A 60-minute duration of chewing on ice did not have any effect on the degree of mucositis the patient experienced (Stokman et al., 2006).

Cryotherapy is a preventive method, appropriate for people receiving chemotherapy, and is effective, inexpensive, and easy to administer. The challenge becomes the discomfort with chewing on ice for 30 minutes (Keefe et al., 2007).

Licorice (root of *Glycyrrhiza glabra*): Licorice is an expectorant used in Ayurvedic medicine (where it is commonly found in tooth powder). It is used topically for aphthous ulcer and oral herpes treatment. Glycyrrhizic acid from licorice is the active ingredient in Gelclair® (EKR Therapeutics, Inc.), now U.S. Food and Drug Administration–approved for mucositis management. Compounds in licorice can be toxic at doses as low as 50 g (2 oz) a day. Caution should be taken with this root, especially when liver dysfunction or hypertension is present. Deglycyrrhizinated licorice has been produced to avoid these toxic side effects (U.S. National Library of Medicine MedlinePlus®, 2010).

Payayor (*Clinacanthus nutans*): Payayor is a medicinal plant preparation from Thailand traditionally used for burns, insect bites, rashes, herpes simplex and zoster, and varicella lesions. It has localized analgesic and anti-inflammatory action. Payayor preparations are available over the counter in Thailand, and it was the first medicinal plant product approved for use in Thai hospitals. A randomized clinical trial by Putwatana et al. (2009) compared glycerin payayor oral drops to benzydamine mouth rinse in 60 patients receiving H&N radiation therapy. The payayor group (n = 30) experienced delayed onset of oral mucositis (at 1.24 weeks versus 0.44 weeks for the benzydamine group) and significantly less weight loss, and xerostomia and taste alteration were delayed in the intervention group. The severity of mucositis was the same in both groups when it occurred.

Traditional Chinese medicine: Indigowood root (*Isatis indigotica Fort.* or Ban Lan Gen) is an herb used in traditional Chinese medicine (TCM) for the removal of toxic heat in the blood and the relief of convulsions. It has been found to contain components that have antiviral, anti-inflammatory, and antipyretic effects. TCM uses mixtures of different, mostly plant, materials in remedies; however, indigowood root was a key ingredient in the following studies. Radiation-related injury is explained in TCM to be "evil fire heat," which injures both yin and qi. In a very small, prospective, double-blind, randomized control arm study of patients receiving H&N radiation, 20 participants were randomized to two groups. The control group (n = 9) used normal saline mouth rinse, and the intervention arm (n = 11) used a prophylactic application using 30 ml indigowood root solution to gargle for three minutes and swallow before meals daily. The study arm showed a significant effect on the severity of mucositis in patients receiving radiation to the oral cavity. Four participants in the intervention arm versus two of the control arm were able to complete treatment without breaks (You, Hsieh, & Huang, 2009).

Randomized controlled trials have reported on two different TCM decoctions (tea, infusion) possible for use in the reduction or prevention of radiation-induced oral mucositis. Wu, Yuan, Liu, and Wang (2007) found that **Qingre Liyan decoction** (QRLYD) was beneficial because of the "use of its function in clearing heat to expel toxin, nourishing yin, and supplementing qi, and activating blood circulation to remove blood stasis" (p. 280). This two-arm study of 60 participants was equally randomized to either a control arm using Dobell's solution (sodium borate, sodium bicarbonate, phenol, and glycerol) or the QRLYD intervention. QRLYD was found to be effective in increasing the concentration of epidermal growth factor in the saliva, which helps to promote the repair process of membrane renewal. The researchers also describe evidence for the TCM effect, which is too complex for the purposes of this chapter. Dai, Li, Wang, Li, and Yang (2009) found that **Yangyin Humo decoction** (YHD) given orally six times a day in addition to the standard, control arm intervention of IV lidocaine, dexamethasone, gentamycin, vitamin B_{12}, and normal saline solution was beneficial. The control arm also had a sodium bicarbonate oral rinse. Forty-two participants were equally randomized to the two arms. The intervention arm experienced delayed reaction of oral mucosal membranes to radiation, lessened severity, and accelerated repair time after a lesion occurred in the group that had the additive. The researchers, however, found that YHD is limited in use alone because prolonged use promoted dampness and injured Pi-wei (yin), as seen in a thick, greasy tongue coating and resultant poor appetite. Pi-wei is understood in TCM as the spleen-stomach network where food is changed to nourish qi. The researchers recommended that TCM medicines be added to strengthen Pi to avoid this limitation.

Interventions That Are Not Harmful and May Be Useful

Aloe vera: Aloe vera (AV) is a plant-based remedy that has a long history of common topical use for mild burns and sunburn. AV juice has been used as a very effective laxative. Two trials have studied the use of AV to treat oral mucositis. Su et al. (2004) studied a total of 58 patients with H&N cancer who received radiation therapy (28 in the AV group and 30 in the placebo group). This study showed no statistically significant differences in the severity or duration of mucositis. Other measures, such as quality of life, weight loss, and use of pain medication, were also comparable.

In Thailand, Puataweepong et al. (2009) performed a double-blind, placebo-controlled study with patients with H&N cancer receiving radiation therapy. Their sample size was 61, with 30 people in the AV group and 31 in the placebo group. The groups were instructed to take 15 ml of solution three times daily during their course of radiation and through the end of the eighth week in follow-up. The study arm used a solution of 80% AV juice with a small amount of preservative, lemon-lime flavoring, and sweetener. The placebo was matched for taste. All were instructed in usual oral care and had supportive care for mucositis available to them. The results showed that the AV juice did not affect the onset of mucositis but did decrease the severity. This study showed that 53% of the AV group experienced severe mucositis compared to 87% in the placebo group. Other measures such as breaks in treatment and weight loss did not have statistically significant differences, but the aloe group did have fewer treatment breaks and less weight loss. The researchers noted that AV does not seem to prevent mucositis but helps to decrease the severity and help with healing. There were differences in the solutions, and this group observed their solution may have had more essential active compounds such as glycoproteins, which are recognized for their healing and anti-inflammatory properties. AV was used in the radiation therapy population of patients with H&N cancer, and because of the small group, additional research is needed. The researchers concluded that AV solution could be a good alternative to treat radiation mucositis, and it is readily accessible and inexpensive to produce.

Honey: Honey has been used medicinally since the time of the Ancient Egyptians and continues to be useful in current wound healing. Derived from flower nectar, honey has been found to have antibacterial action and encourages epithelialization of tissue (Simon et al., 2009). Honey has been found to be useful in mucositis as well, although most studies have been small nonblinded or nonrandomized (Bardy, Slevin, Mais, & Molassiotis, 2008). Honey is inexpensive and readily available. Motallebnejad, Akram, Moghadamnia, Moulana, and Omidi (2008) found, in their randomized trial of 40 patients randomized to honey or saline rinse during H&N field radiation, that the treatment arm showed a significant reduction in mucositis. All patients were treated via cobalt 60 to a total dose of 50–60 Gy over five to six weeks. Participants received usual oral care recommendations and were randomized equally to two arms. The intervention arm swished and slowly swallowed 20 ml pure natural honey 15 minutes before radiation therapy and a 20 ml dose again at 15 minutes and then 6 hours after each radiation treatment. The control arm members rinsed their mouths before and after each radiation treatment with 20 ml normal saline. Weekly evaluations using the Oral Mucositis Assessing Scale were used to score response. Twenty percent (four patients) of the intervention arm had no evidence of mucositis during the length of treatment. Ten patients (50%) in the intervention arm had no weight loss during treatment, whereas the control group's mean weight loss was 2–11 kg.

Another small, well-designed Egyptian study (Rashad, Al-Gezawy, El-Gezawy, & Azzaz, 2009) looked at *Candida* colonization. This study consisted of 40 patients with H&N cancer receiving radiation randomized to usual care with and without prophylactic application of honey. Participants were evaluated weekly to assess for mucositis; aerobic cultures and *Candida* colonization were completed via swabs before and at completion of radiation therapy or when infection was identified. The intervention group had no development of grade 4 mucositis, and three participants (15%) developed grade 3 mucositis. The control group, on the other hand, had 13 patients (65%) with grade 3 or 4 mucositis. Candida colonization was greater in the control group, with 60% versus 15% positive cultures in the intervention group.

Biswal, Zakaria, and Ahmad (2003) performed a randomized controlled study involving 40 patients using topical honey with radiation (treatment) versus radiation therapy alone (control). They hoped to show that the honey would enhance the reepithelialization of the mucosa and decrease morbidity. Patients used 20 ml of honey before radiation, another 20 ml after radiation, and another 20 ml six hours later. They rinsed or swished the honey in their mouth, then slowly swallowed it to allow it to completely coat the oral and pharyngeal mucosa. Both groups had usual instruction for adequate fluid intake, good oral care, and a high-protein diet. All 20 patients in the honey treatment arm completed the course, with results showing a significant reduction in grade 3 and 4 mucositis (p = 0.0058). There was no significant difference between the treatment and control groups in grade 1 and 2 mucositis, but only 20% of the treatment arm had grade 3 and 4 mucositis, while 75% of the control arm had grade 3 and 4 mucositis. As a result, 20% (4 patients) of the control arm had to take a break from radiation, whereas all the patients in the honey treatment arm were able to complete their radiation on time. It was also noted that 55% of the honey treatment patients maintained or gained weight, in contrast to only 25% in the control arm (p = 0.053). Blood sugars were monitored and showed no changes with the use of honey. No adverse events were noted (Biswal et al., 2003). It is recognized that this study is small, and honey would need to be studied against another intervention such as cryotherapy as opposed to no or minimal intervention as has been conducted thus far. To confidently recommend honey would need additional research. Honey treatment also may be effective in chemotherapy-induced mucositis and is simple and inexpensive.

Ratanhia: In Germany, ratanhia and myrrh are used as "phytotherapeutics" for the local treatment of mild inflammation of the oral mucosa. A poorly designed, prospective, single-arm study of proprietary oral products (mouthwash and toothpaste) made by the Swiss herbal manufacturer Weleda, found no negative effects on patients with breast cancer using these products during chemotherapy (Tiemann, Toelg, & Ramos, 2006). The study was unable to differentiate between the effect of good oral hygiene and the use of these products because it lacked a control arm. The study had 49 participants who all insisted on being in the treatment group. Thirty-two out of the 49 participants were able to complete the study. The study included a complete professional dental cleaning. The products were used three times a day for four weeks. Chemotherapy given included carboplatin, cyclophosphamide, epirubicin, and paclitaxel. One of the researchers also worked for Weleda (Tiemann et al., 2006).

Zinc supplementation is used for a variety of immune support situations and has found some use in mucositis. A double-blind, randomized study (N = 97) was carried out to evaluate the effectiveness in improving mucositis and dermatitis after radiation therapy for patients with H&N cancer. Forty-nine patients received capsules containing 25 mg of oral zinc, and the other 48 received a soybean oil capsule placebo. Each group took three capsules daily from the first to the last radiation treatment, including nontreatment days such as weekends. The experimental group had fewer cases of grade 3 mucositis (p = 0.0003) and to a lesser degree (p = 0.003) than the control group. The duration of mucositis was also shorter for the experimental group. Zinc supplementation did not have much effect on those patients receiving concurrent chemotherapy. A standard dose has not been determined, nor has the effect on tumor growth been determined (Lin, Que, Lin, & Lin, 2006).

Management

Relaxation and imagery: Syrjala, Donaldson, Davis, Kippes, and Carr (1995) showed that 94 bone marrow transplant recipients with oral mucositis pain experienced reduced pain when trained in and using relaxation and imagery; adding cognitive-behavioral skills did not provide any further relief. Participants were randomized to four intervention conditions: (1) treatment-as-usual control, (2) therapist support, (3) relaxation and imagery training, and (4) cognitive-behavioral skills training including relaxation and imagery. Clarkson et al. (2007) have criticized this study as not discussing the alternatives to the study available to the subjects.

Interventions With No or Weak Evidence but May Be Useful

Topical capsaicin was used in a very small study (N = 11) and was found to provide temporary reduction of mucositis pain. Capsaicin is the active ingredient in chili pepper, or cayenne. Topical capsaicin had been used previously in studies of postherpetic neuralgia but could be studied further as a possible temporary pain desensitizer if used prior to the onset of mucositis (Berger et al., 1995). All patients verbally rated their pain on a 0–10 scale. The capsaicin was placed in taffy. Taffy was considered a good medium because the sucrose and the oral manipulation in chewing the candy lessened the burning of the capsaicin. All 11 participants reported clinical pain relief but required four to six candies over two to four days for pain relief. Two participants ultimately discontinued the use of the candy, one because of nausea and the other because of a recurrence of burning hemorrhoids. There have not been further studies of capsaicin on mucositis pain.

Chamomile (*Matricaria recutita L.*): Chamomile is a flower traditionally made into tea for stomach ailments and anxiety. Chamomile is found to have anti-inflammatory action. Mazokopakis, Vrentzos, Papadakis, Babalis, and Ganotakis (2005) reported in a case study that chamomile mouthwash was used effectively by a patient with oral mucositis from methotrexate for rheumatoid arthritis.

A larger, phase III, randomized, double-blind study of patients on fluorouracil-based regimens over a 14-day period found no difference between the chamomile mouthwash and the placebo mouthwash (Fidler et al., 1996). The researchers studied 165 participants receiving fluorouracil chemotherapy in a placebo-controlled trial. All participants used cryotherapy for 30 minutes before chemotherapy administration and then were randomized to either a chamomile or placebo mouthwash to be used three times a day for 14 days. The solution consisted of 100 ml water mixed with 30 drops of either chamomile or placebo mixture. Participants swished the solution around their mouth for approximately one minute and spat it out. This was repeated until all of the 100 ml was used. Participants repeated the procedure three times a day. At the conclusion, no statistical difference was seen between the two groups regarding the severity of mucositis. Of interest was the fact that men seemed to have less mucositis than women, for no explained reason. There was no evidence that chamomile caused any toxicity.

Oren-gedoku-to: Oren-gedoku-to (Huang-Lian-Jie-Du-Tang in TCM), a Japanese herbal antioxidant, was compared to a placebo mouthwash of allopurinol, sodium gualenate, and povidone-iodine in patients with leukemia. The researchers found a decrease in mucositis of almost two-thirds in the treatment arm (Yuki, Kawaguchi, Hazemoto, & Asou, 2003).

Slippery elm (*Ulmus rubra* or *Ulmus fulva*): The leaves of this North American tree contain mucilage that becomes a gel when mixed with water. It is commonly used for ailments soothed by coating with this gel, such as sore throat, cough, gastroesophageal reflux disease, Crohn disease, or ulcerative colitis, and topically for burns, wounds, or rashes. There are no studies on slippery elm for oral mucositis; however, it is a common herbal product traditionally used as listed previously ("Slippery Elm," 2010).

Syousaikotou: Syousaikotou is a Japanese herbal medication used for chemotherapy-induced oral mucositis in the form of a gargle. A study comparing syousaikotou to a povidone-iodine and amphotericin B mixture found that the study arm experienced a significantly decreased incidence and severity of stomatitis. The lingering question would be regarding the rationale for the control arm gargle, which is known to be unpleasant. The research was published in Japanese, and the rationale is not included in the abstract (Matsuoka et al., 2004).

Traumeel S® (Heel, Inc.) is a proprietary homeopathic remedy that has shown some success in treating mucositis. Homeopathy is based on the principle of treating like with like—something that can cause a symptom in a healthy person is used to treat a person that has a similar symptom. For example, *Apis mellifica* is derived from bees and used to treat a person with symptoms similar to a bee sting (acute onset, swelling, pain relieved with cold compress). The treatments are solutions that have varying degrees of dilution, with the thought that the more dilute, the stronger the treatment. Homeopathy is considered safe, with few interactions with other agents and few side effects. Homeopathy is different from herbal medications, which need to be used more cautiously with usual cancer treatments (Kassab, Cummings, Berkovitz, van Haselen, & Fisher, 2009). Review of the data shows that many of the studies were more successful with those receiving radiation therapy than those receiving chemotherapy (Worthington, Clarkson, & Eden, 2007).

Sencer et al. (2009) piloted a study of Traumeel S for mucositis in Israel in the pediatric bone marrow transplant population and found no evidence of effect on mucositis treatment. The study included 190 pediatric stem cell transplant recipients. Participants would swish and swallow the solution five times a day from day 1 of chemotherapy until the mucositis was resolved. No statistical difference was seen between the group using Traumeel S and the placebo group. (This study has been praised as a large, rigorous clinical trial using a CAM therapy carried out using conventional methods of study, despite proving the null.)

Interventions That Are Not Recommended

L-glutamine as a preventive or management systemic treatment for mucositis is currently not recommended by the 2007 Multinational Association of Supportive Care in Cancer/International Society for Oral Oncology mucositis guidelines (Keefe et al., 2007). The reviewers specifically cited a well-designed study (Pytlík et al., 2002) of 40 bone marrow transplant recipients where not only a higher severity of mucositis occurred in the glutamine group but also an increased rate of disease recurrence after two years. A Cochrane review is currently reviewing glutamine supplementation and mucositis in colorectal cancer (Pinto de Lemos, Lemos, Atallah, & Soares, 2004).

However, glutamine has a long history of being used for mucositis and has been viewed as a conditionally essential amino acid in the case of illness or injury. It is necessary for cell mitosis, especially in those cells with rapid turnover, as in the mucosal cells lining the gastrointestinal system. The amino acid is found in the skeletal muscle, mucosa, and plasma. When the body is under stress, such as with chemotherapy treatment, the glutamine is pulled from the skeletal muscle into the gastrointestinal mucosa to assist with cellular regeneration. However, a shortage will develop with the draining of the glutamine, resulting in the initiation of the inflammatory reaction and potential ulcers (Keefe et al., 2007; Noé, 2009; Stokman et al., 2006).

Huang et al. (2000) found that oral glutamine may be effective in reducing the severity or duration of oral mucositis greater than grade 3. The researchers found that oral glutamine was effective in those patients receiving H&N radiation therapy.

Anderson, Schroeder, and Skubitz (1998) studied the effect of glutamine on 24 patients (mostly children) who had experienced moderate to severe oral mucositis during at least one cycle of chemotherapy. They had a twice-daily dose of glutamine suspension, 2 g/m^2 in 4 ml/m^2, days 1–14 of the chemotherapy cycle. Patients swished and swallowed the suspension in the morning and evening. If the mucositis was too painful for swallowing, patients were allowed to swish and spit out the suspension. Statistically significant results showed patients using the glutamine solution experienced 4.5 fewer days of mouth pain than those who used the placebo.

The next challenge was to identify the dosage needed. In Anderson et al.'s (1998) research, doses of glutamine varied from 0.13 g/kg/day to 2 g/m², twice daily. According to Noé's (2009) meta-analysis, the ideal dosing is 20–30 g in divided dosing, thus exposing the gastrointestinal tract to the glutamine more often and enabling cellular regeneration. The inconsistent dosing presents a challenge for healthcare providers.

Oral glutamine is easy to administer, using suspension fluid with a sweetener, and the patient will ideally swish and swallow 10 g three times a day. It is important that as much of the mucosa comes in contact with the glutamine as possible to enable cellular regeneration (Noé, 2009).

Interventions for Orofacial Pain (Excluding Oral Mucositis)

The orofacial region is highly innervated, and necessary motor functions such as speaking, chewing, swallowing, and others are unavoidable triggers if there is pain (Epstein, Elad, Eliav, Jurevic, & Benoliel, 2007). CAM approaches such as hypnosis have been used as a complement to usual pain management but have not been specifically studied to learn their direct effect on orofacial pain.

Interventions for Xerostomia

Xerostomia, or the subjective sensation of dry mouth, is caused by a disruption in the production of saliva or the balance of components of oral saliva. The effects of radiation or surgery on the salivary glands are, therefore, likely to be permanent. It is important for the oncology nurse to recognize that xerostomia that is caused by cancer treatment can be compounded by common non-cancer medications that cause dry mouth as well (such as antihypertensives and antidepressants). Xerostomia is associated with interference with speaking, chewing and swallowing, oral pain or discomfort, infection, and poor dental outcomes, all of which have a significant impact on quality of life (Schiff et al., 2009).

Research-Based Interventions

Acupuncture: Many randomized controlled trials have shown acupuncture to be helpful in the relief of xerostomia. In reviewing six studies using acupuncture for cancer symptoms, Lu (2005) found that acupuncture is used for chemotherapy-induced nausea and vomiting and cancer pain. Other studies point to acupuncture being possibly effective in chemotherapy-induced leukopenia, postchemotherapy fatigue, radiation-induced xerostomia, insomnia, and anxiety. Lu's concern was that despite both the evidence and preliminary evidence, acupuncture remains grossly underutilized, which she saw as a possible quality-of-care issue. A review by Deng, Vickers, Yeung, and Cassileth (2006) of 60 articles supported Lu's analysis and concerns regarding underutilization of a potentially effective CAM intervention. These reviewers furthered the argument that acupuncture has a good safety record, which should support its wider use. Standish, Kozak, and Congdon (2008) found 27 randomized controlled clinical trials of acupuncture used with dyspnea, nausea and vomiting, pain, and xerostomia. Twenty-three of these studies reported statistically significant results in favor of the acupuncture intervention. Once again, these researchers noted that despite its safety, evidence of clinical effectiveness for common symptoms, and being reimbursable, acupuncture remains underutilized in the United States even though it is becoming well integrated into standard palliative care in the United Kingdom.

For the purpose of this chapter, two studies of acupuncture's effect on xerostomia will be described. Cho et al. (2008) conducted a very small pilot quality-of-life study of 12 patients with H&N cancer with radiation-induced xerostomia. The participants were randomized into two groups, one to have real acupuncture and the other to have a sham. Both interventions were conducted twice a week for six weeks in a single-blind setting (the provider knew who was having real versus sham acupuncture). Whole salivary flow rates, both stimulated and unstimulated, were measured. Participants completed a questionnaire to measure subjective symptoms before treatment and at three and six weeks after acupuncture treatment. Both groups showed a slight increase in whole salivary flow rates with no significant difference between the groups. However, the real acupuncture group had markedly increased unstimulated salivary flow and improved scores on the subjective questionnaires (2.33 versus 0.33 in the sham control group).

Meidell and Rasmussen (2009) studied mitigation of xerostomia in hospice patients with cancer. Over two years, the researchers assessed 117 patients for xerostomia; 82 patients had moderate xerostomia, and out of these, 67 met the inclusion criteria. Fourteen participants agreed to the study, but only eight completed it. The researchers found that after using a visual analog scale and measuring saliva production before and after completion of the acupuncture treatment series, dry mouth was alleviated. The problem with their study was with the design, as many hospice patients are not likely to be able to complete a five-week study when they are close to death.

Hypnosis: Schiff et al. (2009) conducted a small but intriguing pilot study of hypnosis on radiation-induced xerostomia in patients with H&N cancer. Twelve participants completed the single-arm, single-intervention study. Each study subject participated in one hypnosis session but was provided with a recording of the session that he or she would listen to at home twice a day for one month. Salivary flow measurements were completed after the first live hypnosis session. Nine patients (75%) had increased salivary flow following hypnosis. Eight patients (66%) reported overall improvement at 12 weeks. The researchers found no correlation between salivary flow rate measurements and subjective reporting (Spearman correlation coefficient $r = 0.134$). However, symptomatic improvement correlated significantly with the number of times the participant listened to the recording. Participants completed a validated questionnaire at 1, 4, and 12 weeks after the hypnosis session. The researchers found that the suggestion of increased salivary triggers using food imagery, such as recall of secretory responses to pleasurable food smells, and relaxation exercises could temper negative expectations of the effect of radiation on saliva ($r = 0.714$, $p = 0.009$). These triggers might optimize the physiological environment for salivation. The researchers commented that even if the rate of salivation was not improved, this was not a predictor of treatment failure. Although the study was very limited in size, the results are intriguing and may help oncology nurses to consider ways to teach patients about changes in salivation more positively. The researchers suggested that presentation of the potential problem can counteract negative expectations or a "nocebo" effect.

Interventions With No Research but May Be Helpful

Oral moisturizers and lubricants: Butter, margarine, or other liquid food oils are available in most home kitchens, and any of these can be applied directly to the surfaces of the oral cavity to help with lubrication. Margarine has been reported to this author as the longest lasting.

Oral sprays: Food oil sprays using light olive, corn, or other light-density food oils in 5 ml of oil to 100 ml of water has been recommended anecdotally. This mixture can be kept in a small spray bottle and sprayed into the mouth as needed to provide moisture and lessen friction. Another suggestion is saline solutions of less than 2 mg of table salt in 1 liter of water, brought to a boil and cooled prior to use. Patients can fill a pocket-sized spray bottle with this solution for frequent use in the mouth.

Xylitol: Xylitol is a natural sweetener that is commonly used in oral hygiene to prevent the development of dental caries (Peldyak & Makinen, 2002). Xylitol is used in many so-called sugarless chewing gums. Although xylitol has not been studied for its effect on cancer-related xerostomia, it is commonly recommended for overall dental health. The act of chewing itself is known to help stimulate the production of saliva (American Dental Association, 1995–2011).

Conclusion

As patients look for assistance in treating oral symptoms of cancer and cancer treatment with CAM therapies, oncology nurses have a key role in helping them learn and decide about appropriate therapies. The initial step for a healthcare practitioner is to evaluate one's own personal and professional beliefs and knowledge level about CAM. A key skill is to learn about evidence-based practice and how to assess the information that is provided for accuracy and validity. This will assist the nurse in learning about the various therapies and will assist patients in their decision making (Decker, 2008).

Nurses have a role in being able to listen to patients in a supportive way, to learn about the treatments they are using or are interested in using, and to educate patients on how to verify practitioner skills and qualifications. Nurses can easily ask patients and families about other treatments or supplements they are using, encouraging them to share any information to help with their care planning. As a part of the interdisciplinary team, nurses can facilitate the discussion and plan of care between the integrative therapies, physicians, and the patient. Finally, opportunities exist for nursing research to improve supportive care in oral symptoms, utilizing some of these remedies that are potentially inexpensive and effective but relatively unknown.

References

American Dental Association. (1995–2011). Chewing gum. Retrieved from http://www.ada.org/1315.aspx

Anderson, P.M., Schroeder, G., & Skubitz, K.M. (1998). Oral glutamine reduces the duration and severity of stomatitis after cytotoxic cancer chemotherapy. *Cancer, 83,* 1433–1439. doi:10.1002/(SICI)1097-0142(19981001)83:7<1433::AID-CNCR22>3.0.CO;2-4

Association of Community Cancer Centers. (2009). *Cancer program guidelines.* Rockville, MD: Author.

Bardy, J., Slevin, N.J., Mais, K.L., & Molassiotis, A. (2008). A systematic review of honey uses and its potential value within oncology care. *Journal of Clinical Nursing, 17,* 2604–2623. doi:10.1111/j.1365-2702.2008.02304.x

Barnes, P., Bloom, B., & Nahin, R. (2008). *Complementary and alternative medicine use among adults and children: United States* (National Health Statistics Reports, No. 12). Hyattsville, MD: National Center for Health Statistics.

Berger, A., Henderson, M., Nadoolman, W., Duffy, V., Cooper, D., Saberski, L., & Bartoshuk, L. (1995). Oral capsaicin provides temporary relief for oral mucositis secondary to chemotherapy/radiation therapy. *Journal of Pain and Symptom Management, 10,* 243–248. doi:10.1016/0885-3924(94)00130-D

Biswal, B., Zakaria, A., & Ahmad, N. (2003). Topical application of honey in the management of radiation mucositis: A preliminary study. *Supportive Care in Cancer, 11,* 242–248. doi:10.1007s00520-003-0443-y

Cassileth, B.R., & Deng, G. (2004). Complementary and alternative therapies for cancer. *Oncologist, 9,* 80–89.

Cassileth, B.R., Deng, G.E., Jorge, E.E., Johnstone, P.A., Kumar, N., & Vickers, A.J. (2007). Complementary therapies and integrative oncology in lung cancer: ACCP evidence-based clinical practice guidelines (2nd edition). *Chest, 132*(Suppl. 3), 340S–354S. doi:10.1378/chest.07-1389

Chiappelli, F. (2005). The molecular immunology of mucositis: Implications for evidence-based research in alternative and complementary palliative treatments. *Evidence-Based Complementary and Alternative Medicine, 2,* 489–494. doi:10.1093/ecam/neh129

Cho, J.H., Chung, W.K., Kang, W., Choi, S.M., Cho, C.K., & Son, C.G. (2008). Manual acupuncture improved quality of life in cancer patients with radiation-induced xerostomia. *Journal of Alternative and Complementary Medicine, 14,* 523–526. doi:10.1089/acm.2007.0793

Clarkson, J.E., Worthington, H.V., Furness, S., McCabe, M., Khalid, T., & Meyer, S. (2010). Interventions for treating oral mucositis for patients with cancer receiving treatment. *Cochrane Database of Systematic Reviews* 2010, Issue 8. Art. No.: CD001973. doi:10.1002/14651858.CD001973.pub4

Dai, A.W., Li, Z.Y., Wang, L.H., Li, S.Y., & Yang, H. (2009). Effect of Yangyin Humo Decoction on oral mucomembranous reaction to radiotherapy. *Chinese Journal of Integrative Medicine, 15,* 303–306. doi:10.1007/s11655-009-0303-9

Decker, G.M. (2008). The marriage of conventional cancer treatments and alternative cancer therapies. *Nursing Clinics of North America, 43,* 221–241. doi:10.1016/j.cnur.2008.02.006

Deng, G., Vickers, A., Yeung, K.S., & Cassileth, B.R. (2006). Acupuncture: Integration into cancer care. *Journal of the Society for Integrative Oncology, 4,* 86–92.

Epstein, J.B., Elad, S., Eliav, E., Jurevic, R., & Benoliel, R. (2007). Orofacial pain in cancer: Part II—Clinical perspectives and management. *Journal of Dental Research, 86,* 506–518. doi:10.1177/154405910708600605

Fidler, P., Loprinzi, C.L., O'Fallon, J.R., Leitch, J.M., Lee, J.K., Hayes, D.L., … Michalak, J.C. (1996). Prospective evaluation of a chamomile mouthwash for prevention of 5-FU-induced oral mucositis. *Cancer, 77,* 522–525. doi:10.1002/(SICI)1097-0142(19960201)77:3<522::AID-CNCR14>3.0.CO;2-6

Halyard, M.Y., Jatoi, A., Sloan, J.A., Bearden, J.D., III, Vora, S.A., Atherton, P.J., … & Loprinzi, C.L. (2007). Does zinc sulfate prevent therapy-induced taste alterations in head and neck cancer patients? Results of phase III double-blind, placebo-controlled trial from the North Central Cancer Treatment Group (N01C4). *International Journal of Radiation Oncology, Biology, Physics, 67,* 1318–1322. doi:10.1016/j.ijrobp.2006.10.046

Huang, E.Y., Leung, S.W., Wang, C.J., Chen, H.C., Sun, L.M., Fang, F.M., … Hsiung, C.Y. (2000). Oral glutamine to alleviate radiation-induced oral mucositis: A pilot randomized trial. *International Journal of Radiation Oncology, Biology, Physics, 46,* 535–539. doi:10.1016/S0360-3016(99)00402-2

Humpel, N., & Jones, S.C. (2006). Gaining insight into the what, why and where of complementary and alternative medicine use by cancer patients and survivors. *European Journal of Cancer Care, 15,* 362–368. doi:10.1111/j.1365-2354.2006.00667.x

Kassab, S., Cummings, M., Berkovitz, S., van Haselen, R., & Fisher, P. (2009). Homeopathic medicines for adverse effects of cancer treatments. *Cochrane Database of Systematic Reviews* 2009, Issue 2. Art. No.: CD004845. doi:10.1002/14651858.CD004845.pub2

Keefe, D.M., Schubert, M.M., Elting, L.S., Sonis, S.T., Epstein, J.B., Raber-Durlacher, J.E., … Peterson, D.E. (2007). Updated clinical practice guidelines for the prevention and treatment of mucositis. *Cancer, 109,* 820–831. doi:10.1002/cncr.22484

Lin, L.C., Que, J., Lin, L.K., & Lin, F.C. (2006). Zinc supplementation to improve mucositis and dermatitis in patients after radiotherapy for head-and-neck cancers: A double-blind, randomized study. *International Journal of Radiation Oncology, Biology, Physics, 65,* 745–750. doi:10.1016/j.ijrobp.2006.01.015

Lu, W. (2005). Acupuncture for side effects of chemoradiation therapy in cancer patients. *Seminars in Oncology Nursing, 21,* 190–195. doi:10.1016/j.soncn.2005.04.008

Matsuoka, H., Mizushima, Y., Kawano, M., Tachibana, N., Sawada, Y., Kato, S., … Tadanobu, K. (2004). Clinical availability of the herbal medicine, Syousaikotou, as a gargling agent for prevention and treatment of chemotherapy-induced stomatitis [Abstract]. *Gan To Kagaku Ryoho, 31,* 2017–2020.

Mazokopakis, E.E., Vrentzos, G.E., Papadakis, J.A., Babalis, D.E., & Ganotakis, E.S. (2005). Wild chamomile (Matricaria recutita L.) mouthwashes in methotrexate-induced oral mucositis. *Phytomedicine, 12,* 25–27.

Meidell, L., & Rasmussen, B.H. (2009). Acupuncture as an optional treatment for hospice patients with xerostomia: An intervention study. *International Journal of Palliative Nursing, 15,* 12–20.

Migliorati, C.A., Oberle-Edwards, L., & Schubert, M. (2006). The role of alternative and natural agents, cryotherapy, and/or laser for management of alimentary mucositis. *Supportive Care in Cancer, 14,* 533–540. doi:10.1007/s00520-006-0049-2

Molassiotis, A., Fernadez-Ortega, P., Pud, D., Ozden, G., Scott, J.A., Panteli, V., ... Patiraki, E. (2005). Use of complementary and alternative medicine in cancer patients: A European survey. *Annals of Oncology, 16,* 655–663. doi:10.1093/annonc/mdi110

Motallebnejad, M., Akram, S., Moghadamnia, A., Moulana, Z., & Omidi, S. (2008). The effect of topical application of pure honey on radiation-induced mucositis: A randomized clinical trial. *Journal of Contemporary Dental Practice, 9*(3), 40–47.

National Center for Complementary and Alternative Medicine. (2010, April). What is complementary and alternative medicine? Retrieved from http://nccam.nih.gov/health/whatiscam

Noé, J.E. (2009). L-glutamine use in the treatment and prevention of mucositis and cachexia: A naturopathic perspective. *Integrative Cancer Therapies, 8,* 409–415. doi:10.1177/1534735409348865

Oncology Nursing Society. (2009). The use of complementary, alternative, and integrative therapies in cancer care [Position statement]. Retrieved from http://www.ons.org/Publications/Positions/CAM

Peldyak, J., & Makinen, K. (2002). Xylitol for caries prevention. *Journal of Dental Hygiene, 76,* 276–285.

Pinto de Lemos, H., Lemos, A., Atallah, Á., & Soares, B. (2004). Glutamine supplementation in enteral or parenteral nutrition for the incidence of mucositis in colorectal cancer (Protocol). *Cochrane Database of Systematic Reviews,* Issue 1. Art. No.: CD004650. doi:10.1002/14651858.CD004650

Pytlík, R., Benes, P., Patorková, M., Chocenská, E., Gregora, E., Procházka, B., & Kozák, T. (2002). Standardized parenteral alanyl-glutamine dipeptide supplementation is not beneficial in autologous transplant patients: A randomized, double-blind, placebo controlled study. *Bone Marrow Transplantation, 30,* 953–961.

Puataweepong, P., Dhanachai, M., Dangprasert, S., Sithatani, C., Swangsilp, T., Narkwong, L., ... Intragumtornchai, T. (2009). The efficacy of oral aloe vera juice for radiation induced mucositis in head and neck cancer patients: A double-blind placebo-controlled study. *Asian Biomedicine, 3,* 375–382.

Putwatana, P., Sanmanowong, P., Oonprasertpong, L., Junda, T., Pitiporn, S., & Narkwong, L. (2009). Relief of radiation-induced oral mucositis in head and neck cancer. *Cancer Nursing, 32,* 82–87. doi:10.1097/01.NCC.0000343362.68129.ed

Rashad, U.M., Al-Gezawy, S.M., El-Gezawy, E., & Azzaz, A.N. (2009). Honey as topical prophylaxis against radiochemotherapy-induced mucositis in head and neck cancer. *Journal of Laryngology and Otology, 123,* 223 –228. doi:10.1017/S0022215108002478

Ravasco, P. (2005). Aspects of taste and compliance in patients with cancer. *European Journal of Oncology Nursing, 9*(Suppl. 2), S84–S91. doi:10.1016/j.ejon.2005.09.003

Rubenstein, E.B., Peterson, D.E., Schubert, M., Keefe, D., McGuire, D., Epstein, J., ... Sonis, S.T. (2004). Clinical practice guidelines for the prevention and treatment of cancer therapy-induced oral and gastrointestinal mucositis. *Cancer, 100*(Suppl. 9), 2026–2046. doi:10.1002/cncr.20163

Rubira, C.M., Devides, N.J., Ubeda, L.T., Bortulucci, A.G., Jr., Lauris, J.R., Rubira-Bullen, I.R., & Damante, J.H. (2007). Evaluation of some oral postradiotherapy sequelae in patients treated for head and neck tumors. *Brazilian Oral Research, 21,* 272–277. doi:10.1590/S1806-83242007000300014

Schiff, E., Mogilner, J.G., Sella, E., Doweck, I., Hershko, O., Ben-Arye, E., & Yarom, N. (2009). Hypnosis for postradiation xerostomia in head and neck cancer patients: A pilot study. *Journal of Pain and Symptom Management, 37,* 1086–1092. doi:10.1016/j.jpainsymman.2008.07.005

Sencer, S., Zhou, T., Oberbaum, M., Freedman, L., McLean, T., Sahdev, I., & Ives, J. (2009, April 24). *The efficacy of the homeopathic agent Traumeel S® in the prevention and treatment of mucositis in children undergoing stem cell transplantation.* Abstract presented at the American Society of Pediatric Hematology/Oncology. Retrieved from http://aspho.confex.com/aspho/2009/webprogram/paper2380.html

Shen, J., Anderson, R., Albert, P.S., Wenger, N., Glaspy, J., Cole, M., & Shekelle, P. (2008). Use of complementary/alternative therapies by women with advanced stage breast cancer. *BMC Complementary Alternative Medicine, 2,* 8. doi:10.1186/1472-6882-2-8

Simon, A., Traynor, K., Santos, K., Blaser, G., Bode, U., & Molan, P. (2007). Medical honey for wound care—Still the 'latest resort'? *Evidence-Based Complementary and Alternative Medicine, 6,* 165–173. doi:10.1093/ecam/nem175

Slippery elm. (2010). Retrieved January 21, 2010, from Epocrates [Software]. San Mateo, CA: Epocrates, Inc.

Smith, W.B., Olaku, O., Michie, J., & White, J.D. (2008). Survey of cancer researchers regarding complementary and alternative medicine. *Journal of the Society for Integrative Oncology, 6,* 2–12.

Standish, L.J., Kozak, L., & Congdon, S. (2008). Acupuncture is underutilized in hospice and palliative medicine. *American Journal of Hospice and Palliative Care, 25,* 298–308. doi:10.1177/1049909108315916

Stokman, M.A., Spijkervet, F.K., Boezen, H.M., Schouten, J.P., Roodenburg, J.L., & de Vries, E.G. (2006). Preventive intervention possibilities in radiotherapy- and chemotherapy-induced oral mucositis: Results of meta-analyses. *Journal of Dental Research, 85,* 690–700. doi:10.1177/154405910608500802

Su, C.K., Mehta, V., Ravikumar, L., Shah, R., Pinto, H., Halpern, J., ... Le, Q.T. (2004). Phase II double-blind randomized study comparing oral aloe vera versus placebo to prevent radiation-related mucositis in patients with head-and-neck neoplasms. *International Journal of Radiation Oncology, Biology, Physics, 60,* 171–177. doi:10.1016/j.ijrobp.2004.02.012

Syrjala, K.L., Donaldson, G.W., Davis, M.W., Kippes, M.E., & Carr, J.E. (1995). Relaxation and imagery and cognitive-behavioral training reduce pain during cancer treatment: A controlled clinical trial. *Pain, 63,* 189–198. doi:10.1016/0304-3959(95)00039-U

Tascilar, M., de Jong, F.A., Verweij, J., & Mathijssen, R.H. (2006). Complementary and alternative medicine during cancer treatment: Beyond innocence. *Oncologist, 11,* 732–741. doi:10.1634/theoncologist.11-7-732

Tiemann, P., Toelg, M., & Ramos, M.H. (2006). Administration of Ratanhia-based herbal oral care products for the prophylaxis of oral mucositis in cancer chemotherapy patients: A clinical trial. *Evidence-Based Alternative and Complementary Medicine, 4,* 361–366. doi:10.1093/ecam/nel070

U.S. National Library of Medicine MedlinePlus®. (2010, July 20). Licorice (*Glycyrrhiza glabra L.*) and DGL (deglycyrrhizinated licorice). Retrieved from http://www.nlm.nih.gov/medlineplus/druginfo/natural/patient-licorice.html

Worthington, H.V., Clarkson, J.E., & Eden, T.O.B. (2007). Interventions for preventing oral mucositis for patients with cancer receiving treatment. *Cochrane Database of Systematic Reviews* 2007, Issue 4. Art. No.: CD000978. doi:10.1002/14651858.CD000978.pub3

Wu, M.H., Yuan, B., Liu, Q.F., & Wang, Q. (2007). Study of qingre liyan decoction in treating and preventing acute radioactive oral mucositis. *Chinese Journal of Integrative Medicine, 13,* 280–284. doi:10.1007/s11655-007-0280-9

You, W.C., Hsieh, C.C., & Huang, J.T. (2009). Effect of extracts from indigowood root (*Isatis indigotica Fort.*) on immune responses in radiation-induced mucositis. *Journal of Alternative and Complementary Medicine, 15,* 771–778. doi:10.1089/acm.2008.03

Yuki, F., Kawaguchi, T., Hazemoto, K., & Asou, N. (2003). Preventive effects of oren-gedoku-to on mucositis caused by anticancer agents in patients with acute leukemia [Abstract]. *Gan To Kagaku Ryoho, 30,* 1303–1307.

CHAPTER 10

Developing a Nursing-Centered "Spray and Weigh" Program

Marilyn L. Haas, PhD, CNS, ANP-BC

One of the most effective interventions nursing can provide to patients receiving therapy for oral cancers is a daily oral evaluation and treatment. We call this, 'A weigh and a spray . . . everyday'! A nurse weighs the patient, examines the mouth, and sprays their oral cavity with saline. Benefits include detecting new infections, management of pain and related symptoms, not to mention the psychological support it offers patients, which is crucial in their completing treatment.
—Elise Carper, RN, MA, ANP-BC, AOCN®,
Director of Nursing, Radiation Oncology Nurse Practitioner at
Continuum Cancer Centers of New York

As part of a comprehensive head and neck chemoradiation supportive care program, the daily 'spray and weigh program' cleanses the oral cavity and assists with secretion removal. Perhaps more importantly, it provides the opportunity for daily assessment of all facets of the patient's condition, from oral mucositis and pain, to nutrition and resource management. Patient feedback indicates the spray is soothing and the daily interaction is comforting during this difficult therapy. Providers believe that patients are more attentive to self-care at home and that early intervention for side effects of therapy will help achieve the primary goal: avoidance of treatment breaks.
—Colleen Lambertz, MBA, MSN, FNP,
Nurse Practitioner, Radiation Oncology St. Luke's Mountain
States Tumor Institute, Boise, Idaho

Introduction

Oral health is vital to a person's general health, level of nutrition, and quality of life and is significant in holistic care. Unfortunately, many patients present with poor oral health (e.g., dental caries, gingivitis) at the time of their cancer diagnosis. A systematic review of dental disease in patients undergoing cancer therapy conducted by Hong et al. (2010) found that 28% of patients had dental caries at the beginning of therapy and 9% experienced caries following radiotherapy. Hence, for individuals who are diagnosed with oral cancers and begin chemotherapy, radiation, or combined-modality therapy, dental evaluations are strongly recommended before beginning treatment.

The oral health needs of patients with cancer of the oral cavity are challenging, and nursing care and patient education become integral parts of the plan of care. Efforts to improve oral hygiene during and after therapy will help individuals with the physical discomfort of oral side effects (Hogan, 2009).

Developed by radiation oncology nurses/nurse practitioners, the spray and weigh program helps with overall patient comfort and emotional support and addresses other problems that patients may face while going through chemoradiation for oral cancers. Many nurses in radiation therapy departments are adopting this oral care program to help patients cope with their oral oncology treatments. The same principles and practices can be applied by medical oncology nurses for their patients who are at high risk for developing oral mucositis.

Clinical components of the spray and weigh program include assessing the oral cavity, performing oral saline spray either before or after radiation treatments, monitoring the patient's weight, teaching and reinforcing oral motor exercises, assessing for side effects, and teaching patients oral hygiene for home care. All of these components are performed during the daily nursing visits. Anecdotally, radiation oncology nurses have shared numerous patient cases about the positive benefits of a spray and weigh program (personal communication with Oncology Nursing Society Radiation Special Interest Group members, 2010). Hopefully, future research will support what radiation oncology nurses are experiencing in their clinical practice regarding the benefits and patient outcomes with this program. The purpose of this chapter is to explain how to develop and implement a spray and weigh program.

Oral Cavity Assessment

Reviewing the oral cavity's anatomy is important to assist in understanding the examination (refer back to Figure 1-1 in Chapter 1). The major structures include the lips, cheeks, buccal mucosa, teeth, upper and lower gingiva, tongue, and hard and soft palates, along with the salivary glands. All of these structures perform important roles in speech, swallowing, mastication, and respirations.

Oral assessments should be performed at every patient visit. Bright lighting is required for inspection of the lips, tongue, floor of the mouth, retromolar trigone, tonsillar pillars, buccal mucosa, hard and soft palates, gingiva, and teeth. Assess for discoloration of the teeth and mucous membranes, unusual lesions, asymmetry of structures, salivary flow, infection, or dental caries. Any odors should be noted. Trismus should be assessed at the beginning and completion of therapy. The nurse can measure how wide the patient can open his or her mouth by using devices, such as the TheraBite® (Atos Medical) individual plastic measurement device, or by using disposable rulers and measuring the opening between the upper and lower front teeth.

Clinicians should document the oral examination using standardized tools. One popular tool is the Common Terminology Criteria for Adverse Events (CTCAE) symptom grading scale (National Cancer Institute Cancer Therapy Evaluation Program, 2009). The CTCAE scale is based on grades 1–5:

1—mild; asymptomatic or mild symptoms where interventions are not indicated

2—moderate; minimal, local, or noninvasive interventions are taken

3—severe but not immediately life threatening; requires hospitalizations for interventions

4—life-threatening consequences; urgent interventions must be taken

5—death related to the adverse event.

The CTCAE related to oral therapies is included in Table 10-1. Note that some adverse events are limited to grades 1–3. Table 10-2 outlines oral mucositis grading.

Daily Saline Sprays

Radiation to the oral cavity or specific chemotherapy agents place patients at high risk for oral mucositis; these patients could benefit from daily oral saline sprays. Oral saline sprays improve hygiene, comfort, and early detection of oral infections. Secondarily, oral saline sprays facilitate nurse-patient interactions in which other symptoms can be prophylactically managed and early interventions can be prescribed.

Equipment required for this procedure is minimal and can be easily assembled by nursing departments. The procedure requires purchasing spraying equipment, saline, emesis basins, and protective outerwear for nurses and patients, which is not a major financial investment (see Table 10-3). The nurse can prepare the equipment prior to seeing the patient by plugging in the compressor and attaching the tubing, filling the atomizer with normal saline, and attaching the pipette to the atomizer, securing the metal tip to the glass container (see Figure 10-1). The glass container can be kept in the warm bath until ready to use that day. The nurse should put on protective gear before beginning the procedure.

Table 10-1. Adverse Events Related to Oral Therapy

Adverse Event	Grade				
	1	2	3	4	5
Dry mouth	Symptomatic (e.g., dry or thick saliva) without significant dietary alteration; unstimulated saliva flow greater than 0.2 ml/min	Moderate symptoms; oral intake alterations (e.g., copious water, other lubricants, diet limited to purees and/or soft, moist foods); unstimulated saliva 0.1–0.2 ml/min	Inability to adequately aliment orally; tube feeding or TPN indicated; unstimulated saliva less than 0.1 ml/min	–	–
Dysphagia	Symptomatic, able to eat regular diet	Symptomatic and altered eating/swallowing	Severely altered eating/swallowing; tube feeding or TPN or hospitalization indicated	Life-threatening consequences; urgent intervention indicated	Death
Oral dysesthesia	Mild discomfort; not interfering with oral intake	Moderate pain; interfering with oral intake	Disabling pain; tube feeding or TPN indicated	–	–
Oral pain	Mild pain	Moderate pain; limiting instrumental ADL	Severe pain; limiting self-care ADL	–	–

ADL—activities of daily living; TPN—total parenteral nutrition

Note. From *Common Terminology Criteria for Adverse Events* [v.4.0], by National Cancer Institute Cancer Therapy Evaluation Program, 2009. Retrieved from http://evs.nci.nih.gov/ftp1/CTCAE/CTCAE_4.03 _2010-06-14_QuickReference_5x7.pdf.

Table 10-2. In-Depth Grading for Oral Mucositis

Grade	Clinical Description
1	Asymptomatic or mild symptoms; intervention not indicated
2	Moderate pain; not interfering with oral intake; modified diet indicated
3	Severe pain; interfering with oral intake
4	Life-threatening consequences; urgent intervention indicated
5	Death

Note. From *Common Terminology Criteria for Adverse Events* [v.4.0], by National Cancer Institute Cancer Therapy Evaluation Program, 2009. Retrieved from http://evs.nci.nih.gov/ftp1/CTCAE/CTCAE_4.03 _2010-06-14_QuickReference_5x7.pdf.

Table 10-3. Equipment for Spray and Weigh Program	
Equipment	**Use**
Spraying equipment: • DeVilbiss® (DeVilbiss Healthcare) Pul-mo-Aide® Compact Compressor Nebulizer Model 3655D • DeVilbiss Atomizer Model 163, glass pipette, and metal tip • Plastic tubing	Assemble and follow manufacturer guidelines. A low-pressure atomizer is used so not to cause any damage to tissues.
Saline (sodium chloride 0.9%) bottles	Use for the oral irrigation solution
Water bath	Warms saline (optional)
Emesis basin	Label each disposable basin with patient's name (with permanent ink marker) and store in plastic bag for daily use or can use disposable cups.
Towel and washcloth	Place towel over patient's neck/chest to protect clothing, and use washcloth to wipe patient's mouth.
Examination gloves	Protect personnel
Safety goggles	Protect personnel

For the saline spray procedure, the patient should sit comfortably in a chair with a towel draped over the neck and chest, holding the emesis basin under his or her lips (see Figure 10-2). The washcloth can be kept on the patient's knees to be used during treatment for any excess rinse or drooling outside the mouth. Before the procedure, the nurse should inquire about any symptoms experienced since the last visit and inspect the oral cavity before spraying with the normal saline solution. The nurse should grade the degree of oral mucositis and xerostomia and assess for odor, possible lesions, infections, or any other complications. During the examination, the nurse can assess how well the patient is performing oral hygiene. This interaction allows the nurse to offer the patient support and education and to proactively intervene with any symptom management.

Cleaning the equipment is the final step. Equipment can be cleaned in the department or sent to a sterile supply department. Always clean according to the manufacturer's specifications. General recommendations include the following.

1. Compressor: Turn the off/on button to the off position and unplug. Disconnect the tubing from the air inlet. Wipe the outside of compressor and tubing with a sanitizer cloth. Place the tubing in a bag labeled with the patient's name.

Figure 10-1. Spray and Weigh Program Equipment

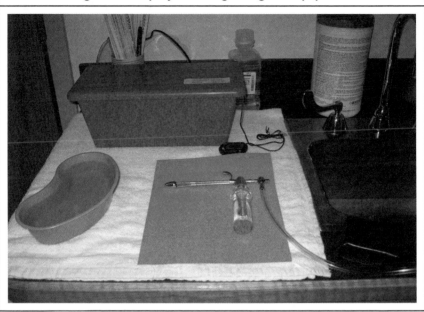

Note. Photo courtesy of Mountain Radiation Oncology. Used with permission.

Figure 10-2. Patient Setup for Saline Spray

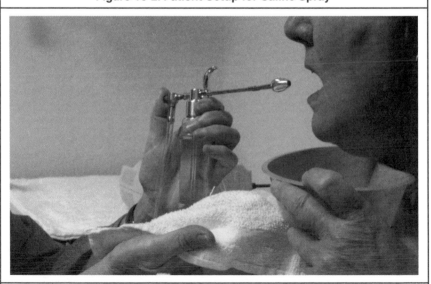

Note. Photo courtesy of Mountain Radiation Oncology. Used with permission.

2. Atomizer, pipette, metal tip, cutoff assembly, and gaskets: Soak in Enzol® (Civco Medical Solutions) (10 minutes), shake thoroughly; Cidex® (Civco Medical Solutions) (45 minutes), shake thoroughly; and sterile water (15 minutes). Dry with a clean cloth and store in a clean, covered container.
3. Patients can reuse their own emesis basin. The nurse should ensure that patient's name is written on the side and that the basin is rinsed and stored in the patient's bag.

Weight

Before or after the oral saline spray, the patient should be weighed. Maintaining weight throughout treatment is optimal, and good nutrition can improve the clinical course, outcomes, and quality of life (Bauer & Capra, 2004). Patients are weighed every day to monitor for any weight loss, and nurses can expect to see fluctuations. Monitoring their weight allows patients to become an active participant in their daily care. Feeding tubes may be required if the patient is not able to eat.

Dietary habits should be reviewed. High-protein and high-caloric diets should be encouraged. Sweets and sugars should be limited to prevent further tooth decay. The patient's ability to chew and swallow foods should be assessed. Facial muscles may be affected by the tumor or from radiation treatments to the point where chewing foods becomes difficult for the patient. High-protein shakes (e.g., Boost® [Nestlé HealthCare Nutrition, Inc.], Ensure® [Abbott Laboratories], Scandishake® [Axcan Pharma Inc.]) are good sources of protein and other nutrients. Thickening agents, tapioca, instant mashed potatoes, or infant rice to thicken fluids may be helpful when swallowing becomes an issue, along with instructions to be upright and sit at a table for meals. Flavoring basic vanilla or chocolate supplements can help the palatability of these shakes or nutritional supplements (see Figure 10-3).

Figure 10-3. Nutritional Supplement Recipes

Apple-Grape Juven® (Abbott Laboratories): 8–10 oz apple juice with 1 packet of grape Juven

Banana Delight: 8 oz vanilla supplement with ½ teaspoon of banana extract

Chocolate-Covered Almond: 8 oz chocolate supplement with ½ teaspoon of almond extract

Chocolate-Covered Banana: 8 oz chocolate supplement with ½ teaspoon of banana extract

Chocolate Mint: 8 oz vanilla supplement with ¼ teaspoon peppermint extract

Cran-Grape Juven: 8–10 oz light cranberry juice with 1 packet of grape Juven

Cran-Orange Juven: 8–10 oz light cranberry juice with 1 packet of orange Juven

Nutty Strawberry: 8 oz strawberry supplement with ½ teaspoon of almond extract

Orange-Apple Juven: 8–10 oz apple juice with 1 packet of orange Juven

Simply Almond: 8 oz vanilla supplement with ½ teaspoon of almond extract

Strawberry Banana Yum: 8 oz strawberry supplement with ½ teaspoon of banana extract

Oral Motor Exercises

It is important to discuss oral motor exercises during therapy, as most patients have a tendency to reduce the use of their muscles to talk, eat, or speak because of pain or fatigue. Teaching patients to perform oral exercises can help them maintain muscle functioning during therapy and have a head start in the recovery phase. Patients can perform these exercises two to three times a day. Starting the exercises at the beginning of therapy can help (see Figure 10-4).

Figure 10-4. Oral Motor Exercises			
Gross Oral Movements (Avoids Muscle Stiffness)	**Facial Exercises (Strengthens Oral Musculature)**	**Lip Exercises**	**Tongue Exercises**
• Open and close mouth (stretch comfortably; avoid overstretching). • Round lips and try to throw kiss. • Protrude tongue, moving side-to-side. • Protrude tongue and lick lower lip; repeat to upper lip.	• Smile and pucker lips. • Puff up cheeks with air (holding 5 seconds) and then blow out. • Suck in cheeks (holding 5 seconds) and then relax. • Puff up cheeks, move air from one cheek to the other without letting air escape out the lips, and repeat side-to-side.	• Throw a kiss. • Close lips tightly as if you are saying "mmm." • Say "ma, ma, ma" as fast as you can. • Say "me, me, me" as fast as you can.	• Protrude tongue, then retract. • Move tongue from side to side, pushing against inside of each cheek. • Protrude tongue and elevate toward nose and down toward chin. • Practice tongue-tip sounds: – La, la, la – Lee, lee, lee – Tea, tea, tea – Top, top, top – Tip, tip, tip.

Symptom Assessment

Acute symptoms from therapies should be addressed at every visit. Patients should be taught the importance of reporting symptoms to their practitioner to possibly avoid complications later in therapy. Common symptoms that patients can experience are oral pain, dry mouth (xerostomia), difficulty swallowing (dysphagia), distortion of taste (dysgeusia), painful swallowing (odynophagia), dehydration, and weight loss. Management of these symptoms is discussed in previous chapters.

Dental Health

Previous chapters outlined detailed patient efforts to maintain oral health once they have been diagnosed with cancer. Patients should seek an evaluation by their dentist or oral surgeon before beginning any radiation or chemotherapy. Dental work should be done prior to any therapy, which would include any teeth extraction, filling any cavities, and dental varnishes. Teeth extraction after radiation only increases the risk of osteoradionecrosis (Reuther, Schuster, Mende, & Kübler, 2003). Protecting the teeth from the effects of xerostomia with dental varnishes will help prevent dental carries (Hogan, 2009; Rankin et al., 2009).

Oral Hygiene at Home

During the initial patient education session, oncology nurses should teach proper oral hygiene for home care before beginning oncology treatments. This would include brushing teeth, flossing, using oral rinses, and performing daily inspection. Patients should use a soft toothbrush because gums may become sore and irritated from treatments. Bleeding and tender gums are common problems in patients undergoing chemoradiation for oral tumors (Pavlatos & Gilliam, 2010). Nonfluoride toothpastes (i.e., Biotene® [GlaxoSmithKline]) help to soothe irritated gums. For comfort and healing, patients can mix together a salt and baking soda oral rinse (Tipton, 2009). The recipe is ¼ teaspoon of baking soda and ¼ teaspoon of salt in 8 ounces of water. Depending on patient preference, the mixture can be kept cold in the refrigerator or slightly heated under water or warmed in the microwave to aid further comfort. Patients can carry the oral rinse in a spray bottle, which can be used more frequently during the day. Rinsing with an alcohol-based over-the-counter oral rinse (i.e., Listerine® [McNeil-PPC, Inc.]) should be discouraged, as this can burn the tissues and cause more discomfort.

Conclusion

Oral health care is important for all patients, particularly those with oral cancers and receiving chemoradiation. Nurses can take an active part in their patients' oral care during therapy by offering a spray and weigh program. The program is simple to begin and does not require a large financial investment. The oral rinse intervention can offer patients physical and emotional support during treatment. The program will require more research to demonstrate the level of evidence for the investment in staff time and improvement in patient satisfaction and symptom control. Initial reports cited by oncology nurses report positive feedback (personal communication, E. Carper and C. Lambertz, February 1, 2010).

The responsibility of healthcare professionals is to reduce the incidence and severity of oral cancer side effects as much as possible. One intervention toward accomplishing this goal is to implement a basic oral hygiene protocol. Nurses and other healthcare professionals can positively influence patient care by incorporating the evidence-based practices of oral care protocols. Incorporating the spray and weigh program can help patients through their therapy and provide daily nutrition and symptom management.

References

Bauer, J.D., & Capra, S. (2004). Nutrition intervention improves outcomes in patients with cancer cachexia receiving chemotherapy—A pilot study. *Supportive Care in Cancer, 13,* 270–274. doi:10.1007/s00520-004-0746-7

Hogan, R. (2009). Implementation of an oral care protocol and its effects on oral mucositis. *Journal of Pediatric Oncology Nursing, 26,* 125–135. doi:10.1177/1043454209334356

Hong, C.H., Napeñas, J.J., Hodgson, B.D., Stokman, M.A., Mathers-Stauffer, V., Elting, L.S., … Brennan, M.T. (2010). A systematic review of dental disease in patients undergoing cancer therapy. *Supportive Care in Cancer, 18,* 1007–1021. doi:10.1007/s00520-010-0873-2

National Cancer Institute Cancer Therapy Evaluation Program. (2009). *Common terminology criteria for adverse events* [v.4.0]. Retrieved from http://evs.nci.nih.gov/ftp1/CTCAE/CTCAE_4.02_2009-09-15_QuickReference_5x7.pdf

Pavlatos, J., & Gilliam, K.K. (2008). Oral care protocols for patients undergoing cancer therapy. *General Dentistry, 56,* 464–478.

Rankin, K.V., Epstein, J., Huber, M.A., Peterson, D.E., Plemons, J.M., Redding, S.S., … Sonis, S.T. (2009). Oral health in cancer therapy. *Texas Dental Journal, 126,* 389–397, 406–419, 422–437.

Reuther, T., Schuster, T., Mende, U., & Kübler, A. (2003). Osteoradionecrosis of the jaws as a side effect of radiotherapy of head and neck tumour patients—A report of a thirty year retrospective review. *International Journal of Oral and Maxillofacial Surgery, 32,* 289–295. doi:10.1054/ijom.2002.0332

Tipton, J.M. (2009). Mucositis. In L.H. Eaton & J.M. Tipton (Eds.), *Putting evidence into practice: Improving oncology patient outcomes* (pp. 193–200). Pittsburgh, PA: Oncology Nursing Society.

CHAPTER 11

Sexuality and Quality of Life

Miranda J. Kramer, RN, MS, ACNP, CNS

Introduction

Despite the high prevalence of cancer and cancer treatment–related issues that could affect a patient's sexual well-being, there is a paucity of well-designed research that elucidates patients' symptoms and guides practitioners. The World Health Organization (WHO) defines sexual health as follows:

> Sexual health is a state of physical, emotional, mental, and social well-being in relation to sexuality; it is not merely the absence of disease, dysfunction, or infirmity. Sexual health requires a positive and respectful approach to sexuality and sexual relationships, as well as the possibility of having pleasurable and safe sexual experiences, free of coercion, discrimination, and violence. (WHO, 2006, p. 5)

Cancer and cancer treatment can affect all aspects of an individual's sexuality, including sexual desire and physical and psychological sexual function. Yet, medical practitioners often omit or avoid assessing their patients' sexual health concerns because of lack of time, experience in assessment and treatment, and knowledge about the resources available for their patients. Sexuality is a complex issue that focuses on the physical, psychological, interpersonal, and behavioral aspects of a patient and his or her partner (Gilbert, Ussher, & Perz, 2010; Hordern, 2008; Hordern & Street, 2007b; Hughes, 2009; Juraskova et al., 2003; Mick, 2007).

Factors in Sexuality

Sexuality is related to gender identity, self-esteem, and personal interactions on many levels. Sexuality is interrelated with ethnicity, culture, upbringing, social class, education, generation, and life circumstances. Thus, the nurse needs to understand and relate the patient's challenges with the diagnosis and treatments within the patient's personal framework. In evaluating a patient for sexual dysfunction, most texts address problems related to the physical or functional elements of human sexual behavior. However, this approach only represents a fraction of the overall issue of sexual health. Barton, Wilwerding, Carpenter, and Loprinzi (2004) presented a schematic of the various concepts involved in sexual health and functioning (see Figure 11-1). Barton et al. described the general factors surrounding sexual health as related to the concepts of interest, function, and satisfaction. Within each of these concepts, emotion plays an integral role. Treatment side effects affect each of the individual categories. The patient must be assessed for symptoms related to each category (physical, emotional, lifestyle, etc.) when a possible sexual problem is identified through a detailed interview with the patient alone or with the patient and partner.

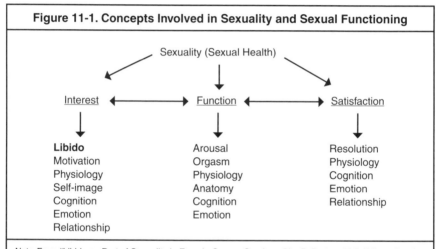

Figure 11-1. Concepts Involved in Sexuality and Sexual Functioning

Note. From "Libido as Part of Sexuality in Female Cancer Survivors," by D. Barton, M.B. Wilwerding, L. Carpenter, and C. Loprinzi, 2004, *Oncology Nursing Forum, 31,* p. 600. Copyright 2004 by the Oncology Nursing Society. Reprinted with permission.

Patient Oral Symptoms and Their Effects on Sexuality and Intimacy

Mucositis

Severe oral mucositis has been demonstrated to increase the length of hospital stay. Sonis et al. (2001) found that patients with oral mucositis and ulceration remained hospitalized longer than their counterparts with less severe mucositis. In general, increased hospitalization decreases the amount of time the patient and partner have to be intimate. Intimacy is related to having adequate opportunity, environment, and time to express oneself. The regimen of hospital life, the sterile environment, and lack of privacy do not encourage intimacy between the patient and partner. The addition of discomfort due to oral mucositis and the patient's underlying disease process compound the risks to intimacy. Additionally, patients who develop mucositis have significantly increased rates of mood disturbance, depression, and anger (Dodd et al., 2001). Patients' concerns about their body image, appearance, or disfigurement as a result of their treatment can have a devastating impact on their social interactions.

Pain

Pain decreases one's ability to not only speak or eat but also to participate in intimate or sexual interactions, such as kissing and performing oral sex.

Xerostomia, Ageusia, and Trismus

Concomitant issues such as xerostomia or trismus further impair the patient's ability to interact with his or her partner. These symptoms affect interpersonal interaction, potential loss of the ability to kiss, loss of saliva production, and loss of taste sensation (ageusia).

Infectious Disease

Infections of the oral cavity can complicate the course of patients with oral mucositis. Patients need to know that infections are common while undergoing chemotherapy and radiation therapy. If infectious agents are present, infection or superinfection can be passed between partners. The fragility of the oral mucosa during mucositis puts patients at greater risk for developing infectious lesions. Herpes simplex virus, candidiasis, human papillomavirus (HPV), and bacterial infections are all common in patients with oral mucositis. The patient should understand the process of developing mucositis and that local infections can lead to systemic infections and sepsis. Safe sex practices (i.e., use of barriers such as condoms or dental dams) to safeguard patients from preventable infection are essential. Secondary infections with viral agents such as hepatitis and HPV are related to development of the cancers themselves.

During the phases of the biologic process of mucositis (see Figure 3-2 in Chapter 3), the most painful stage is the ulcerative/microbiologic stage (Brown & Wingard, 2004; Dose, 1995; Sonis, 2004, 2009). This stage poses the greatest risk for systemic infection and potential sepsis for the patient because of breakdown of the mucosal barrier, which allows pathogens to break through normal defense mechanisms. Any type of pathogen may pose a risk, including bacteria, viruses, and fungi and yeast. Oral herpes simplex virus is a very common organism in the general population. In a cohort of patients undergoing chemotherapy, 40%–70% of all oral lesions cultured were positive for HSV (Greenberg et al., 1987). Candida superinfections following chemotherapy or chemoradiotherapy are not uncommon (Yeo, Alvarado, Fainstein, & Bodey, 1985). Bacterial infections including gram-negative rods and anaerobes also are common but are difficult to separate from the variety of organisms that inhabit the oral cavity.

Dental Disease

Poorly fitting dental appliances, such as bridges or dentures, can inhibit patients' ability to interact with their partner. Acute weight loss secondary to decreased oral intake can cause dental appliances to not fit well and become a potential source of increased irritation. In such cases, patients should see their dentist so that adjustments can be made to improve the fit of the appliance and maintain adequate nutrition. In turn, patients feel better about their appearance and ability to maintain social interactions.

Assessing Sexual Health

Most texts that address sexual health focus on impairment of the ability to enjoy sexual intercourse or attempt to quantify physical dysfunction. These studies typically assess impairment of arousal, interferences with sexual response, climactic problems, or the sequelae of these events. Sexual dysfunction remains a common long-term complication following cancer treatment in both men and women (Ananth, Jones, King, & Tookman, 2003). Tools used in assessment include the Oral Mucositis Daily Questionnaire (OMDQ) and the Mouth and Throat Soreness (MTS) questionnaire. The OMDQ assesses 10 items while the MTS assesses for pain and other quality-of-life indicators, but neither assesses intimacy or sexual health issues. Thus, sexual health is a separate but related diagnosis to oral health. Patients typically underreport difficulties in sexual health (Cox, Jenkins, Catt, Langridge, & Fallowfield, 2006; Hordern & Street, 2007a; Hughes, 2000). Yet, understanding that a patient has sexual dysfunction coupled with oral side effects points to an increased potential for further impairments to intimacy.

Provider Issues

In assessing a patient's sexual health, it is important for the provider to understand his or her own sexuality. This provides a framework for a therapeutic conversation between the patient and provider. Although issues and ideas may arise that the provider is uncomfortable with, these concerns are important to the client and need to be respected. In asking for education or advice regarding sexual health, the patient is reaching out for help and guidance. Remaining professional, not making light of the issue, and taking the patient's concerns seriously while employing techniques in therapeutic communication will benefit both the patient and the provider. Providers often take the stance that sexuality is of lesser concern than survival. Patients often are looking for practical advice on dealing with issues of sexuality and intimacy and finding a new state of normalcy in the face of a cancer diagnosis (Hordern & Street, 2007b).

Partner Issues

The patient's partner also is at risk for altered sexual health related to a cancer diagnosis. The experience of the patient is also the life experience of the partner. Both individuals in the relationship need to cope with emotions such as fear and anxiety and require education. Thus, assessment of sexual health of the patient should include the partner when possible. The partner will likely have the role of primary caregiver as well, which could lead to increased anxiety, fear, loss of control, and fatigue. Quality of partner interaction has been found to be more significant than marital status itself. It is additionally correlated with a lower morbidity of a variety of diseases (Ren, 1997). Morgan (2009) presented an excellent review of the literature of patient-partner communication in cancer care, including communication, coping patterns, and strategies.

Domestic violence has an increased incidence in medically vulnerable populations. Schmidt, Woods, and Stewart (2006) postulated that a cancer diagnosis itself may be a risk factor for domestic violence. The identification of patients with cancer who are at risk for any of the forms of domestic violence (physical, psychological, or sexual) is currently being researched.

Assessments and Interventions

Many simple assessments and interventions can be performed by the nurse to identify patients with altered sexual health.
- Identify risk factors for the development of oral side effects of treatment, including the following (Pico, Avila-Garavito, & Naccache, 1998).
  - Patients with hematologic malignancies (rather than solid tumors)
  - Patients younger than 20 years of age
  - Patients with poor baseline oral hygiene
  - Patients receiving chemotherapy regimens with high incidence of mucositis
  - Patients receiving radiation (greater than 20 Gy to the treatment field) to the head and neck region
- Identify comorbid disease related to sexual dysfunction.
  - Depression
  - Preexisting diagnosis of sexual dysfunction

- Cardiopulmonary disease
- Exercise intolerance
- Neuromuscular disease
- During patient teaching sessions, include education regarding oral sexual health.
  - Educate patients that their oral mucosa may be more fragile and prone to trauma because of their treatment. Oral sex should be performed with caution because of impaired resistance, risk of infection, slower wound healing, trauma potentially causing increased oral pain, and bleeding.
  - For xerostomia, keep oral lubricants available (e.g., a glass of water, lip balm, artificial saliva products).
  - If oral ulcers cause pain with kissing or other activities, a physician or nurse practitioner can prescribe topical agents to cover the ulcer and alleviate pain.
- Assess the need for medical intervention to palliate symptoms. This includes systemic pain medications, topical agents (topical lidocaine rinses), and sialogogues (medications that stimulate saliva flow).
- Continue encouraging meticulous dental hygiene. This will promote good oral health, improve breath odor, prevent dental caries, and improve self-image. Instruct use of fluoride gels as prescribed.
- Provide referral for professional counseling and support services as needed.
- Employ the BETTER model to promote a conversation about the patient's sexual health (Mick, Hughes, & Cohen, 2004). This tool was developed for oncology nurses to assess and communicate with their patients about sexuality. BETTER stands for
  - **B**ring up the topic.
  - **E**xplain that sexuality is a part of quality of life and that the patient should be aware that the healthcare team is open to discussing these issues.
  - **T**ell the patient about the resources that will provide help, or assist the individual in finding some.
  - **T**ime the discussion to the patient's preference.
  - **E**ducate the patient on the impact of the cancer treatment on sexuality.
  - **R**ecord the interaction with the patient and that the topic has been discussed.
- Utilize therapeutic communication (Hordern & Street, 2007c; Kotronoulas, Papadopoulou, & Patiraki, 2009; Kruijver, Kerkstra, Bensing, & van de Wiel, 2000; Park, Norris, & Bober, 2009; Sheldon, 2009).
  - Approach the patient's questions in a nonjudgmental manner.
  - Provide privacy to the patient and partner when discussing their sexual health or any other health issue.
  - Ask leading and open-ended questions that prompt conversation, such as "Many of my patients often have questions about mucositis and their sexual health but are afraid to ask. Do you have any questions you would like to discuss?"
  - Be available to answer the patient's questions.

— Be alert for both verbal and nonverbal clues that the patient is concerned about his or her sexual health.

Conclusion

Sexual health is an integral part of each individual's care. It is a complex topic that affects the physical and emotional dimensions of the patient's daily life. The nurse plays an important role in assessing and treating patients who experience oral side effects and have altered sexual health. Including the patient's partner whenever possible is an essential component of holistic care. A host of factors coincide with oral health, including other underlying medical diagnoses, partner interactions, and medication regimens, that confound sexual health issues. Good oral hygiene and use of prescribed medications will improve the patient's self-image and may facilitate the patient's sexual health and intimacy with his or her partner. The oral mucosa is particularly susceptible to trauma during and following treatments for cancer.

Providers rarely discuss sexual health concerns with their patients. Time should be allotted to this endeavor, and addressing the patient's sexual health should be part of the treatment plan. Assess the patient for factors related to oral complications of treatment that diminish sexual health and quality of life. Also, nurses need to understand that sexuality is an issue that concerns patients even in advanced disease and is not dependent on age.

References

Ananth, H., Jones, L., King, M., & Tookman, A. (2003). The impact of cancer on sexual function: A controlled study. *Palliative Medicine, 17,* 202–205. doi:10.1191/0269216303pm759oa

Barton, D., Wilwerding, M., Carpenter, L., & Loprinzi, C. (2004). Libido as part of sexuality in female cancer survivors. *Oncology Nursing Forum, 31,* 599–609. doi:10.1188/04.ONF.599-609

Brown, C.G., & Wingard, J. (2004). Clinical consequences of oral mucositis. *Seminars in Oncology Nursing, 20,* 16–21.

Cox, A., Jenkins, V., Catt, S., Langridge, C., & Fallowfield, L. (2006). Information needs and experiences: An audit of UK cancer patients. *European Journal of Oncology Nursing, 10,* 263–272. doi:10.1016/j.ejon.2005.10.007

Dodd, M.J., Dibble, S., Miaskowski, C., Paul, S., Cho, M., MacPhail, L., ... Shiba, G. (2001). A comparison of the affective state and quality of life of chemotherapy patients who do and do not develop chemotherapy-induced oral mucositis. *Journal of Pain and Symptom Management, 21,* 498–505. doi:10.1016/S0885-3924(01)00277-9

Dose, A.M. (1995). The symptom experience of mucositis, stomatitis, and xerostomia. *Seminars in Oncology Nursing, 11,* 248–255.

Gilbert, E., Ussher, J.M., & Perz, J. (2010). Renegotiating sexuality and intimacy in the context of cancer: The experiences of carers. *Archives of Sexual Behavior, 39,* 998–1009. doi:10.1007/s10508-008-9416-z

Greenberg, M.S., Friedman, H., Cohen, S.G., Oh, S.H., Laster, L., & Starr, S. (1987). A comparative study of herpes simplex infections in renal transplant and leukemic patients. *Journal of Infectious Diseases, 156,* 280–287.

Hordern, A. (2008). Intimacy and sexuality after cancer: A critical review of the literature. *Cancer Nursing, 31*(2), E9–E17. doi:10.1097/01.NCC.0000305695.12873.d5

Hordern, A., & Street, A. (2007a). Communicating about patient sexuality and intimacy after cancer: Mismatched expectations and unmet needs. *Medical Journal of Australia, 186,* 224–227.

Hordern, A., & Street, A. (2007b). Issues of intimacy and sexuality in the face of cancer: The patient perspective. *Cancer Nursing, 30*(6), E11–E18. doi:10.1097/01. NCC.0000300162.13639.f5

Hordern, A., & Street, A. (2007c). Let's talk about sex: Risky business for cancer and palliative care clinicians. *Contemporary Nurse, 27,* 49–60. doi:10.5555/conu.2007.27.1.49

Hughes, M.K. (2000). Sexuality and the cancer survivor: A silent coexistence. *Cancer Nursing, 23,* 477–482.

Hughes, M.K. (2009). Sexuality and cancer: The final frontier for nurses [Online exclusive]. *Oncology Nursing Forum, 36,* E241–E246. doi:10.1188/09.ONF.E241-E246

Juraskova, I., Butow, P., Robertson, R., Sharpe, L., McLeod, C., & Hacker, N. (2003). Post-treatment sexual adjustment following cervical and endometrial cancer: A qualitative insight. *Psycho-Oncology, 12,* 267–279. doi:10.1002/pon.639

Kotronoulas, G., Papadopoulou, C., & Patiraki, E. (2009). Nurses' knowledge, attitudes, and practices regarding provision of sexual health care in patients with cancer: Critical review of the evidence. *Supportive Care in Cancer, 17,* 479–501. doi:10.1007/s00520-008-0563-5

Kruijver, I.P., Kerkstra, A., Bensing, J.M., & van de Wiel, H.B. (2000). Nurse-patient communication in cancer care. A review of the literature. *Cancer Nursing, 23,* 20–31.

Mick, J. (2007). Sexuality assessment: 10 strategies for improvement. *Clinical Journal of Oncology Nursing, 11,* 671–675. doi:10.1188/07.CJON.671-675

Mick, J., Hughes, M., & Cohen, M.Z. (2004). Using the BETTER model to assess sexuality. *Clinical Journal of Oncology Nursing, 8,* 84–86. doi:10.1188/04.CJON.84-86

Morgan, M.A. (2009). Considering the patient-partner relationship in cancer care: Coping strategies for couples. *Clinical Journal of Oncology Nursing, 13,* 65–72. doi:10.1188/09. CJON.65-7

Park, E.R., Norris, R.L., & Bober, S.L. (2009). Sexual health communication during cancer care: Barriers and recommendations. *Cancer Journal, 15,* 74–77. doi:10.1097/ PPO.0b013e31819587dc

Pico, J.-L., Avila-Garavito, A., & Naccache, P. (1998). Mucositis: Its occurrence, consequences and treatment in the oncology setting. *Oncologist, 3,* 446–451.

Ren, X.S. (1997). Marital status and quality of relationships: The impact on health perception. *Social Science and Medicine, 44,* 241–249. doi:10.1016/S0277-9536(96)00158-X

Schmidt, N.K., Woods, T.E., & Stewart, J.A. (2006). Domestic violence against women with cancer: Examples and review of the literature. *Journal of Supportive Oncology, 4,* 24–33.

Sheldon, L.K. (2009). *Communication for nurses: Talking with patients* (2nd ed.). Sudbury, MA: Jones and Bartlett.

Sonis, S.T. (2004). Oral mucositis in cancer therapy. *Journal of Supportive Oncology, 2*(6, Suppl. 3), 3–8.

Sonis, S.T. (2009). Mucositis: The impact, biology and therapeutic opportunities of oral mucositis. *Oral Oncology, 45,* 1015–1020. doi:10.1016/j.oraloncology.2009.08.006

Sonis, S.T., Oster, G., Fuchs, H., Bellm, L., Bradford, W.Z., Edelsberg, J., ... Horowitz, M. (2001). Oral mucositis and the clinical and economic outcomes of hematopoietic stem-cell transplantation. *Journal of Clinical Oncology, 19,* 2201–2205.

World Health Organization. (2006). *Defining sexual health: Report of a technical consultation on sexual health, 28–31 January 2002, Geneva.* Retrieved from http://www.who.int/ reproductivehealth/publications/sexual_health/defining_sexual_health.pdf

Yeo, E., Alvarado, T., Fainstein, V., & Bodey, G.P. (1985). Prophylaxis of oropharyngeal candidiasis with clotrimazole. *Journal of Clinical Oncology, 3,* 1668–1671.

CHAPTER 12

Paradigms of Eating

Maureen B. Huhmann, DCN, RD, CSO

Introduction

According to the National Cancer Institute (NCI), in 2010 there will be close to 10 million cancer survivors in the United States (Horner et al., 2009). NCI defines a cancer survivor as anyone who has been diagnosed with cancer, from the time of diagnosis through the balance of his or her life. As one could imagine, these survivors have a unique set of health issues, including late effects of the cancer treatments. Some of these late effects can affect one's ability to consume and digest adequate nutrients. This chapter will review the impact of some of the oral late effects on nutrition status and oral intake.

Diet Following Chemotherapy

Oral and IV cancer therapies can cause oral complications that can be acute or chronic. Most of the oral complications of chemotherapy are acute. This section will touch on the few chronic side effects of chemotherapy and their impact on oral intake. The high cellular turnover rate of the oral mucosa makes it susceptible to the direct and indirect toxic effects of chemotherapy (Ilgenli, Ören, & Uysal, 2001). A recent study indicated that more than 50% of patients receiving outpatient chemotherapy experienced sore mouth during treatment (Brown et al., 2009).

The implementation of oral care protocols, including basic oral hygiene, can decrease the incidence of some oral complications (Hogan, 2009). The American Academy of Pediatric Dentistry (2008–2009) recommends the following preventive strategies following cancer therapy.

• Oral hygiene (normal brushing and flossing, air-drying of brushes)

- Noncariogenic diet
- Use of fluoride (toothpaste, supplements, gels/rinses, varnish)
- Lip care (lanolin-based creams and ointments)

The Association of Community Cancer Centers outlines in its *Cancer Program Guidelines* the specific recommendations and rationale for nutritional support services in cancer programs (Grant, 2009). These guidelines state that nutritional support services must be provided by registered dietitians (Grant, 2009). A registered dietitian has the training to appropriately assist patients in making modifications to their diet to assist them in maintaining or improving their nutritional status.

Bisphosphonate-Associated Osteonecrosis

Bisphosphonate-associated osteonecrosis (BON) was first reported in 2003 (Marx, 2003). BON is described as avascular necrosis of the jawbones caused by treatment with bisphosphonates. Bisphosphonates are synthetic analogs of pyrophosphate, which has a high affinity for calcium, that accumulate over time within the matrix of bone. The bisphosphonates pamidronate and zoledronic acid are widely used in patients with cancer to treat hypocalcemia and bony metastases (Migliorati, Schubert, Peterson, & Seneda, 2005). BON has been reported as occurring both spontaneously and following dental work, including tooth extraction (Marx, 2003). When compared to the large number of individuals taking bisphosphonates, the incidence of BON is small. However, some lesions can progress to large sizes and cause severe changes in the patient's quality of life. Advanced and nonresponsive infections may require hospitalization, prolonged antibiotic therapy, or even extensive jawbone resection (Migliorati, Casiglia, et al., 2005). Currently, prevention is the best treatment for BON (Migliorati, Casiglia, et al., 2005). Prevention currently includes establishing careful oral hygiene and avoiding risk factors such as trauma to the tissue with unnecessary surgery.

Individuals with BON may need to make adjustments to the consistency of their food to facilitate eating. Solid food may need to be chopped or pureed depending on the extent of the osteonecrosis. The National Dysphagia Diet (see Table 12-1) can be used to describe appropriate consistency based on individual limitations. In situations where the jaw is resected, patients may need to follow a full liquid diet during initial recovery (Goh, Lee, Tideman, & Stoelinga, 2008). Patients often require liquid nutritional supplementation in addition to texture modifications (Silver, 2009). The availability of numerous commercial liquid nutrition supplements allows for more choices.

Stem Cell Transplantation and Oral Development

Stem cell transplantation (SCT) requires myeloablative conditioning and may or may not require total body irradiation. SCT is an effective treatment

| Table 12-1. National Dysphagia Diet ||
Diet Consistency	Description
National Dysphagia Diets	
National Dysphagia Diet 1 (NDD-1) "Dysphagia Pureed"	Foods of pudding-like consistency that are smooth or pureed with no lumps
National Dysphagia Diet 2 (NDD-2) "Dysphagia Mechanically Altered"	Foods that are moist and soft-textured, such as tender ground or finely diced meats, soft-cooked vegetables, soft ripe or canned fruit, and some moistened cereals
National Dysphagia Diet 3 (NDD-3) "Dysphagia Advanced"	Most regular foods except very hard, sticky, or crunchy items Bread, rice, cake, shredded lettuce, and tender, moist meats are allowed.
Liquid Consistencies	
Spoon-thick	Liquids thickened to the consistency of pudding; they remain on the spoon in a soft mass.
Honey-like	Liquids thickened to the consistency of honey; the liquid flows off a spoon in a ribbon, just like actual honey.
Nectar-like	Liquids that have been thickened to a consistency that coats and drips off a spoon, similar to unset gelatin
Thin liquids	Allows all liquids

Note. Based on information from National Dysphagia Diet Task Force, 2002.

for childhood malignancies. These regimens have documented long-term effects on dentition and oral tissue in children, including tooth agenesis (failed tooth development), hypodontia, enamel hypoplasia, and malformed roots (Hölttä, Alaluusua, Saarinen-Pihkala, Peltola, & Hovi, 2005; Hölttä et al., 2002). In a study of children who underwent allogeneic SCT, nearly 100% had dental development issues, including agenesis and distorted root growth (van der Pas-van Voskuilen et al., 2009). Furthermore, 30% of these children were also found to have inadequate oral hygiene and severe gingivitis (van der Pas-van Voskuilen et al., 2009).

Similar to individuals with BON, individuals with abnormal tooth development may require food texture modifications. Liquid nutritional supplements may be helpful in these patients.

Chronic graft-versus-host disease (GVHD) is a complication of allogeneic SCT. Lenssen et al. (1990) found that more than 60% of allogeneic SCT patients exhibited chronic GVHD, resulting in weight loss in 28% of patients

(Lenssen et al., 1990). Oral sensitivity, stomatitis, xerostomia, anorexia, reflux, diarrhea, and dysgeusia were reported as symptoms that contributed to suboptimal nutrition status (Lenssen et al., 1990). Chronic GVHD is thought to occur as a result of immunocompetent donor T cells recognizing the host as foreign and therefore mounting an immune response. Chronic GVHD occurs more than 100 days after transplantation and commonly occurs in the skin, upper gastrointestinal tract, lungs, eyes, and liver (Roberts & Thompson, 2005). Chronic GVHD is treated with immunosuppressive therapy including steroids. Oral chronic GVHD can cause pain and dysphagia, which can interfere with oral intake and lead to weight loss (Jacobsohn, Margolis, Doherty, Anders, & Vogelsang, 2002). Oral chronic GVHD is managed with topical steroids, as well as topical immunosuppressants, antifungals, and sialogogues (NCI, 2010). Topical anesthetics often are essential to control pain associated with eating.

Nutrition interventions in chronic GVHD vary depending on the severity of the disease. Individuals with mouth sores should avoid salty, spicy, acidic, and rough-textured foods. Alcohol, carbonated beverages, and extremes of temperatures also can exacerbate chronic GVHD (Roberts & Thompson, 2005). Patients who are unable to maintain their weight via oral intake may require feeding tube placement and enteral feedings. Initiating enteral feedings early in the SCT period may reduce infections caused by the disruption of the gut mucosal barrier, leading to a decrease in the inflammatory response, which may predispose the patient to GVHD (Lipkin, Lenssen, & Dickson, 2005). However, obtaining enteral access may not be possible in the presence of mucositis, intractable vomiting, or diarrhea. In these cases, parenteral, or IV, nutrition would be indicated (Muscaritoli, Grieco, Capria, Iori, & Fanelli, 2002). It should be noted that parenteral nutrition is associated with an increased risk of infection and mortality in patients with cancer, so this should be considered a last resort (August & Huhmann, 2009).

Diet Following Radiation Therapy

Late oral complications of radiation therapy are chiefly a result of chronic injury to the vasculature, salivary glands, mucosa, connective tissue, and bone. The types and severity of these changes are directly related to the dose and duration of treatment (NCI, 2010). Salivary tissue changes lead to hyposalivation (Schiødt & Hermund, 2002). Interosseous blood vessel damage and decreased remodeling capacity of bone leads to risk for osteonecrosis. Late effects of radiation therapy appear weeks to months after completion of therapy and can be permanent (Barasch, Safford, & Eisenberg, 1998).

Chronic Xerostomia

Radiation may permanently alter the quality and quantity of salivary flow. Chronic xerostomia results from damage to acinar cells, the secretory cells of the salivary gland, and from tissue fibrosis (Cooper, Fu, Marks, & Silverman, 1995). It can range from small decreases in saliva production to complete dryness. Saliva plays a role in preparing food for mastication, swallowing, and normal taste perception. Hyposalivation can cause a decrease in patient quality of life related to inability to easily chew and swallow food, leading to embarrassment with eating in public (Logemann et al., 2003; Rodrigues et al., 2009; van Rij et al., 2008). In the absence of saliva's antimicrobial properties, dental caries also can become an issue. Chronic xerostomia can last months to years (Logemann et al., 2003; Mossman, Shatzman, & Chencharick, 1982).

The best treatment for chronic xerostomia is symptomatic management with use of saliva substitutes or chemical sialogogues; however, these interventions have their limitations, such as limited longevity and the need for frequent reapplication (Cooper et al., 1995; Garg & Malo, 1997). Also, sialogogues are only beneficial in patients with some residual saliva production (Garg & Malo, 1997). Recently, hypnosis and acupuncture have shown some promise in clinical trials, but more research is needed to identify the ideal number of treatments and duration of effect (Garcia et al., 2009; Schiff et al., 2009).

Xerostomia is associated with poor nutrition status and weight loss in patients with cancer (Oates et al., 2007). Patients with xerostomia frequently have difficulty in obtaining proper nutrition because of problems associated with lubricating, masticating, tasting, and swallowing food. Nutrition interventions for xerostomia include adding moisture to assist with these components of eating. Interventions such as using moist foods, adding gravies, and sipping liquids with meals may benefit the patient. One publication suggested using milk as a saliva substitute to assist with eating (Herod, 1994). Patients should be advised to maintain hydration and refrain from consuming alcohol. Sugar-free candy and gum between meals can assist with palliation as well (Garg & Malo, 1997). Patients often complain of thick, "ropey" saliva, which can lead to nausea (Rodrigues et al., 2009). Hydration assists with this to some extent. Anecdotally, patients report some relief from this ropey saliva with frequent rinses with cool, sugar-free seltzer. In the presence of persistent weight loss due to xerostomia, enteral feedings should be considered.

Dysgeusia

Dysgeusia, or distorted taste, can be a distressing late effect of radiation therapy that interferes with eating. Dysgeusia is associated with several factors, including direct neurotoxicity to taste buds, xerostomia, and infection. Changes in taste have been perceived with doses of radiation as low as 200–400 cGy (Conger, 1973). In a study of patients receiving radiation for head and neck cancer, bitter taste was affected the most, and the threshold for sweet was only affected if the tip of the tongue was in the radiation field (Zheng, Inokuchi, Yamamoto, & Komiyama, 2002). Fernando et al. (1995) observed that the degree of taste loss was associated with the proportion of tongue in the radiation field. Dysgeusia is proposed to result from damage to nerve fibers within the tongue as well as to the outer surface of the taste cells (Nelson, 1998). In some cases, taste acuity returns in two to three months after cessation of radiation; however, many patients develop permanent hypogeusia (Chasen & Bhargava, 2009; Nelson, 1998).

Nutrition interventions primarily focus on enhancing the flavor of food with more intense flavors, for example, adding additional spice to a dish while cooking. Marinating with vinegar or fruit juice–based sauces can also improve flavor. Caution should be used with acidic marinades if mouth sores are present. Also, adding strong-flavored foods, such as bacon, garlic, or Swiss cheese, to a dish can improve perception of taste.

Trismus

Trismus refers to difficulty in opening the mouth and has been defined as an interincisal gap of 25 mm or less (Bhatia et al., 2009). This occurs as a consequence of fibrosis, which develops when the muscles of mastication are involved in the treatment field. A reported 45%–50% of patients who receive radiation to the head and neck experience trismus (Bhatia et al., 2009; Kent et al., 2008). Trismus can interfere with oral hygiene, fluoride application, and dental care and is associated with decreased quality of life (Kent et al., 2008; Scott, Butterworth, Lowe, & Rogers, 2008). Speech-language pathologists can instruct patients on interventions, including mandibular stretching exercises and the use of prosthetic aids designed to reduce severity of fibrosis. It is important that these approaches be instituted prior to trismus development (Leonard, 1999). Despite the use of these exercises, some patients still require surgical release of the trismus (Heller et al., 2005).

Oral diets may require texture modifications based on the patient's ability to open the mouth and chew (Scott et al., 2008). Similar to the diet descriptions used for patients with osteonecrosis, the National Dysphagia Diet can be used to describe the oral food modifications appropriate to the individual's needs (National Dysphagia Diet Task Force, 2002).

Edentulism

Saliva plays an integral role in the prevention of dental caries. Without its protective action, acidogenic oral bacteria, such as *Streptococcus mutans* and *Lactobacillus*, colonize (Cooper et al., 1995; Higham, Quek, & Cohen, 2009). Carious lesions, often called radiation caries, may begin to appear within three months of radiation therapy and can progress rapidly (Garg & Malo, 1997). Because of the decrease in healing ability of the tissues from decreases in blood supply, infections to the jaw can be serious. These infections often result from diseased teeth. Extraction of the posterior mandibular teeth may be planned if more than 60 Gy is expected in that field (Cooper et al., 1995). Meticulous oral care, along with fluoride rinses and aggressive management of oral infections, is essential to prevent tooth loss (Sennhenn-Kirchner et al., 2009).

Diet interventions in edentulous patients must be individualized to the patient in terms of texture modifications. Patients with or at risk for tooth loss should be counseled on a noncariogenic, low-simple-carbohydrate diet to deter the development of caries. This diet should exclude regular soda, sugar-sweetened candy and gum, and concentrated juices (Rothwell, 1987).

Osteoradionecrosis

Osteoradionecrosis refers to the osteonecrosis that occurs in the jawbone as a result of damage inflicted by radiation. Chronic changes involving bone and mucosa are a result of the process of vascular inflammation and scarring that in turn result in ulceration and exposure of necrotic bone. This can lead to intolerable pain and, potentially, fracture (Cooper et al., 1995). Osteoradionecrosis has been observed in more than 60% of patients receiving radiation to the head and neck (Bhatia et al., 2009). The incidence varies with the total dose administered to the mandible, with those receiving greater than 75 Gy yielding the larger number. Also, the presence of teeth increases the risk of osteoradionecrosis (Cooper et al., 1995). Dietary interventions in these patients need to be individualized. Diet consistency can range from regular to pureed. Patients with intense pain may require enteral feedings.

Diet Following Surgery: Dysphagia

Dysphagia is a disruption to the swallowing process. It can occur at any point during transit from the oral cavity to the stomach (Gaziano, 2002). Soft tissue fibrosis, surgically induced mandibular discontinuity, and habits associated with emotional stress caused by cancer and its treatment can lead to dysphagia. Postoperative swallowing dysfunction can last more than a year after oral cancer surgery (Tei et al., 2007).

Cough; change in voice tone or quality after swallowing; abnormal movements of the mouth, tongue, or lips; abnormal gag; delayed swallowing; pharyngeal pooling; and delayed or absent trigger of swallow are symptoms of dysphagia (Buchholz, 1997; Groher, 1997; Ravich, 1997). Patients with dysphagia may not exhibit overt signs such as coughing. "Silent aspiration," or aspiration that occurs without a cough, is a common cause of complications. This occurs in more than 40% of patients treated for laryngeal cancer (Hutcheson et al., 2008). These patients require enteral feedings to avoid aspiration pneumonia (Nguyen et al., 2008). The speech-language pathologist is instrumental in the identification and treatment of dysphagia in patients with head and neck cancer (Gaziano, 2002).

The symptoms associated with dysphagia cause decreases in food intake with subsequent results in malnutrition. Patients who experience dysphagia illustrate changes in weight and albumin, indicating malnutrition (Murphy & Gilbert, 2009). This malnutrition commonly occurs secondary to inability to consume an adequate volume of food. Frustrations with the process of feeding and swallowing impede adequate ingestion of food (Gaziano, 2002). The period of adjustment to new dietary restrictions, as well as the length of duration of the rehabilitation period, may affect intake for long periods of time. Malnutrition due to inadequate protein, calorie, and micronutrient intake can significantly impede recovery. Early screening and treatment of dysphagia leads to more cost-effective treatment, improves quality of care, and ensures optimal outcome (Murphy & Gilbert, 2009).

The potential impact of pain and dysphagia on patients' ability to ingest adequate nutrients during and after cancer treatments has prompted many physicians to place prophylactic enteral feeding tubes in patients intraoperatively or prior to the initiation of cancer treatment (Raykher et al., 2009). Patients often rely on these feeding tubes for several months following the completion of their therapy (McLaughlin et al., 2010). A registered dietitian should be involved to manage enteral feedings and hydration in these patients.

Conclusion

The potential late effects of cancer treatments on the oral cavity are numerous. Dietary interventions should be individualized to the patient. A registered dietitian has the training to make recommendations based on individual issues. Referral to a registered dietitian early in the course of treatment can lead to the development of a care plan and early patient education, which leads to a better-educated patient. Educated patients can be advocates for themselves, alerting the medical team of new issues and thus allowing for early treatment.

References

American Academy of Pediatric Dentistry. (2008–2009). Guideline on dental management of pediatric patients receiving chemotherapy, hematopoietic cell transplantation, and/or radiation. *Pediatric Dentistry, 30,* 219–225.

August, D.A., & Huhmann, M.B. (2009). A.S.P.E.N. clinical guidelines: Nutrition support therapy during adult anticancer treatment and in hematopoietic cell transplantation. *Journal of Parenteral and Enteral Nutrition, 33,* 472–500. doi:10.1177/0148607109341804

Barasch, A., Safford, M., & Eisenberg, E. (1998). Oral cancer and oral effects of anticancer therapy. *Mount Sinai Journal of Medicine, 65,* 370–377.

Bhatia, K.S., King, A.D., Paunipagar, B.K., Abrigo, J., Vlantis, A.C., Leung, S.F., & Ahuja, A.T. (2009). MRI findings in patients with severe trismus following radiotherapy for nasopharyngeal carcinoma. *European Radiology, 19,* 2586–2593. doi:10.1007/s00330-009-1445-z

Brown, C.G., McGuire, D.B., Peterson, D.E., Beck, S.L., Dudley, W.N., & Mooney, K.H. (2009). The experience of a sore mouth and associated symptoms in patients with cancer receiving outpatient chemotherapy. *Cancer Nursing, 32,* 259–270. doi:10.1097/NCC.0b013e3181a38fc3

Buchholz, D.W. (1997). Neurologic disorders of swallowing. In M.E. Groher (Ed.), *Dysphagia: Diagnosis and management* (3rd ed., pp. 37–72). Boston, MA: Butterworth-Heinemann.

Chasen, M.R., & Bhargava, R. (2009). A descriptive review of the factors contributing to nutritional compromise in patients with head and neck cancer. *Supportive Care in Cancer, 17,* 1345–1351. doi:10.1007/s00520-009-0684-5

Conger, A.D. (1973). Loss and recovery of taste acuity in patients irradiated to the oral cavity. *Radiation Research, 53,* 338–347.

Cooper, J.S., Fu, K., Marks, J., & Silverman, S. (1995). Late effects of radiation therapy in the head and neck region. *International Journal of Radiation Oncology, Biology, Physics, 31,* 1141–1164. doi:10.1016/0360-3016(94)00421-G

Fernando, I.N., Patel, T., Billingham, L., Hammond, C., Hallmark, S., Glaholm, J., & Henk, J.M. (1995). The effect of head and neck irradiation on taste dysfunction: A prospective study. *Clinical Oncology, 7,* 173–178.

Garcia, M.K., Chiang, J.S., Cohen, L., Liu, M., Palmer, J.L., Rosenthal, D.I., ... Chambers, M.S. (2009). Acupuncture for radiation-induced xerostomia in patients with cancer: A pilot study. *Head and Neck, 31,* 1360–1368. doi:10.1002/hed.21110

Garg, A.K., & Malo, M. (1997). Manifestations and treatment of xerostomia and associated oral effects secondary to head and neck radiation therapy. *Journal of the American Dental Association, 128,* 1128–1133.

Gaziano, J.E. (2002). Evaluation and management of oropharyngeal dysphagia in head and neck cancer. *Cancer Control, 9,* 400–409.

Goh, B.T., Lee, S., Tideman, H., & Stoelinga, P.J. (2008). Mandibular reconstruction in adults: A review. *International Journal of Oral and Maxillofacial Surgery, 37,* 597–605. doi:10.1016/j.ijom.2008.03.002

Grant, B. (2009). CSOs—Certified specialists in oncology nutrition: Taking nutrition care in community cancer centers to new heights. *Oncology Issues, 24*(6), 47–49.

Groher, M.E. (1997). Mechanical disorders of swallowing. In M.E. Groher (Ed.), *Dysphagia: Diagnosis and management* (3rd ed., pp. 73–106). Boston, MA: Butterworth-Heinemann.

Heller, F., Wei, F.-C., Chang, Y.-M., Tsai, C.-Y., Liao, H.-T., Lin, C.-L., & Kuo, Y.-C. (2005). A non-tooth-borne mouth-opening device for postoperative rehabilitation after surgical release of trismus. *Plastic and Reconstructive Surgery, 116,* 1856–1859. doi:10.1097/01.prs.0000191178.21552.7f

Herod, E.L. (1994). The use of milk as a saliva substitute. *Journal of Public Health Dentistry, 54,* 184–189.

Higham, P., Quek, S., & Cohen, H.V. (2009). Dental management for head and neck cancer patients undergoing radiation therapy: Comprehensive patient based planning—A case report. *Journal of the New Jersey Dental Association, 80*(1), 31–33.

Hogan, R. (2009). Implementation of an oral care protocol and its effects on oral mucositis. *Journal of Pediatric Oncology Nursing, 26,* 125–135. doi:10.1177/1043454209334356

Hölttä, P., Alaluusua, S., Saarinen-Pihkala, U.M., Peltola, J., & Hovi, L. (2005). Agenesis and microdontia of permanent teeth as late adverse effects after stem cell transplantation in young children. *Cancer, 103,* 181–190. doi:10.1002/cncr.20762

Hölttä, P., Alaluusua, S., Saarinen-Pihkala, U.M., Wolf, J., Nyström, M., & Hovi, L. (2002). Long-term adverse effects on dentition in children with poor-risk neuroblastoma treated with high-dose chemotherapy and autologous stem cell transplantation with or without total body irradiation. *Bone Marrow Transplantation, 29,* 121–127. doi:10.1038/sj.bmt.1703330

Horner, M., Ries, L., Krapcho, M., Neyman, N., Aminou, R., Howlader, N., Altekruse, S., ... Edwards, B.K. (2009). SEER cancer statistics review, 1975–2006. Retrieved from http://seer.cancer.gov/csr/1975_2006/

Hutcheson, K.A., Barringer, D.A., Rosenthal, D.I., May, A.H., Roberts, D.B., & Lewin, J.S. (2008). Swallowing outcomes after radiotherapy for laryngeal carcinoma. *Archives of Otolaryngology—Head and Neck Surgery, 134,* 178–183. doi:10.1001/archoto.2007.33

Ilgenli, T., Ören, H., & Uysal, K. (2001). The acute effects of chemotherapy upon the oral cavity: Prevention and management. *Turkish Journal of Cancer, 31,* 93–105.

Jacobsohn, D.A., Margolis, J., Doherty, J., Anders, V., & Vogelsang, G.B. (2002). Weight loss and malnutrition in patients with chronic graft-versus-host disease. *Bone Marrow Transplantation, 29,* 231–236. doi:10.1038/sj.bmt.1703352

Kent, M.L., Brennan, M.T., Noll, J.L., Fox, P.C., Burri, S.H., Hunter, J.C., & Lockhart, P.B. (2008). Radiation-induced trismus in head and neck cancer patients. *Supportive Care in Cancer, 16,* 305–309. doi:10.1007/s00520-007-0345-5

Lenssen, P., Sherry, M.E., Cheney, C.L., Nims, J.W., Sullivan, K.M., Stern, J.M., … Aker, S.N. (1990). Prevalence of nutrition-related problems among long-term survivors of allogeneic marrow transplantation. *Journal of the American Dietetic Association, 90,* 835–842.

Leonard, M. (1999). Trismus: What is it, what causes it, and how to treat it. *Dentistry Today, 18*(6), 74–77.

Lipkin, A.C., Lenssen, P., & Dickson, B.J. (2005). Nutrition issues in hematopoietic stem cell transplantation: State of the art. *Nutrition in Clinical Practice, 20,* 423–439. doi:10.1177/0115426505020004423

Logemann, J.A., Pauloski, B.R., Rademaker, A.W., Lazarus, C.L., Mittal, B., Gaziano, J., … Newman, L.A. (2003). Xerostomia: 12-month changes in saliva production and its relationship to perception and performance of swallow function, oral intake, and diet after chemoradiation. *Head and Neck, 25,* 432–437. doi:10.1002/hed.10255

Marx, R.E. (2003). Pamidronate (Aredia) and zoledronate (Zometa) induced avascular necrosis of the jaws: A growing epidemic. *Journal of Oral and Maxillofacial Surgery, 61,* 1115–1117. doi:10.1016/S0278-2391(03)00720-1

McLaughlin, B.T., Gokhale, A.S., Shuai, Y., Diacopoulos, J., Carrau, R., Heron, D.E., … Argiris, A. (2010). Management of patients treated with chemoradiotherapy for head and neck cancer without prophylactic feeding tubes: The University of Pittsburgh experience. *Laryngoscope, 120,* 71–75. doi:10.1002/lary.20697

Migliorati, C.A., Casiglia, J., Epstein, J., Jacobsen, P.L., Siegel, M.A., & Woo, S.B. (2005). Managing the care of patients with bisphosphonate-associated osteonecrosis: An American Academy of Oral Medicine position paper. *Journal of the American Dental Association, 136,* 1658–1668.

Migliorati, C.A., Schubert, M.M., Peterson, D.E., & Seneda, L.M. (2005). Bisphosphonate-associated osteonecrosis of mandibular and maxillary bone: An emerging oral complication of supportive cancer therapy. *Cancer, 104,* 83–93. doi:10.1002/cncr.21130

Mossman, K., Shatzman, A., & Chencharick, J. (1982). Long-term effects of radiotherapy on taste and salivary function in man. *International Journal of Radiation Oncology, Biology, Physics, 8,* 991–997. doi:10.1016/0360-3016(82)90166-3

Murphy, B.A., & Gilbert, J. (2009). Dysphagia in head and neck cancer patients treated with radiation: Assessment, sequelae, and rehabilitation. *Seminars in Radiation Oncology, 19,* 35–42. doi:10.1016/j.semradonc.2008.09.007

Muscaritoli, M., Grieco, G., Capria, S., Iori, A.P., & Fanelli, F.R. (2002). Nutritional and metabolic support in patients undergoing bone marrow transplantation. *American Journal of Clinical Nutrition, 75,* 183–190.

National Cancer Institute. (2010). Oral complications of chemotherapy and head/neck radiation (PDQ®) [Health professional version]. Retrieved from http://www.cancer .gov/cancertopics/pdq/supportivecare/oralcomplications/healthprofessional/ allpages#Section_409

National Dysphagia Diet Task Force. (2002). *National Dysphagia Diet: Standardization for optimal care.* Chicago, IL: American Dietetic Association.

Nelson, G.M. (1998). Biology of taste buds and the clinical problem of taste loss. *Anatomical Record, 253,* 70–78. doi:10.1002/(SICI)1097-0185(199806)253:3<70::AID-AR3>3.0.CO;2-I

Nguyen, N.P., Frank, C., Moltz, C.C., Millar, C., Vos, P., Smith, H.J., … Sallah, S. (2008). Risk of aspiration following radiation for non-nasopharyngeal head and neck cancer. *Journal of Otolaryngology-Head and Neck Surgery, 37,* 225–229.

Oates, J.E., Clark, J.R., Read, J., Reeves, N., Gao, K., Jackson, M., … O'Brien, C.J. (2007). Prospective evaluation of quality of life and nutrition before and after treatment for nasopharyngeal carcinoma. *Archives of Otolaryngology—Head and Neck Surgery, 133,* 533–540. doi:10.1001/archotol.133.6.533

Ravich, W.J. (1997). Esophageal dysphagia. In M.E. Groher (Ed.), *Dysphagia: Diagnosis and management* (3rd ed., pp. 107–130). Boston, MA: Butterworth-Heinemann.

Raykher, A., Correa, L., Russo, L., Brown, P., Lee, N., Pfister, D., … Shike, M. (2009). The role of pretreatment percutaneous endoscopic gastrostomy in facilitating therapy of head and neck cancer and optimizing the body mass index of the obese patient. *Journal of Parenteral and Enteral Nutrition, 33,* 404–410. doi:10.1177/0148607108327525

Roberts, S., & Thompson, J. (2005). Graft-vs-host disease: Nutrition therapy in a challenging condition. *Nutrition in Clinical Practice, 20,* 440–450. doi:10.1177/0115426505020004440

Rodrigues, N.A., Killion, L., Hickey, G., Silver, B., Martin, C., Stevenson, M.A., … Ng, A.K. (2009). A prospective study of salivary gland function in lymphoma patients receiving head and neck irradiation. *International Journal of Radiation Oncology, Biology, Physics, 75,* 1079–1083. doi:10.1016/j.ijrobp.2008.12.053

Rothwell, B.R. (1987). Prevention and treatment of the orofacial complications of radiotherapy. *Journal of the American Dental Association, 114,* 316–322.

Schiff, E., Mogilner, J.G., Sella, E., Doweck, I., Hershko, O., Ben-Arye, E., & Yarom, N. (2009). Hypnosis for postradiation xerostomia in head and neck cancer patients: A pilot study. *Journal of Pain and Symptom Management, 37,* 1086–1092.e1. doi:10.1016/j.jpainsymman.2008.07.005

Schiødt, M., & Hermund, N.U. (2002). Management of oral disease prior to radiation therapy. *Supportive Care in Cancer, 10,* 40–43.

Scott, B., Butterworth, C., Lowe, D., & Rogers, S.N. (2008). Factors associated with restricted mouth opening and its relationship to health-related quality of life in patients attending a maxillofacial oncology clinic. *Oral Oncology, 44,* 430–438. doi:10.1016/j.oraloncology.2007.06.015

Sennhenn-Kirchner, S., Freund, F., Grundmann, S., Martin, A., Borg-von Zepelin, M., Christiansen, H., … Jacobs, H.G. (2009). Dental therapy before and after radiotherapy—An evaluation on patients with head and neck malignancies. *Clinical Oral Investigations, 13,* 157–164. doi:10.1007/s00784-008-0229-1

Silver, H.J. (2009). Food modification versus oral liquid nutrition supplementation. *Nestlé Nutrition Institute Workshop Series: Clinical and Performance Programme, 12,* 79–93. doi:10.1159/000235670

Tei, K., Maekawa, K., Kitada, H., Ohiro, Y., Yamazaki, Y., & Totsuka, Y. (2007). Recovery from postsurgical swallowing dysfunction in patients with oral cancer. *Journal of Oral and Maxillofacial Surgery, 65,* 1077–1083. doi:10.1016/j.joms.2005.12.082

van der Pas-van Voskuilen, I.G., Veerkamp, J.S., Raber-Durlacher, J.E., Bresters, D., van Wijk, A.J., Barasch, A., … Gortzak, R.A. (2009). Long-term adverse effects of hematopoietic stem cell transplantation on dental development in children. *Supportive Care in Cancer, 17,* 1169–1175. doi:10.1007/s00520-008-0567-1

van Rij, C.M., Oughlane-Heemsbergen, W.D., Ackerstaff, A.H., Lamers, E.A., Balm, A.J., & Rasch, C.R. (2008). Parotid gland sparing IMRT for head and neck cancer improves xerostomia related quality of life. *Radiation Oncology, 3,* 41. doi:10.1186/1748-717X-3-41

Zheng, W.K., Inokuchi, A., Yamamoto, T., & Komiyama, S. (2002). Taste dysfunction in irradiated patients with head and neck cancer. *Fukuoka Igaku Zasshi, 93*(4), 64–76.

CHAPTER 13

Psychosocial Challenges

Erika Schroeder, RN, MS, OCN®, CNL, and Mary Ellyn Witt, RN, MS, AOCN®

Introduction

> Psychosocial and social problems created or exacerbated by cancer—including depression and other emotional problems; lack of information or skills needed to manage illness; lack of transportation or other resources; and disruptions in work, school, and family life—cause additional suffering, weaken adherence to prescribed treatments, and threaten patients' return to health.
> —From Institute of Medicine [IOM], 2008, p.1

The opening quote summarizes the findings of a 2008 report from IOM titled *Cancer Care for the Whole Patient: Meeting Psychosocial Health Needs*. The National Institutes of Health and IOM convened the project to study what psychosocial services are needed for patients with cancer, how they are delivered, and what improvements the healthcare system should make to address these issues. The report recommended that all patients who receive cancer care are entitled to appropriate psychosocial health services. In short, addressing psychosocial health needs is an "integral part of quality cancer care" (IOM, 2008, p. 8).

The IOM report and many advocates in cancer care have beseeched clinicians to appreciate the interrelatedness of cancer, its treatment, and the economic, societal, and psychosocial impacts that a cancer diagnosis can impart (see Figure 13-1). Even so, nearly 3 in 10 (28%) patients and families polled in the National Survey of Households Affected by Cancer, conducted jointly by *USA Today*, the Kaiser Family Foundation, and the Harvard School of Public Health (Kaiser Family Foundation, 2006), said they do not have a doctor who pays attention to factors outside of their direct medical care, such as

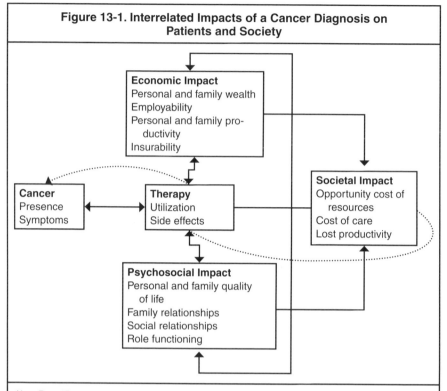

Figure 13-1. Interrelated Impacts of a Cancer Diagnosis on Patients and Society

Note. From "Psychosocial and Economic Impact of Cancer," by L.S. Elting, E.B.C. Avritscher, C.D. Cooksley, M. Cardenas-Turanzas, A.S. Garden, and M.S. Chambers, 2008, *Dental Clinics of North America, 52,* p. 232. Copyright 2008 by Elsevier. Reprinted with permission.

their support network for dealing with cancer. Furthermore, one-third of respondents said that the experience of having cancer caused someone in their household to have emotional or psychological problems (Kaiser Family Foundation, 2006). Patients with cancer with oral complications are not immune to this gap in care, and the psychosocial impact of cancer may actually be greater in these patients for a number of reasons. Patients with oral complications as a result of surgery, chemotherapy, or radiotherapy may have altered vital functions, such as chewing and swallowing, and disfigurement. Changes in the dental integrity can also impair speaking. These visible deformities can greatly affect a person's body image and interaction with society. For these reasons, head and neck (H&N) cancer specifically has been described as a "psychologically highly traumatic cancer type" (De Boer, McCormick, Pruyn, Ryckman, & van den Borne, 1999). Patients with H&N cancer are reported to experience the highest rates of major depressive disorder of all patients with cancer (Lydiatt, Moran, & Burke, 2009). A recent study involving patients with oral chronic graft-versus-host disease (cGVHD) following hematopoietic stem cell transplantation found that subjects with moderate to severe oral dryness tended to report the poorest overall health-related quality of life. Subjects with more severe oral cGVHD manifestations reported significantly lower scores in the social and family well-being domains on the Functional Assessment of Cancer Therapy–General (Fall-Dickson et al., 2010). These findings support the role for an intense psychosocial monitoring and intervention plan in patients with oral complications. This chapter will highlight the unique needs of this population along with tools and references to aid oncology nurses in providing high-quality psychosocial services to their patients.

Oral Complications of Survivorship

Nurses are educated to recognize and manage symptoms along the entire treatment trajectory, from diagnosis to long-term and late effects of cancer treatments. Patients deserve more than just a prescription to treat the life-altering side effects they may experience; they deserve the recognition of how these chronic symptoms affect relationships within and outside the home, their financial stability, and the psychosocial adjustments they must make throughout their experience.

What are the chronic complications that may affect adjustment? Xerostomia (dry mouth), trismus (inability to open the mouth), taste changes, impaired nutrition, alterations in breathing and appearance, and unrelieved pain may affect a patient's quality of life for many years after treatment has ended. Xerostomia, or salivary hypofunction, is associated with oral discomfort and pain, increased rates of dental caries and oral infection, difficulty speaking and swallowing, and, in severe cases, decreased oral intake and weight loss (Chambers, Garden, Kies, & Martin, 2004). Although it often is thought of in the context of H&N radiation, severe xerostomia has been found to be a distressing symptom for patients receiving chemotherapy, analgesics, and antidepressants. While the symptoms of mild xerostomia may be ameliorated with inexpensive sugarless gum, severe and prolonged xerostomia can contribute to the need for costly medications and expensive dental care for the prevention and extraction of caries (Elting et al., 2008).

Trismus may develop because of tumor invasion of the masticator muscles or the temporomandibular joint (TMJ) or as a side effect of treatment if these areas are in the radiation field. Survivors may experience this complication as a result of muscle fibrosis in the ligaments around the TMJ and scarring of the muscle (Vissink, Jansma, Spijkervet, Burlage, & Coppes, 2003). Dental treatment and intraoral examination can be difficult and may result in chronic pain (Melchers et al., 2009).

A variety of rehabilitation aids are available that can help maintain and restore function of the jaw following treatment. Dynasplint® (Dynasplint Systems, Inc.), TheraBite® (Altos Medical), OraStretch® (CranioMandibular Rehab, Inc.), and other devices are available to assist in the rehabilitation process. Insurance will often cover the cost of a device to aid in improving the effects of trismus. However, research by Melchers et al. (2009) revealed that insurance coverage and teaching a patient to use the device does not guarantee a good outcome. Their research explored factors that influenced exercise adherence with the use of TheraBite. Internal motivation to exercise, perceiving a positive effect, self-discipline, and having a clear exercise goal positively influenced exercise adherence. Perceiving no effect, limitations in TheraBite opening range, and reaching the exercise goal or a plateau in mouth opening were negative influences. Pain and anxiety could influence using the device both positively and negatively (Melchers et al., 2009).

Alterations in taste can result from chemotherapy and radiation to the oral cavity. Subjective recovery can be appreciated within months after treatment, but with more aggressive treatment, taste changes have a slower recovery time and may never return to pretreatment function. Disappointment when eating can lead to weight loss and the use of costly supplements to maintain weight (Rydholm & Strang, 2002; Specht, 2002).

Dysphagia, or difficulty swallowing, may be a temporary survivorship challenge or one that may last a lifetime. Patients often are unprepared for the emotions they encounter when mealtime consumption is altered. The inability to participate in mealtimes and dining out can be isolating. Increased mealtimes, limited food choices, special food preparation methods, and untidy consumption contribute to avoidance of social food consumption (Gaziano, 2002).

Survivors may experience stress related to returning to work and the alterations of the food process. Use of tube feedings, diet modifications, adaptive equipment, or rehabilitative strategies for safe and adequate intake may attract unwanted attention and become a source of anxiety for the patient (Gaziano, 2002).

Facial and neck disfigurement has long been viewed as one of the most potentially distressing aspects of H&N cancer because of the vital importance of the facial region to self-concept, interpersonal relationships, and communication, and the fact that disfigurement in the face and neck is highly visible. Katz, Irish, Devins, Rodin, and Gullane (2003) reported that women with disfigurement reported higher intensities of depressive symptoms than men. On the other hand, women with disfigurement experienced more benefit from social support than men with disfigurement.

Chronic pain in a survivor may be the result of damage from the tumor that started before treatment or a complication from surgery or radiation. Scharpf, Karnell, Chistensen, and Funk (2009) reported that 10% of patients treated for H&N cancer reported severe pain 12 months after diagnosis. Pain often is accompanied by fatigue, nausea, and insomnia, which can affect physical health. Chronic pain can lead to feelings of agitation, anger, and hopelessness and can influence overall mental health (Scharpf et al., 2009). Living in chronic pain can take away many of life's pleasures that were once enjoyed. Patients and families may not admit to the healthcare provider how their life has changed and how they are coping with these alterations. It becomes the nurse's role to take the time to assess the psychosocial ramifications and work with the patient and family to improve quality of life during survivorship.

In conclusion, survivors with oral complications may experience limitations with eating, speaking, and oral hygiene. These limitations can greatly affect their body image and may cause them to withdraw from social interactions. Because a good support network has been shown to improve health-related quality of life in patients with H&N cancer (Llewellyn, McGurk, & Weinman, 2005), it is vital to address body image issues with patients before they arise and during treatment. It also is key to recognize the effect that depression may have on patients and their treatment. It has been shown that depressed patients take more treatment breaks and require a longer time period to complete their prescribed therapy (Lydiatt et al., 2009). Early intervention to screen for and diagnose depression is vital in this vulnerable population.

Financial Challenges

A significant portion of patients receiving treatment for cancer report that their illness has a substantial impact on their finances, with almost half of those people questioned in a national survey saying that the cost of cancer care was a significant burden to their families (Kaiser Family Foundation, 2006). Treatment-related costs, time off of work, the cost of medication, and other expenses can severely burden patients, especially those who have limited means before their illness and those without health insurance. Financial struggles cause significant stress in patients undergoing cancer treatment. As one researcher stated, "the complex financial issues associated with a cancer diagnosis within the family are often hidden from friends and health professionals as families struggle to make decisions, manage emotions, and preserve the family unit" (Bennett et al., 2008, p. 1058). It is unknown whether the entire cohort of patients with cancer with oral complications suffers more or less with financial issues than the general cancer population. Studies have, however, reported that low socioeconomic status is associated with an increased risk of oral cancer (Conway et al., 2008) and that patients with H&N cancer who are living in areas of high poverty have higher rates of mortality from their disease (Molina et al., 2008). These observations highlight the interrelatedness of socioeconomic status and cancer and should be a consideration in the plan of care for a patient with oral complications.

Patients may be reluctant to ask for financial assistance, but nurses can support their patients by assessing their level of need, providing them with information, and connecting them to community resources. Social workers, case managers, and nurse navigators typically have more expertise in navigating insurance coverage for patients and connecting them with local and national resources. A referral to these professionals may be appropriate for patients who have extraordinary financial burdens that have worsened as a result of their cancer. On the other hand, a large portion of patients with cancer may feel that they do not require financial assistance but could benefit from financial counseling to budget for their planned and unplanned financial expenses in light of their cancer diagnosis. The American Cancer Society and the Lance Armstrong Foundation both provide excellent resources for financial planning and budgeting on their Web sites (see Table 13-1). Providing in-

Table 13-1. Resources for Financial Assistance for Patients With Cancer		
Resource	**Type of Assistance**	**Web Address**
American Cancer Society	Provides a number of insurance and financial resources to educate patients and caregivers. A section titled "Taking Care of Money Matters" includes guidance on how to budget in case cancer occurs in the family and coping financially when a loved one dies of cancer.	www.cancer.org/Treatment/ FindingandPayingforTreatment/index
Livestrong, the Lance Armstrong Foundation	Section titled "Practical Effects of Cancer" provides information and links to resources on topics including assistance programs, employment, finances, and healthcare planning.	www.livestrong.org/Get-Help/Learn -About-Cancer/Cancer-Support -Topics/Practical-Effects-of-Cancer
National Cancer Institute	Maintains a database that can be searched for financial resources from both government and nonprofit agencies. The database is searchable by type of financial assistance and by keyword.	https://cissecure.nci.nih.gov/ factsheet/FactsheetSearch8_3.aspx
NeedyMeds	Provides links to patient assistance programs that help with paying for the cost of medicines. The site provides Web links and step-by-step instructions on how to apply for a number of these programs. A comprehensive list of medications, listed by brand and generic name, can be queried to find assistance programs linked to a specific drug.	www.needymeds.org

formation about financial resources can be one way to increase the sense of control a patient feels in dealing with the illness.

It is estimated that approximately half of all patients with cancer are employed or available for employment at the time of diagnosis (Rasmussen & Elverdam, 2008). Remaining employed is important to cancer survivors for a variety of reasons, including financial status, quality of life, and self-esteem (Buckwalter, Karnell, Smith, Christensen, & Funk, 2007; Verdonck-de Leeuw, van Bleek, Leemans, & de Bree, 2010). Reasons for not returning to work after cancer treatment may not always be related to the cancer or treatment. Patients who are older at the time of diagnosis or have multiple comorbidities may choose to retire at the time of diagnosis.

The cancer survivor's ability to return to work is associated with a number of variables. Survivors with advanced cancer at diagnosis, those who received treatment that included chemotherapy, and those with a history of alcohol use typically encounter more barriers with returning to work. The patient's type of work, workplace support, education level, and income can influence the decision to return to work. Pain and fatigue resulting from the cancer or treatment also have been shown to cause patients to discontinue employment (Verdonck-de Leeuw et al., 2010).

Physical changes to the oral cavity may influence a patient's return to employment and ability to maintain employment. Anxiety, along with oral dysfunctions, such as xerostomia, trismus, sticky saliva, problems with teeth, loss of appetite, and problems with social eating and social contacts, can affect the patient's ability to feel comfortable and function in the work environment (Verdonck-de Leeuw et al., 2010). Buckwalter et al. (2007) reported in a study of patients with H&N cancer that of 239 patients who were employed at the time of diagnosis, 38.1% discontinued work because of their cancer and treatment. Five factors were significant for not returning to work: fatigue, change in speech, change in eating, pain or discomfort, and change in appearance.

McKee-Ryan, Song, Wanberg, and Kinicki (2005) reported that the way in which an individual copes with unemployment will affect overall adjustment during this life change. Personal resources, physical health, and financial resources contribute to adjustment with unemployment. Personal resources are internal resources that an individual will draw on when faced with a stressful life event. Simply phrased, an individual's personality can affect his or her psychological well-being during unemployment. Individuals with higher self-esteem, higher perceived control, and higher levels of optimism generally cope more effectively (McKee-Ryan et al., 2005).

Survivors dealing with physical limitations, especially exhaustion, may have higher levels of depression, irritability, anxiety, and difficulty with mastering a job change or unemployment. They may start to engage in high-risk behavior and could be at risk for abusing alcohol. Nurses can identify patients who could benefit from intensive rehabilitation after treatment completion. Rehabilitation focuses not only on the physical symptoms but also psychosocial support for patient and caregivers. This may involve referral to a support group or recommending an individual or family for counseling (McKee-Ryan et al., 2005; Vartanian, Carvalho, Toyota, Kowalski, & Kowalski, 2006). Family counseling may be beneficial in certain situations because unemployment will cause role changes within the family structure. Patient finances influence the patient's ability to follow through on a referral for counseling. For patients who cannot afford to pay for counseling on their own, being aware of community resources can lessen their stress when counseling and rehabilitation are recommended.

Assessment Tools

Screening patients for psychosocial problems and referring them to resources may or may not be a routine part of the oncology nurse's clinical practice. The 2008 IOM report *Cancer Care for the Whole Patient: Meeting Psychosocial Health Needs* confirmed that screening for psychosocial needs using validated instruments is not routine practice in oncology. In a national survey of 1,000 randomly selected members of the American Society of Clinical Oncology, only 14% of those interviewed reported that they screened for psychosocial distress using a standardized tool (Jacobsen & Ransom, 2007). The reasons cited for not screening included lack of time, a perception of limited resources, and a belief that patients would be unwilling to discuss their distress with the provider (Jacobsen & Ransom, 2007). In response, IOM recommended that all providers of cancer care must design and implement plans to identify each patient's psychosocial health needs (IOM, 2008). Ambiguity exists surrounding which screening tool is the most sensitive and specific in identifying patients who could receive the most benefit from screening and referral; however, well-validated tools are available that need to be implemented and evaluated in practice. The following section will provide a brief summary of some screening tools along with how long each one takes to administer. Each of these tools are evidence based and have been validated, but it will take more research in the entire oncology community, and especially in individual practices, to see which tool is best suited for clinical practice. For more information on screening tools, the reader is referred to a systematic review conducted by Wen and Gustafson (2004) on needs assessment tools and a review by Vodermaier, Linden, and Siu (2009) that looked specifically at assessment screening tools for emotional distress in patients with cancer.

Distress Thermometer

The National Comprehensive Cancer Network (NCCN) publishes clinical practice guidelines to provide evidence-based cancer treatment and symptom management recommendations to clinicians. Their toolkit includes a guideline for distress management in patients with cancer. The panel that created these guidelines specifically addresses their intention behind using the word *distress* as opposed to *psychiatric, psychosocial*, or *emotional* management of patients. They stated that the term *distress* is less stigmatizing than the aforementioned words and may be less embarrassing and more acceptable to both clinicians and patients alike (NCCN, 2010). The tool that the NCCN endorses is termed the distress thermometer (DT). This tool asks patients to provide a rating of their level of distress over the past week on a scale of 0 (no distress) to 10 (extreme distress). A 36-item problem list also accompanies it, in which patients can identify problems in specific categories: practical, family, emotional, spiritual/religious, and physical (see Figure 13-2). A distress score of

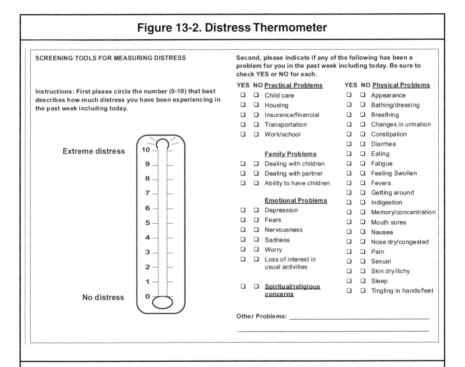

Figure 13-2. Distress Thermometer

4 or higher suggests a clinically significant finding that should be addressed. The advantages of the DT include that the tool can be completed by the patient independently; it takes no more than a few minutes to complete; and it has shown good sensitivity and specificity in identifying patients with distress (NCCN, 2010). After studying the DT alongside several other screening tools, Clover, Carter, Mackinnon, and Adams (2009) concluded that using the DT as part of a two-stage screening algorithm minimized the burden on patients and staff while maximizing screening effectiveness. Patients who scored 4 or higher on the DT were given a second screening tool with a written copy of the results generated for their oncologist. Patients whose distress fell below the level of clinical significance (71% of patients in this study) on the DT received no further intervention. This method of screening falls in line with the general principle cited in the 2008 IOM report and the NCCN guidelines— that no patient with distress goes unrecognized and untreated.

The optimal schedule for evaluating distress has not been identified, but NCCN recommends that patients be screened at the initial visit and as clinically indicated, especially if changes occur that make a patient more vulnerable in the cancer journey. Figure 13-3 highlights periods of increased vulnerability along with patient characteristics that may place the patient at an increased risk for ineffective coping.

Hospital Anxiety and Depression Scale

The Hospital Anxiety and Depression Scale (HADS) (Zigmond & Snaith, 1983) is a tool widely used in oncology that is specific to identifying states of anxiety and depression. It is a 14-question self-screening questionnaire for patients that includes seven questions for anxiety and seven for depression. A study by Singer et al. (2008) compared six screening instruments for mental disorders in patients with laryngeal cancer. Although all of the tools were highly accurate, the HADS was the most specific and sensitive in picking up these disorders in this patient population. The assessment can be completed by the patient in the waiting room and takes less than five minutes to complete.

Screening Tools for Patients With Oral Complications

No uniform screening tool exists for all patients with cancer who have oral complications. Site- and treatment-specific assessments are available, however, that provide oncology nurses and providers with a glimpse of a particular patient's health-related quality of life at a point in time. Murphy, Ridner, Wells, and Dietrich (2007) found 10 quality-of-life instruments for patients with H&N cancer in their review, while an earlier study done by De Boer et al. (1999) found 14 measures specific to these patients. The Functional Assessment of Cancer Therapy–Head and Neck scale, the European Organisation for Research and Treatment of Cancer Quality of Life Questionnaire–Head and Neck-35, and the University of Washington Quality of Life Questionnaire are popular assessment tools used specifically in patients with H&N cancer. In hematopoietic stem cell and bone marrow transplan-

---

Figure 13-3. Psychosocial Distress Patient Characteristics[a]

Patients at Increased Risk for Distress[b]
- History of psychiatric disorder/substance abuse
- History of depression/suicide attempt
- Cognitive impairment
- Communication barriers[c]
- Severe comorbid illnesses
- Social problems
- Family/caregiver conflicts
  - Inadequate social support
  - Living alone
  - Financial problems
  - Limited access to medical care
  - Young or dependent children
  - Younger age; woman
  - History of abuse (physical, sexual)
  - Other stressors
- Spiritual/religious concerns

Periods of Increased Vulnerability
- Finding a suspicious symptom
- During workup
- Finding out the diagnosis
- Awaiting treatment
- Change in treatment modality
- End of treatment
- Discharge from hospital following treatment
- Stresses of survivorship
- Medical follow-up and surveillance
- Treatment failure
- Recurrence/progression
- Advanced cancer
- End of life

[a] For site-specific symptoms with major psychosocial consequences, see Holland, JC, Greenberg, DB, Hughes, MD, et al. Quick Reference for Oncology Clinicians: The Psychiatric and Psychological Dimensions of Cancer Symptom Management. (Based on the NCCN Distress Management Guidelines). IPOS Press, 2006. Available at www.apos-society.org.

[b] From the NCCN Palliative Care Clinical Practice Guidelines in Oncology. Available at www.nccn.org.

[c] Communication barriers include language, literacy, and physical barriers.

Note: All recommendations are category 2A unless otherwise indicated.

Clinical Trials: The NCCN believes that the best management of any cancer patient is in a clinical trial. Participation in clinical trials is especially encouraged.

Note. Reproduced with permission from The NCCN 1.2010 Distress Management Clinical Practice Guidelines in Oncology. ©National Comprehensive Cancer Network, 2010. Available at http://www.nccn.org. Accessed January 7, 2010. To view the most recent and complete version of the guideline, go online to www.nccn.org.

These Guidelines are a work in progress that will be refined as often as new significant data becomes available.

The NCCN Guidelines are a statement of consensus of its authors regarding their views of currently accepted approaches to treatment. Any clinician seeking to apply or consult any NCCN guideline is expected to use independent medical judgment in the context of individual clinical circumstances to determine any patient's care or treatment. The National Comprehensive Cancer Network makes no warranties of any kind whatsoever regarding their content, use or application and disclaims any responsibility for their application or use in any way.

These Guidelines are copyrighted by the National Comprehensive Cancer Network. All rights reserved. These Guidelines and illustrations herein may not be reproduced in any form for any purpose without the express written permission of the NCCN.

tation, the Functional Assessment of Cancer Therapy–Bone Marrow Transplantation frequently is used to follow health-related quality of life during and after transplantation.

It is beyond the scope of this chapter to discuss which quality-of-life measurement is best suited for patients with oral complications; however, picking an instrument and piloting it in practice could be the first step in providing better psychosocial care to patients.

Interventions

When a patient screens positive for clinically significant distress or an unmet need for psychosocial services is identified, referral to the appropriate service is necessary. The NCCN (2010) clinical practice guidelines for distress management consist of a number of algorithms to guide treatment for the entire spectrum of distress that a patient may experience. The guidelines provide evidence-based treatment recommendations for a variety of distressing symptoms, from the very common feelings of hopelessness and isolation to less common experiences such as mood disorders and delirium. Referral to an appropriate service will depend on the diagnosis and may include social workers, nurse navigators, chaplains, psychiatrists, and other members of the oncology team. The NCCN guidelines can be accessed for free at www.nccn.org.

Pharmacologic interventions are indicated for people experiencing severe distress, clinical depression, and other mental disorders. For the majority of patients with mild to moderate distress, six nonpharmacologic evidence-based interventions are used: cognitive-behavioral therapy, stress reduction exercises, problem-solving techniques (COPE), exercise, support groups, and complementary therapies (American Psychosocial Oncology Society, 2006). Unfortunately, the intervention that a patient chooses to try may depend on the services available in his or her area as well as financial coverage by an insurance company; however, many support groups are free and various nonprofit agencies around the country have stepped in to provide these services. In 2009, the Wellness Community and Gilda's Club merged to provide psychosocial services to patients with cancer at no cost; the combined organization comprises 50 local affiliates, 12 affiliates in development, and more than 100 satellite locations. Together the organizations provide professionally led support groups, educational workshops, nutrition and exercise programs, and stress-reduction classes to patients with cancer and their caregivers. These groups see the 2008 IOM report on psychosocial cancer care as defining affirmation of the work of both the Wellness Community and Gilda's Club (Cancer Support Community, n.d.). The American Cancer Society, the Leukemia and Lymphoma Foundation, and many other groups are committed to lessening the psychosocial burden of a cancer diagnosis. Putting patients in contact with a nonprofit resource could be invaluable to help them cope with their disease.

Education

Education is another important nursing intervention for all patients with oral complications. A systematic review by Harrison, Young, Price, Butow, and Solomon (2009) showed that information was one of the most frequently reported unmet supportive care needs in patients with cancer. In support of providing education, a review by De Boer et al. (1999) reached the conclusion that information and support have a positive influence on the rehabilitation of patients with H&N cancer. Nurses need to continually educate themselves on symptom management strategies, new treatment regimens, and disease pathology so that they can be ready to answer questions from their patients. The National Cancer Institute has a number of educational pamphlets available. These booklets can be ordered at no cost, or the material can be viewed online at www.cancer.gov.

Alcohol and Tobacco Cessation

The main risk factors for H&N cancers are alcohol consumption and tobacco smoking and, when combined, account for approximately 75% of disease incidence (Marron et al., 2009). Quitting tobacco smoking has been shown to provide a beneficial effect on the risk of all H&N cancer subsites within 1–4 years after quitting; however, it takes 20 years or more to see a benefit from alcohol cessation (Marron et al., 2009). A number of support programs are available to assist patients with their commitment to quitting smoking and ending their dependence on alcohol, as well as pharmacologic agents to reduce anxiety and cravings and nicotine replacement therapy (nicotine patches and inhalers). Providing patients with information on the risks of continued smoking or excessive alcohol consumption is necessary to help them make an informed decision to quit. It is also prudent to screen patients for symptoms of alcohol withdrawal when they are admitted for surgery or other procedures.

Additional Resources

The American Psychosocial Oncology Society (2006) has published a pocket-sized reference for clinicians attending to the psychiatric and psychological needs of patients with cancer titled *Quick Reference for Oncology Clinicians: The Psychiatric and Psychological Dimensions of Cancer Symptom Management.* This reference book guides clinicians on appropriate dosing of pharmacologic treatments for patients as well as nonpharmacologic interventions. Even more impressive is a chapter in this book that defines common psychosocial issues specific to cancer site. Common site-specific symptoms and problems appear in a table on the left-hand side of the page along with treatment recommendations on the right. For patients with H&N cancer, the book lists interventions for problems such as "trouble swallowing psychotropic medications" (American Psychosocial Oncology Society, 2006, p. 137) along with a list of drugs that can be given sublingually or swallowed more easily.

Conclusion

A diagnosis of cancer can be a significant psychosocial challenge for anyone. However, many resources are available to assist patients with achieving balance in their lives, from diagnosis through survivorship. The DT (NCCN, 2010) and HADS (Zigmond & Snaith, 1983) are available to serve as evidence-based methods of screening for psychosocial distress. In addition, site- and treatment-specific assessments provide oncology nurses and providers with a glimpse of a particular patient's health-related quality of life at a point in time. These tools can provide insight into the psychosocial challenges that a patient is facing and serve as an opportunity for the nurse to make a referral to the appropriate service.

Finances, including maintaining employment and insurance coverage, can be a significant stressor for patients with oral complications. Changes in body image and function may place additional stress on patients. Fortunately, many healthcare systems and nonprofit organizations have begun to offer services to address the varied needs of these patients.

Nurses must remember to focus on the entire person when caring for someone with cancer and try to implement changes in their practice to address the patient's individual psychosocial needs. Screening for psychosocial challenges should be a routine part of oncology nursing practice. It is an instrumental part of providing comprehensive cancer care for all patients undergoing treatment and progressing through survivorship.

References

American Psychosocial Oncology Society. (2006). Issues specific to the cancer site. In J.C. Holland, D.B. Greenberg, & M.K. Hughes (Eds.), *Quick reference for oncology clinicians: The psychiatric and psychological dimensions of cancer symptom management* (pp. 135–138). Charlottesville, VA: IPOS Press.

Bennett, J.A., Brown, P., Cameron, L., Whitehead, L.C., Porter, D., & McPherson, K.M. (2008). Changes in employment and household income during the 24 months following a cancer diagnosis. *Supportive Care in Cancer, 17*, 1057–1064. doi:10.1007/s00520-008-0540-z

Buckwalter, A.E., Karnell, L.H., Smith, R.B., Christensen, A.J., & Funk, G.F. (2007). Patient-reported factors associated with discontinuing employment following head and neck cancer treatment. *Archives of Otolaryngology—Head and Neck Surgery, 133*, 464–470.

Cancer Support Community. (n.d.). CSC fact sheet: About the Cancer Support Community. Retrieved from http://www.thewellnesscommunity.org/fm/About/TWC-Fact-Sheet_1.aspx

Chambers, M.S., Garden, A.S., Kies, M.S., & Martin, J.W. (2004). Radiation-induced xerostomia in patients with head and neck cancer: Pathogenesis, impact on quality of life, and management. *Head and Neck, 26*, 796–807. doi:10.1002/hed.20045

Clover, K., Carter, G.L., Mackinnon, A., & Adams, C. (2009). Is my patient suffering clinically significant emotional distress? Demonstration of a probabilities approach to evaluating algorithms for screening for distress. *Supportive Care in Cancer, 17*, 1455–1462. doi:10.1007/s00520-009-0606-6

Conway, D.I., Petticrew, M., Marlborough, H., Berthiller, J., Hashibe, M., & Macpherson, L.M. (2008). Socioeconomic inequalities and oral cancer risk: A systematic review and meta-analysis of case-control studies. *International Journal of Cancer, 122*, 2811–2819. doi:10.1002/ijc.23430

De Boer, M.F., McCormick, L.K., Pruyn, J.F., Ryckman, R.M., & van den Borne, B.W. (1999). Physical and psychosocial correlates of head and neck cancer: A review of the literature. *Otolaryngology—Head and Neck Surgery, 120*, 427–436. doi:10.1016/S0194-5998(99)70287-1

Elting, L.S., Avritscher, E.B.C., Cooksley, C.D., Cardenas-Turanzas, M., Garden, A.S., & Chambers, M.S. (2008). Psychosocial and economic impact of cancer. *Dental Clinics of North America, 52*, 231–252. doi:10.1016/j.cden.2007.09.001

Fall-Dickson, J.M., Mitchell, S.A., Marden, S., Ramsay, E.S., Guadagnini, J.-P., Wu, T., … Pavletic, S.Z. (2010). Oral symptom intensity, health-related quality of life, and correlative salivary cytokines in adult survivors of hematopoietic stem cell transplantation with oral chronic graft-versus-host disease. *Biology of Blood and Marrow Transplantation, 16*, 948–956. doi:10.1016/j.bbmt.2010.01.017

Gaziano, J.E. (2002). Evaluation and management of oropharyngeal dysphagia in head and neck cancer. *Cancer Control, 9*, 400–409.

Harrison, J.D., Young, J.M., Price, M.A., Butow, P.N., & Solomon, M.J. (2009). What are the unmet supportive care needs of people with cancer? A systematic review. *Supportive Care in Cancer, 17*, 1117–1128. doi:10.1007/s00520-009-0615-5

Institute of Medicine. (2008). *Cancer care for the whole patient: Meeting psychosocial health needs.* Washington, DC: National Academies Press.

Jacobsen, P.B., & Ransom, S. (2007). Implementation of NCCN distress management guidelines by member institutions. *Journal of the National Comprehensive Cancer Network, 5*, 99–103. Retrieved from http://www.cas.usf.edu/~jacobsen/Jacobsen%20NCCN.pdf

Kaiser Family Foundation. (2006). USA Today/Kaiser Family Foundation/Harvard School of Public Health national survey of households affected by cancer. Retrieved from http://www.kff.org/kaiserpolls/pomr112006pkg.cfm

Katz, M.R., Irish, J.C., Devins, G.M., Rodin, G.M., & Gullane, P.J. (2003). Psychosocial adjustment in head and neck cancer: The impact of disfigurement, gender, and social support. *Head and Neck, 25*, 103–112. doi:10.1002/hed.10174

Llewellyn, C.D., McGurk, M., & Weinman, J. (2005). Are psycho-social and behavioural factors related to health related-quality of life in patients with head and neck cancer? A systematic review. *Oral Oncology, 41*, 440–454. doi:10.1016/j.oraloncology.2004.12.006

Lydiatt, W.M., Moran, J., & Burke, W.J. (2009). A review of depression in the head and neck cancer patient. *Clinical Advances in Hematology and Oncology, 7*, 397–403. Retrieved from http://www.clinicaladvances.com/article_pdfs/ho-article-200906-lydiatt.pdf

Marron, M., Boffetta, P., Zhang, Z.-F., Zaridze, D., Wünsch-Filho, V., Winn, D.M., … Hashibe, M. (2009). Cessation of alcohol drinking, tobacco smoking and the reversal of head and neck cancer risk. *International Journal of Epidemiology, 39*, 182–196. doi:10.1093/ije/dyp291

McKee-Ryan, F., Song, Z., Wanberg, C.R., & Kinicki, A.J. (2005). Psychological and physical well-being during unemployment: A meta-analytic study. *Journal of Applied Psychology, 90*, 53–76. doi:10.1037/0021-9010.90.1.53

Melchers, L.J., Van Weert, E., Beurskens, C.H.G., Reintsema, H., Slagter, A.P., Roodenburg, J.L.N., & Dijkstra, P.U. (2009). Exercise adherence in patients with trismus due to head and neck oncology: A qualitative study into the use of the Therabite®. *International Journal of Oral and Maxillofacial Surgery, 38*, 947–954. doi:10.1016/j.ijom.2009.04.003

Molina, M.A., Cheung, M.C., Perez, E.A., Byrne, M.M., Franceschi, D., Moffat, F.L., ... Koniaris, L.G. (2008). African American and poor patients have a dramatically worse prognosis for head and neck cancer. *Cancer, 113,* 2797–2806. doi:10.1002/cncr.23889

Murphy, B.A., Ridner, S., Wells, N., & Dietrich, M. (2007). Quality of life research in head and neck cancer: A review of the current state of science. *Critical Reviews in Oncology/Hematology, 62,* 251–267. doi:10.1016/j.critrevonc.2006.07.005

National Comprehensive Cancer Network. (2010, January 22). *NCCN Clinical Practice Guidelines in Oncology™: Distress management* [v.1.2010]. Retrieved from http://www.nccn.org/professionals/physician_gls/PDF/distress.pdf

Rasmussen, D.M., & Elverdam, B. (2008). The meaning of work and working life after cancer: An interview study. *Psycho-Oncology, 17,* 1232–1238. doi:10.1002/pon.1354

Rydholm, M., & Strang, P. (2002). Physical and psychosocial impact of xerostomia in palliative cancer care: A qualitative interview study. *International Journal of Palliative Nursing, 8,* 318–323.

Scharpf, J., Karnell, L.H., Chistensen, A.J., & Funk, G.G. (2009). The role of pain in head and neck cancer recurrence and survivorship. *Archives of Otolaryngology—Head and Neck Surgery, 135,* 789–794. doi:10.1001/archoto.2009.107

Singer, S., Danker, H., Dietz, A., Hornemann, B., Koscielny, S., Oeken, J., Matthäus, C., ... Krauss, O. (2008). Screening for mental disorders in laryngeal cancer patients: A comparison of 6 methods. *Psycho-Oncology, 17,* 280–286. doi:10.1002/pon.1229

Specht, L. (2002). Oral complications in the head and neck radiation patient: Introduction and scope of the problem. *Supportive Care in Cancer, 10,* 36–39. doi:10.1007/s005200100283

Vartanian, J.G., Carvalho, A.L., Toyota, J., Kowalski, I.S.G., & Kowalski, L.P. (2006). Socioeconomic effects of and risk factors for disability in long-term survivors of head and neck cancer. *Archives of Otolaryngology—Head and Neck Surgery, 132,* 32–35.

Verdonck-de Leeuw, I.M., van Bleek, W.-J., Leemans, C.R., & de Bree, R. (2010). Employment and return to work in head and neck cancer survivors. *Oral Oncology, 46,* 56–60. doi:10.1016/j.oraloncology.2009.11.001

Vissink, A., Jansma, J., Spijkervet, F.K.L., Burlage, F.R., & Coppes, R.P. (2003). Oral sequelae of head and neck radiotherapy. *Critical Reviews in Oral Biology and Medicine, 14,* 199–212. doi:10.1177/154411130301400305

Vodermaier, A., Linden, W., & Siu, C. (2009). Screening for emotional distress in cancer patients: A systematic review of assessment instruments. *Journal of the National Cancer Institute, 101,* 1464–1488. doi:10.1093/jnci/djp336

Wen, K.-Y., & Gustafson, D.H. (2004). Needs assessment for cancer patients and their families. *Health and Quality of Life Outcomes, 2,* 11. doi:10.1186/1477-7525-2-11

Zigmond, A.S., & Snaith, R.P. (1983). The Hospital Anxiety and Depression Scale. *Acta Psychiatrica Scandinavica, 67,* 361–370.

CHAPTER 14

Considerations for Older Cancer Survivors—Aging, Comorbidity, and Cancer Treatment

Sarah H. Kagan, PhD, RN, AOCN®, and Kristen W. Maloney, MSN, RN, AOCNS®

Introduction

Oral health is an important consideration for older adults that is made more prominent by the effects of cancer treatment. Community-dwelling older adults experience a range of oral health and dental problems that may limit function and quality of life (Chalmers & Ettinger, 2008; Smith, 2008; Turner & Ship, 2007). Conditions of concern in late life include coronal and root caries, xerostomia, gingival and periodontal disease, and the functional consequences of tooth loss and edentulism resulting in problems in mastication and deglutition (swallowing). These problems are mirrored by those resulting from treatment for head and neck (H&N) cancers. Additionally, the acute problem of mucositis affects older adults treated with chemotherapy or chemoradiation for an array of cancers. Consequently, older cancer survivors are faced with more complicated pretreatment needs, the need for frequent dental care during treatment, and the likelihood of more numerous and potentially debilitating acute and chronic oral health problems. While the risk of these oral health concerns varies by cancer site and treatment modalities, the impact on function and quality of daily living for cross-cutting concerns such as xerostomia and edentulism is profound (Dirix, Nuyts, Vander Poorten, Delaere, & Van den Bogaert, 2008; Ikebe et al., 2007; Orellana et al., 2006; Turner & Ship, 2007).

Alterations in oral health that amplify the effects of cancer treatment for older adults stem from common age-related changes, comorbid disease, and treatment of chronic conditions with medications that have oral side effects. Age-related changes encompass the risks of edentulism, the prevalence of which has declined in past decades (Chalmers & Ettinger, 2008), and the common problems of dental caries and gingival disease, along with salivary dysfunction, which may affect a third or more of community-dwelling older adults (Chalmers & Ettinger, 2008; Grisius, 2001; Turner & Ship, 2007). Comorbid diseases, such as primary salivary diseases, autoimmune diseases, Alzheimer disease, Parkinson disease, and osteoarthritis, further alter oral health (Turner & Ship, 2007). Alterations in oral health may occur because of direct effects on salivary function or on capacity to maintain oral hygiene. Many medications that are prescribed or taken as over-the-counter preparations, especially those with anticholinergic effects, further compromise oral health, largely through xerostomia (Chalmers & Ettinger, 2008; Turner & Ship, 2007).

This chapter addresses oral health and treatment effects in older cancer survivors as a foundation for nursing practice that addresses the special needs of these individuals and their families. The chapter begins with a brief summary of the demographics of aging in America coupled with a review of age-related concerns and comorbid conditions that influence oral health. A detailed review of the oral effects of treatment for H&N cancer forms the body of the chapter. Consideration of oral effects of treatments for other cancers follows, centering primarily on mucositis. The next section explores considerations in oral assessment and intervention for older cancer survivors and emphasizes coordination of the interdisciplinary team. The chapter concludes with a summary of highlights for nursing practice.

Oral Health and the Aging Population

The U.S. population demographics have changed dramatically during the past century and are projected to shift even more sharply toward longer life expectancy and increasing proportions of people older than 65 years of age (Chalmers & Ettinger, 2008; Olshansky, Goldman, Zheng, & Rowe, 2009). The proportion of the population older than 65 is currently just under 15% will reach 20% as we near mid-century with life expectancy reaching well into the ninth decade of life (Institute of Medicine, 2008; Olshansky et al., 2009). Older adults are more likely than younger individuals to experience comorbid and chronic health conditions and to use more health services (Chalmers & Ettinger, 2008; Olshansky et al., 2009). Oral health among older adults is improving in some dimensions, such as edentulism, but tooth retention and increased longevity increase the risk of dental caries, gingival and mucosal disease, and conditions such as xerostomia (Chalmers & Ettinger, 2008). Consequently, oral health and dental care for the United States' aging population are increasingly identified as a public health concern (Chalmers & Ettinger, 2008; Smith, 2008).

Oral Health Problems Among Older Adults

Primary oral health concerns among older adults center on tooth retention, dental caries, and gingival and mucosal integrity (Chalmers & Ettinger, 2008). Among both community-dwelling and institutionalized older adults, Smith (2008) posited marked improvement in edentulism, even among vulnerable institutionalized older adults, from 33% to 18% in 2004. These heartening figures reveal commensurate improvement in functional dentition to almost half of all nursing home residents as the most at-risk older adults in the nation. Smith built her case using detailed statewide data on dental care for nursing home residents from Minnesota and national data on edentulism, which involves about one out of four adults (Smith, 2008). In doing so, she paints a picture of increasingly orally functional older adults, most of whom live in the community and have the capacity to access dental care. However, with improved tooth retention and functional dentition, older adults are at risk for coronal and root caries, as well as gingival and periodontal disease. These risks are, of course, absent in edentulism. Such risk commonly necessitates more frequent dental care than many older adults find possible, especially those with limited financial resources. In general, Chalmers and Ettinger (2008) pointed to a lower risk of caries for those who have higher income, better education, and do not smoke. Disparities in dental care are conferred by sex and ethnicity, resulting in untreated caries and periodontal disease severe enough to cause loss of tooth attachment. Older men, older African Americans, and older Hispanic Americans all suffer disproportionate risk for caries, gingival disease, tooth loss, and lack of treatment for these conditions (Chalmers & Ettinger, 2008).

Secondary oral health concerns for older adults include significant xerostomia and oral mucosal disease (Chalmers & Ettinger, 2008; Smith, 2008; Turner & Ship, 2007). Turner and Ship (2007) suggested that in excess of one-third of older adults may experience xerostomia. Furthermore, specific groups of older adults, such as those with diseases that create dry mouth (e.g., Sjögren syndrome) or those undergoing therapies that affect salivary flow (e.g., radiation involving the salivary glands, chronic antihistamine use), are even more profoundly affected by this debilitating condition. Incidence approaches 100% in those who have Sjögren syndrome or who have received radiation therapy (Turner & Ship, 2007; von Bültzingslöwen et al., 2007). Turner and Ship (2007) detailed aspects of primary xerostomia, arising from salivary dysfunction and oral effects of systemic diseases in late life, and secondary causes of dry mouth, including side effects from drug therapies and radiation therapy. They noted the manifold consequences of xerostomia. These range from the sensation of dryness, stretching from the lips to the pharynx, and affecting chemosensation, mastication, deglutition, and speech, to an increased risk of caries and gingivitis that result in tooth loss, halitosis, and oral infections like candidiasis (Turner & Ship, 2007). Oral mucosal disease, while not as widespread as xerostomia, disproportionately affects older adults, who may have greater cumulative exposure to risk factors (Chalmers & Ettinger, 2008). Tobacco and alcohol consumption confer cocarcinogenic risk and often result in premalignant lesions like erythroplakia and leukoplakia that antedate diagnosis of a malignancy by months or years (Petersen, Bourgeois, Ogawa, Estupinan-Day, & Ndiaye, 2005; Shah & Gil, 2009; Warnakulasuriya, Sutherland, & Scully, 2005). In addition, older adults may also experience idiopathic lesions such as lichen planus, which carries some risk of oral malignancy.

Needs for and Access to Dental Care

Oral health concerns experienced by older adults create an intricate cycle of disease, treatment, side effects, and impaired function. This cycle, where one problem begets another with the concomitant risk of absent or limited access to dental care, is promoted by the threat of stigmatization, self-imposed social isolation, and further barriers to dental care. Older adults who have xerostomia, whether related to cancer treatment or a comorbid condition or treatment, for example, are likely to experience diminished quality of life and the manifold implications of anxiety, depression, and social isolation (Dirix et al., 2008; Rogers, Ahad, & Murphy, 2007; Turner & Ship, 2007). Despite the epidemiology of oral health problems and the general availability of dental care, older adults face significant barriers to accessing this care (Chalmers & Ettinger, 2008; Turner & Ship, 2007; Wiseman, 2006). Medicare and many other forms of health insurance offer no routine dental coverage and do not cover treatments and prosthetics. Thus, financial concerns and residential settings, as well as functional capacity, impinge upon access to dental care, resulting in frequent lack of care or undertreatment.

Intersections of Oral Health and Cancer for Older Adults

Cancer remains the leading cause of morbidity for men and women ages 40–79 years and the second leading cause of death, after cardiovascular disease, for those older than 80 (Jemal, Siegel, Xu, & Ward, 2010). More than 60% of all cancers are diagnosed in those individuals age 65 and older, creating a profound burden of disease and necessitating extensive, ongoing care (Jemal et al., 2010). Cancer therapies—both for cancers that directly involve oral and oropharyngeal structures and those involving adjacent structures, as well as those for sites distant to the mouth—affect oral health through a variety of side effects. Cancer treatment initiates interactions among baseline oral health concerns, the impact of comorbid conditions and chronic medications, functional capacity to perform oral hygiene, and the effects of cancer treatment on oral health and related functional abilities. These manifold interactions result in risks of tooth loss with associated concerns of infection, gingival and mucosal disease exacerbations that may present systemic infection risk, and persistent and disabling xerostomia compounded by acute mucositis. Subsequent risks for impaired swallowing, malnutrition, and diminished well-being and quality of life further jeopardize older survivors. Oncology nurses caring for older cancer survivors over the course of the cancer trajectory, from diagnosis through long-term survivorship, play a key role in identifying these risks and assessing alterations in oral health to achieve necessary education, self-care by the older adult and family members, appropriate referrals for advanced care, and integrated interdisciplinary follow-up.

Oral Treatment Effects in Head and Neck Cancer

H&N cancers, and the known carcinogenetic agents implicated in development of these squamous cell malignancies, directly affect oral health. Fundamentally, oral cancers are a manifestation of oral health (Chalmers & Ettinger, 2008). Their diagnosis may culminate a months- or years-long surveillance for chronic premalignant lesions, including leukoplakia, erythroplakia, and lichen planus (Reddi & Shafer, 2006). Cancers of adjacent anatomic structures such as the pharynx and larynx, while they may not be manifestations of oral health, commonly involve substance use and often impinge upon oral hygiene and oral as well as overall health. Older adults and those who have used substances that contain carcinogens known to affect the oral cavity, oropharynx, and larynx are at risk for poor oral health, premalignant lesions, and cancers of these tissues (Petersen et al., 2005; Reddi & Shafer, 2006; Shah & Gil, 2009). Long-term use of tobacco products, including those packed into the buccal cavity, chewed, and mixed with other agents like lime and betel nut, create deleterious effects on dental health and oral hygiene in addition to initiating carcinogenesis (Petersen, 2003, 2009; Petersen et al., 2005; Shah & Gil, 2009; Warnakulasuriya et al., 2005). Consumption of alcohol exacerbates these effects, defining it as a significant cocarcinogen for oral and other squamous cell H&N cancers (Petersen, 2009; Reddi & Shafer, 2006; Shah & Gil, 2009). Thus, older adults diagnosed with oral and other H&N cancers are more likely to have extant oral health problems and may have poor oral hygiene practices and limited access to dental care. These oral health problems can arise from multiple etiologies—as with gingival disease arising from primary xerostomia and tobacco use—and side effects of cancer treatment may further exacerbate them.

Treatment for any H&N cancer affects oral health directly and indirectly through side effects, depending on modality. As H&N cancer treatment evolves, the use of multimodality therapy has created a complex array of oral health effects (Kagan, 2006; Rogers, Ahad, et al., 2007; Rogers, Thomson, O'Toole, & Lowe, 2007; Shah & Gil, 2009). Treatment protocols are rapidly advancing and have moved from surgery as a mainstay of therapy toward a multimodality approach that encompasses primary and salvage surgery, primary and adjuvant radiotherapy, chemoradiotherapy, and targeted therapies, of which cetuximab—an epidermal growth factor receptor inhibitor—is the most used agent (Kagan, 2006; Shah & Gil, 2009). Oral effects of treatment for H&N cancer, regardless of the causative modality, include those occurring acutely and those that are persistent or delayed, creating a chronic concern.

Older adults are at risk for complex presentation, delayed or complicated recovery, or both because of oral conditions that existed before cancer treatment. Treatment modalities may result in predictable acute treatment effects, as with postsurgical pain or mucositis arising from radiation or chemoradiation therapy. In this case, the temporal nature of the effect and introduction of focused preventive or symptom management strategies deployed to improve comfort and limit tissue involvement may reassure the older survivor and family members. Individualized care and successful management rely on evidence-based care and adequate treatment. Evidence-based care is achieved through thoughtful adherence to published guidelines, such as those discussed earlier in Chapters 3 and 4 and in guidelines set forth in published literature specific to side effects and to care of older adults (Barkin, Barkin, & Barkin, 2005; Keefe et al., 2007). Furthermore, evidence-based care requires avoiding ageist assumptions and actions in order to meet the needs of the individual (Happ, Williams, Strumpf, & Burger, 1996; Kagan, 2008). Avoiding undertreatment, especially in managing pain, and promoting function to complete oral hygiene and regain mobility and instrumental tasks will reduce distress and limit complications, as with all symptoms experienced by older cancer survivors (Kagan, 2008, 2009).

The presentation and severity of oral effects vary by cancer treatment modality. Thus, consideration of the modality should refine surveillance, assessment, and intervention patterns and their application among individual older patients. For example, growing evidence and clinical experience points to a greater severity of acute side effects, such as mucositis, in chemoradiation (Eilers & Million, 2007; Keefe et al., 2007; Rogers, Ahad, et al., 2007). Conversely, innovations in radiation delivery techniques, such as intensity-modulated radiation therapy, mitigate side effects (Keefe et al., 2007). Here, however, older adults may have more complex presentation of mucositis and other symptoms if preexisting oral health conditions are involved, and they may endure slowed recovery in light of senescent processes and those preexisting conditions (Gironés, Torregrosa, & Díaz-Beveridge, 2010; Marinello et al., 2008; Percival, 2009; Sanabria et al., 2007). Finally, etiologic factors may be difficult to distinguish in light of preexisting oral health conditions as, for example, with mucositis in a patient who has preexisting conditions such as xerostomia or lichen planus.

Acute treatment effects are likely to distress older adults, as they do young adults, if they are unfamiliar with them or feel unprepared. Older adults may or may not feel greater distress at a worsening condition and be concerned about the outcome of this additive effect (Borggreven et al., 2007). Even older adults who do not have preexisting conditions may experience frustration or despair of recovery if oral effects of H&N cancer treatment become especially severe, or if pain or other distressing and functionally limiting manifestations become uncontrolled or sustained. Here, attention to adequate treatment and mitigation of clinical judgments predicated on ageist assumptions rather than current evidence is critical to parity in caring for older survivors (Kagan, 2008).

As with acute treatment effects, older adults experiencing chronic oral treatment effects after H&N cancer may have complex presentations and complicated treatment needs. This more intricate clinical picture emerges given the interactions of other oral health problems and the likelihood of oral effects from treatment for other comorbid diseases (Scully & Ettinger, 2007; Turner & Ship, 2007). Xerostomia among older adults is well documented and studied. Other chronic effects, including dysphagia, pain, trismus, lymphedema, osteonecrosis, and oral infection, are less well explored but no less consequential to oral and general health, function, and well-being.

Xerostomia, given its prevalence in approximately one-third of older adults and nearly all people treated with any protocol employing radiation therapy for H&N cancer, is the foremost chronic oral effect of cancer treatment (Borggreven et al., 2007; Smith, 2008; Turner & Ship, 2007). Xerostomia is difficult to manage (Shiboski, Hodgson, Ship, & Schiødt, 2007; von Bültzingslöwen et al., 2007), regardless of the etiology, and creates a cascade of secondary conditions that necessitates further management (Shiboski et al., 2007; Turner & Ship, 2007). Older adults with xerostomia that antedates cancer treatment may experience more pronounced or persistent secondary effects, such as dysgeusia and dysphagia, in addition to having individualized responses to the presentation and severity of the compound presentation of xerostomia itself.

Dysphagia generates both acute and—more distressingly—chronic impairment for older survivors of H&N cancer (Raykher et al., 2007). Murphy and Gilbert (2009) provide a thorough and current analysis of dysphagia in H&N cancer, describing its manifold and intersecting etiologies and presentations. In addition to emerging as a result of the acute treatment effects of inflammation and edema, permanent tissue changes, including fibrosis and neuromuscular damage, alter all phases of deglutition (Murphy & Gilbert, 2009). Preexisting dental problems, such as tooth loss and xerostomia, may influence the oral preparatory phase and oral phase of swallowing, while xerostomia can further limit the pharyngeal phase. Additionally, comorbid neurologic and neuromuscular diseases such as stroke, Parkinson disease, and Alzheimer disease, all of which may affect the phases and coordination of swallowing, present complex actual and potential interactions with dysphagia resulting from cancer treatment. Rehabilitation for dysphagia is complex, requiring interdisciplinary intervention and sustained self-care and engagement in therapeutic exercise (Murphy & Gilbert, 2009). Older adults who incur sustained deconditioning of the muscles involved in swallowing or who become fearful of swallowing because of pain or sensations of food "sticking" are at risk for poor rehabilitation from acute dysphagia and potential long-term enteral feeding (Murphy & Gilbert, 2009; Rogers, Thomson, et al., 2007).

Oral and H&N pain holds the double-edged character of being a warning sign of cancer and other oral health problems such as abscessed teeth, as well as a lasting reminder of cancer treatment (Clark & Ram, 2008). Clark and Ram (2008) offer a thorough and useful review of the etiologies, presentations, and treatment of pain in H&N cancer. However, their attention to the unique needs of older adults is scant, and thus, the synthesis provided by Barkin et al. (2005) completes the immediate resources necessary to support older survivors in preventing chronic pain to the greatest extent possible and managing remaining pain optimally. Ageism remains a concern in pain assessment and management for older adults (Barkin et al., 2005; Kagan, 2008). Older adults are more likely to be assessed incompletely and receive less than optimal treatment for acute and chronic pain. Thus, Barkin et al.'s principles of preventing pain; relying on polymodal polypharmacy (i.e., using combinations of analgesics and modalities of analgesia simultaneously); using timed dosing and accounting for pharmacokinetic and pharmacodynamic changes with age; and addressing sensory and emotional needs form a substantive foundation for treating chronic oral pain in older cancer survivors (Barkin et al., 2005; Mercadante & Arcuri, 2007). Importantly, Clark and Ram (2008) contended that pain is often a presenting symptom of H&N cancer. This dual nature of H&N pain reinforces the need for patient education that attends to changes in pain patterns. H&N cancer survivors are at increased risk for metachronous cancers, often termed *field cancerization* (Roesch-Ely et al., 2007). Older adults generally are at increased risk for cancer. Therefore, older adult H&N cancer survivors must remain vigilant for subsequent cancers.

Trismus (decreased excursion of the mandible), like xerostomia, is a distressing and debilitating symptom in and of itself, while concomitantly generating a cascade of secondary effects. Trismus commonly results in poor oral hygiene, impaired speech and swallowing, and potentially deleterious effects on nutrition if an enteral feeding plan is not in place. Trismus and its secondary effects interact with oral health concerns for which older adults are generally at risk, amplifying effects and multiplying potential consequences. Unlike other acute and chronic oral effects of cancer treatment, trismus is poorly studied in general, and specifically among older adults. Management relies largely on physical therapy of the temporomandibular joint (TMJ), using everything from repurposed tongue depressors to specially designed devices to increase extension of the TMJ. Older adults may have variable, clinically altered presentation of trismus and response to this therapy. The TMJ in older adults may be affected by preexisting damage to the joint. Furthermore, the comorbid presentation of other conditions, such as osteoarthritis or mild cognitive impairment, may affect the capacity of older adults to participate in physical therapy. Research in hyperbaric oxygen and pharmacologic prevention and treatment of fibrosis are poorly explored, and practically unexplored specifically in older adult populations (Delanian & Lefaix,

2007). Limiting the radiation dose to normal tissues and adjacent anatomic structures, along with advances in lymph node dissection, appears to limit the extent of fibrosis and lymphedema (O'Sullivan & Levin, 2003; Shah & Gil, 2009). Nonetheless, physical therapy remains a mainstay of management for trismus and lymphedema that occur as a result of H&N cancer treatment (Delanian & Lefaix, 2007; O'Sullivan & Levin, 2003).

Lymphedema profoundly affects the anatomy and physiology of tissues and structures, along with appearance and functional performance, among H&N cancer survivors (Withey, Pracy, Vaz, & Rhys-Evans, 2001). Surgery, radiation, and chemoradiation alone or in combination remove or alter lymphatic structures and, in the case of radiation, result in fibrosis. This complex of soft tissue and lymphatic changes results in a range of edematous changes that are difficult to predict and challenging to manage (Delanian & Lefaix, 2007; Murphy & Gilbert, 2009; O'Sullivan & Levin, 2003). The influence of normative aging changes and pathologies common in later life are unexplored, and clinical variation is difficult to discern by age. As with trismus, which results from some of the same changes in tissue elasticity and is often compounded by lymphedema, only techniques designed to limit tissue damage in surgery and radiation have proved promising in preventing lymphedema. Management continues to rely on manual manipulation, compression, and exercise, requiring the attention of specially trained lymphedema therapists and particularly those familiar with the special needs of H&N cancer survivors both young and old.

Osteonecrosis presents in two forms relevant to older survivors of H&N cancer treatment. Those older adults who were treated with radiation or chemoradiation in a field that included the mandible are at risk for osteoradionecrosis. Older adults receiving these therapies should be treated prophylactically with extractions of abscessed or damaged teeth, which appear to promote necrosis (Miller & Quinn, 2006). Older adults taking bisphosphonates as treatment for osteoporosis may incur osteonecrosis as a side effect of this treatment (Body et al., 2007; Ripamonti et al., 2009). Although these conditions are rare, they are life altering, necessitating extensive therapies including hyperbaric oxygen and reconstructive surgery (Delanian & Lefaix, 2007; O'Sullivan & Levin, 2003). However, just how risk, presentation, experience, and response to therapy differ in older adults compared to younger individuals is poorly understood.

Oral infection may occur more often in older cancer survivors. These infections may result from alterations in the microflora as a result of both age- and cancer-related events, such as use of dental prosthetics and conditions like xerostomia or malnutrition (Migliorati & Madrid, 2007; Percival, 2009). Percival (2009) provides a comprehensive review of effects on microflora and oral manifestations of host defenses. As with most treatment effects experienced by older survivors, concerns about infection arise in the interactions of relevant age- and cancer-related conditions that create additive risk (Percival, 2009). Additive risk in an older individual is difficult to predict in

230 MANAGING THE ORAL EFFECTS OF CANCER TREATMENT: DIAGNOSIS TO SURVIVORSHIP

terms of timing, manifestation, and consequences. Absent the ability to predict actual risk of infection, older adults require meticulous attention to factors such as pain, mucositis, xerostomia, oral hygiene, and dental prosthetics that may alter the oral environment and predispose them to infection (Migliorati & Madrid, 2007).

Oral Treatment Effects in Survivors of Other Cancers

Oral treatment effects experienced by older survivors who have cancers outside the H&N include oral manifestations of systemic therapies, such as mucositis, or consequences of them, such as oral candidiasis in the case of altered host defenses (Epstein, 2007; Keefe et al., 2007; Maschmeyer & Haas, 2008). Most of these oral effects are acute in presentation and temporary in duration if given optimal treatment. Both assessment and treatment are essentially similar to those performed with H&N cancer survivors. However, assessment parameters must include attention to dimensions of systemic therapies, such as dose and schedule. Additionally, intervention should rely on current specific evidence that accounts for causative agents, as in mucositis (Keefe et al., 2007), and addresses specific considerations in comorbid disease and functional capacity relevant to older adults.

Beyond well-explored oral effects lies the relatively unstudied challenge of dysgeusia (altered sense of taste), often accompanied by dysphagia, that affects older H&N cancer survivors as well as those who have been treated for other cancers with chemotherapy and chemoradiation (Bernhardson, Tishelman, & Rutqvist, 2007; Dirix et al., 2008; Genden et al., 2005; Hutton, Baracos, & Wismer, 2007; Kaplan, Zuk-Paz, & Wolff, 2008; Murphy & Gilbert, 2009). Many older survivors report experiencing persistent chemosensory changes and clinical dysgeusia during and after chemotherapy and chemoradiation in fields outside the H&N (Bernhardson et al., 2007; Bernhardson, Tishelman, & Rutqvist, 2008; Hutton et al., 2007). Those who did not receive radiation to the oral cavity generally experienced restored taste and smell within several months after the end of therapy (Bernhardson et al., 2007, 2008). Those who received oral radiation may not recover chemosensation, and the absence of normal taste and smell is commonly compounded by xerostomia (Dirix et al., 2008). Additionally, patients with advanced cancer are likely to experience dysgeusia, generally as part of the syndrome of cachexia (Hutton et al., 2007). As with other oral effects, older survivors are doubly at risk for chemosensory changes and dysgeusia because they occur more often in late life and may be harbingers of other diseases, including Alzheimer disease, or effects of concurrent medications for comorbid conditions (Schiffman & Graham, 2000). The interactions of age-related changes with those resulting from cancer treatment are, however, unexplored. Comprehensive assessment and thoughtful, individualized intervention are fundamentally important in dysgeusia, especially absent substantial evidence to guide assessment and intervention.

Considerations in Assessment and Intervention for Oral Effects in Older Survivors

Assessment of the oral effects of cancer treatment in older adults is ideally a continuous and interdisciplinary process. Older adults and their family members, and other people who provide support, benefit from understanding how cancer treatment affects oral health and interacts with extant oral conditions and disease. Consequently, baseline assessment of oral health grounds a plan of care. That assessment includes components performed by nonspecialist providers, such as oncology nurses and oncologists, and by specialist providers, including a general dentist and dental subspecialists, such as a maxillofacial prosthodontist, who may lead dental care for patients with oral cancers, and a speech-language pathologist.

Fundamentally, understanding alterations in oral health for individual older survivors is a multifaceted process in which members of the interdisciplinary team share information about oral and systemic health, cancer and other diseases and conditions, and cancer therapies and other medications (Raykher et al., 2007; Scully & Ettinger, 2007). Shared information and careful attention to changes over time enable targeted intervention coupled with generally applicable strategies such as optimizing oral hygiene and maintaining oral and enteral nutrition (Raykher et al., 2007). The complexity of oral health in later life necessitates a broadly inclusive interdisciplinary team along with advance planning where possible. For example, older adults should receive ongoing generalist and specialist dental assessment and dental prophylaxis throughout treatment and survivorship along with any necessary treatment or extraction before beginning cancer treatment to limit the risk of complications such as osteoradionecrosis (Miller & Quinn, 2006).

Intervention for oral health issues among older cancer survivors relies on creative use of the interdisciplinary team (Scully & Ettinger, 2007). Specialist members unique to the type of cancer or treatment modality should be engaged in the care of patients from diagnosis, if possible, or as early as a problem appears to be a potential threat. For example, every older adult diagnosed with H&N cancer should see a speech-language pathologist and a registered dietitian experienced in H&N cancer treatment. Similarly, older adults who show early signs of lymphedema should be referred to a certified lymphedema therapist at that time. The best available evidence provides a preferred platform for the plan of care; nevertheless, many discrete problems of oral health for older cancer survivors lack substantive evidence. As a result, clinical judgment should be combined, as always, with detailed knowledge of the individual to enact best practices and create individualized care that accounts for the needs and preferences of the particular older adult patient (Happ et al., 1996).

Referral to an oncology or geriatric social worker is paramount for almost all older cancer survivors. Medicare often does not cover therapies for oral effects of cancer treatment, and other health insurance may offer limited support as well. As Chalmers and Ettinger (2008) noted, older adults with limited resources, as well as those facing barriers to access because of ethnicity, are already at risk for poorer oral health before cancer is diagnosed, amplifying their needs and impinging on their access to specialist care (Chalmers & Ettinger, 2008). Finally, care that addresses the unique needs of older survivors in the context of comprehensive cancer care and integrated health care is only complete with well-structured, continuous education for the older survivor, the family members, and others who provide instrumental, emotional, and spiritual support for that person. Nurses are ideally positioned to coordinate the interdisciplinary plan of care, support access to appropriate generalist and specialist care, and provide education throughout survivorship.

Conclusion

As oral health declines in older adults, those faced with cancer and its treatment have more severe concerns related to their oral effects. Edentulism is declining among older adults while functional dentition is rising, resulting in greater risk of dental caries and gingival disease. Many older adults suffer from xerostomia, which greatly affects function and quality of life. Oral mucosal disease disproportionately affects older adults who have used tobacco and alcohol.

H&N cancers have notable and sustained effects on oral health. Oral effects among older H&N cancer survivors vary by treatment and preexisting oral health problems. Effects commonly include mucositis acutely, as well as chronic concerns of dysphagia, pain, trismus, lymphedema, osteonecrosis, and oral infection. Xerostomia remains a common problem.

Oral effects may arise from the treatment of other cancers. These most often include mucositis and oral candidiasis or other infections, which present acutely and, with best treatment, are only temporary. Dysgeusia is a complex concern arising from cancer and its treatments, among those who are treated for H&N and other types of cancer. Additionally, dysgeusia may present in advanced cancer as part of cachexia.

Managing oral effects requires a robust interdisciplinary team, which should include oncology nurses and physicians as well as a dentist, maxillofacial prosthodontist, speech-language pathologist, registered dietitian, certified lymphedema therapist, and oncology or geriatric social worker, among others, to effectively support older adult cancer survivors.

References

Barkin, R.L., Barkin, S.J., & Barkin, D.S. (2005). Perception, assessment, treatment, and management of pain in the elderly. *Clinics in Geriatric Medicine, 21,* 465–490. doi:10.1016/j.cger.2005.02.006

Bernhardson, B.M., Tishelman, C., & Rutqvist, L.E. (2007). Chemosensory changes experienced by patients undergoing cancer chemotherapy: A qualitative interview study. *Journal of Pain and Symptom Management, 34,* 403–412. doi:10.1016/j.jpainsymman.2006.12.010

Bernhardson, B.M., Tishelman, C., & Rutqvist, L.E. (2008). Self-reported taste and smell changes during cancer chemotherapy. *Supportive Care in Cancer, 16,* 275–283. doi:10.1007/s00520-007-0319-7

Body, J.-J., Coleman, R., Clezardin, P., Ripamonti, C., Rizzoli, R., & Aapro, M. (2007). International Society of Geriatric Oncology (SIOG) clinical practice recommendations for the use of bisphosphonates in elderly patients. *European Journal of Cancer, 43,* 852–858. doi:10.1016/j.ejca.2006.12.006

Borggreven, P., Verdonck-de Leeuw, I.M., Muller, M.J., Heiligers, M.L.C.H., de Bree, R., Aaronson, N.K., & Leemans, C.R. (2007). Quality of life and functional status in patients with cancer of the oral cavity and oropharynx: Pretreatment values of a prospective study. *European Archives of Oto-Rhino-Laryngology, 264,* 651–657. doi:10.1007/s00405-007-0249-5

Chalmers, J.M., & Ettinger, R.L. (2008). Public health issues in geriatric dentistry in the United States. *Dental Clinics of North America, 52,* 423–446. doi:10.1016/j.cden.2007.12.004

Clark, G.T., & Ram, S. (2008). Orofacial pain and neurosensory disorders and dysfunction in cancer patients. *Dental Clinics of North America, 52,* 183–202. doi:10.1016/j.cden.2007.09.003

Delanian, S., & Lefaix, J.L. (2007). Current management for late normal tissue injury: Radiation-induced fibrosis and necrosis. *Seminars in Radiation Oncology, 17,* 99–107. doi:10.1016/j.semradonc.2006.11.006

Dirix, P., Nuyts, S., Vander Poorten, V., Delaere, P., & Van den Bogaert, W. (2008). The influence of xerostomia after radiotherapy on quality of life. *Supportive Care in Cancer, 16,* 171–179. doi:10.1007/s00520-007-0300-5

Eilers, J., & Million, R. (2007). Prevention and management of oral mucositis in patients with cancer. *Seminars in Oncology Nursing, 23,* 201–212. doi:10.1016/j.soncn.2007.05.005

Epstein, J.B. (2007). Mucositis in the cancer patient and immunosuppressed host. *Infectious Disease Clinics of North America, 21,* 503–522. doi:10.1016/j.idc.2007.03.003

Genden, E.M., Rinaldo, A., Shaha, A.R., Clayman, G.L., Werner, J.A., Suárez, C., & Ferlito, A. (2005). Treatment considerations for head and neck cancer in the elderly. *Journal of Laryngology and Otology, 119,* 169–174.

Gironés, R., Torregrosa, D., & Díaz-Beveridge, R. (2010). Comorbidity, disability and geriatric syndromes in elderly breast cancer survivors. Results of a single-center experience. *Critical Reviews in Oncology/Hematology, 73,* 236–245. doi:10.1016/j.critrevonc.2009.08.002

Grisius, M.M. (2001). Salivary gland dysfunction: A review of systemic therapies. *Oral Surgery, Oral Medicine, Oral Pathology, Oral Radiology, and Endodontology, 92,* 156–162. doi:10.1067/moe.2001.116601

Happ, M.B., Williams, C.C., Strumpf, N.E., & Burger, S.G. (1996). Individualized care for frail elders: Theory and practice. *Journal of Gerontological Nursing, 22*(3), 6–14.

Hutton, J.L., Baracos, V.E., & Wismer, W.V. (2007). Chemosensory dysfunction is a primary factor in the evolution of declining nutritional status and quality of life in patients with advanced cancer. *Journal of Pain and Symptom Management, 33,* 156–165. doi:10.1016/j.jpainsymman.2006.07.017

Ikebe, K., Matsuda, K., Morii, K., Wada, M., Hazeyama, T., Nokubi, T., & Ettinger, R.L. (2007). Impact of dry mouth and hyposalivation on oral health-related quality of life of elderly Japanese. *Oral Surgery, Oral Medicine, Oral Pathology, Oral Radiology, and Endodontology, 103,* 216–222. doi:10.1016/j.tripleo.2005.12.001

Institute of Medicine. (2008). *Retooling for an aging America: Building the health care workforce.* Washington, DC: National Academies Press.

Jemal, A., Siegel, R., Xu, J., & Ward, E. (2010). Cancer statistics, 2010. *CA: A Cancer Journal for Clinicians, 60,* 277–300. doi:10.3322/caac.20073

Kagan, S.H. (2006). The older adult with head and neck cancer. In D.G. Cope & A.M. Reb (Eds.), *An evidence-based approach to the treatment and care of the older adult with cancer* (pp. 167–183). Pittsburgh, PA: Oncology Nursing Society.

Kagan, S.H. (2008). Ageism in cancer care. *Seminars in Oncology Nursing, 24,* 246–253. doi:10.1016/j.soncn.2008.08.004

Kagan, S.H. (2009). The influence of nursing in head and neck cancer management. *Current Opinion in Oncology, 21,* 248–253. doi:10.1097/CCO.0b013e328329b819

Kaplan, I., Zuk-Paz, L., & Wolff, A. (2008). Association between salivary flow rates, oral symptoms, and oral mucosal status. *Oral Surgery, Oral Medicine, Oral Pathology, Oral Radiology, and Endodontology, 106,* 235–241. doi:10.1016/j.tripleo.2007.11.029

Keefe, D.M., Schubert, M.M., Elting, L.S., Sonis, S.T., Epstein, J.B., Raber-Durlacher, J.E., … Peterson, D.E. (2007). Updated clinical practice guidelines for the prevention and treatment of mucositis. *Cancer, 109,* 820–831. doi:10.1002/cncr.22484

Marinello, R., Marenco, D., Roglia, D., Stasi, M.F., Ferrando, A., Ceccarelli, M., … Ciccone, E. (2008). Predictors of treatment failures during chemotherapy: A prospective study on 110 older cancer patients. *Archives of Gerontology and Geriatrics, 48,* 222–226. doi:10.1016/j.archger.2008.01.011

Maschmeyer, G., & Haas, A. (2008). The epidemiology and treatment of infections in cancer patients. *International Journal of Antimicrobial Agents, 31,* 193–197. doi:10.1016/j.ijantimicag.2007.06.014

Mercadante, S., & Arcuri, E. (2007). Pharmacological management of cancer pain in the elderly. *Drugs and Aging, 24,* 761–776.

Migliorati, C.A., & Madrid, C. (2007). The interface between oral and systemic health: The need for more collaboration. *Clinical Microbiology and Infection, 13*(Suppl. 4), 11–16. doi:10.1111/j.1469-0691.2007.01799.x

Miller, E.H., & Quinn, A.I. (2006). Dental considerations in the management of head and neck cancer patients. *Otolaryngologic Clinics of North America, 39,* 319–329. doi:10.1016/j.otc.2005.11.011

Murphy, B.A., & Gilbert, J. (2009). Dysphagia in head and neck cancer patients treated with radiation: Assessment, sequelae, and rehabilitation. *Seminars in Radiation Oncology, 19,* 35–42. doi:10.1016/j.semradonc.2008.09.007

O'Sullivan, B., & Levin, W. (2003). Late radiation-related fibrosis: Pathogenesis, manifestations, and current management. *Seminars in Radiation Oncology, 13,* 274–289. doi:10.1016/S1053-4296(03)00037-7

Olshansky, S.J., Goldman, D.P., Zheng, Y., & Rowe, J.W. (2009). Aging in America in the twenty-first century: Demographic forecasts from the MacArthur Foundation Research Network on an Aging Society. *Milbank Quarterly, 87,* 842–862.

Orellana, M.F., Lagravère, M.O., Boychuk, D.G., Major, P.W., Flores-Mir, C., & Ortho, C. (2006). Prevalence of xerostomia in population-based samples: A systematic review. *Journal of Public Health Dentistry, 66,* 152–158.

Percival, R.S. (2009). Changes in oral microflora and host defences with advanced age. In S.L. Percival (Ed.), *Microbiology and aging: Clinical manifestations* (pp. 131–152). New York, NY: Springer. doi:10.1007/978-1-59745-327-1_7

Petersen, P.E. (2003). The World Oral Health Report 2003: Continuous improvement of oral health in the 21st century—The approach of the WHO Global Oral Health Programme. *Community Dentistry and Oral Epidemiology, 31,* 3–24. doi:10.1046/j..2003.com122.x

Petersen, P.E. (2009). Oral cancer prevention and control—The approach of the World Health Organization. *Oral Oncology Supplement, 3,* 8. doi:10.1016/j.oos.2009.06.006

Petersen, P.E., Bourgeois, D., Ogawa, H., Estupinan-Day, S., & Ndiaye, C. (2005). The global burden of oral diseases and risks to oral health. *Bulletin of the World Health Organization, 83,* 661–669.

Raykher, A., Russo, L., Schattner, M., Schwartz, L., Scott, B., & Shike, M. (2007). Enteral nutrition support of head and neck cancer patients. *Nutrition in Clinical Practice, 22,* 68–73.

Reddi, S.P., & Shafer, A.T. (2006). Oral premalignant lesions: Management considerations. *Oral and Maxillofacial Surgery Clinics of North America, 18*, 425–433. doi:10.1016/j.coms.2006.08.002

Ripamonti, C.I., Maniezzo, M., Campa, T., Fagnoni, E., Brunelli, C., Saibene, G., … Cislaghi, E. (2009). Decreased occurrence of osteonecrosis of the jaw after implementation of dental preventive measures in solid tumour patients with bone metastases treated with bisphosphonates. The experience of the National Cancer Institute of Milan. *Annals of Oncology, 20*, 137–145. doi:10.1093/annonc/mdn526

Roesch-Ely, M., Nees, M., Karsai, S., Ruess, A., Bogumil, R., Warnken, U., … Bosch, F.X. (2007). Proteomic analysis reveals successive aberrations in protein expression from healthy mucosa to invasive head and neck cancer. *Oncogene, 26*, 54–64. doi:10.1038/sj.onc.1209770

Rogers, S.N., Ahad, S.A., & Murphy, A.P. (2007). A structured review and theme analysis of papers published on 'quality of life' in head and neck cancer: 2000–2005. *Oral Oncology, 43*, 843–868. doi:10.1016/j.oraloncology.2007.02.006

Rogers, S.N., Thomson, R., O'Toole, P., & Lowe, D. (2007). Patients experience with long-term percutaneous endoscopic gastrostomy feeding following primary surgery for oral and oropharyngeal cancer. *Oral Oncology, 43*, 499–507. doi:10.1016/j.oraloncology.2006.05.002

Sanabria, A., Carvalho, A., Vartanian, J., Magrin, J., Ikeda, M., & Kowalski, L. (2007). Co-morbidity is a prognostic factor in elderly patients with head and neck cancer. *Annals of Surgical Oncology, 14*, 1449–1457. doi:10.1245/s10434-006-9296-1

Schiffman, S.S., & Graham, B.G. (2000). Taste and smell perception affect appetite and immunity in the elderly. *European Journal of Clinical Nutrition, 54*(Suppl. 3), S54–S63.

Scully, C., & Ettinger, R.L. (2007). The influence of systemic diseases on oral health care in older adults. *Journal of the American Dental Association, 138*(Suppl. 1), 7S–14S.

Shah, J.P., & Gil, Z. (2009). Current concepts in management of oral cancer—Surgery. *Oral Oncology, 45*, 394–401. doi:10.1016/j.oraloncology.2008.05.017

Shiboski, C.H., Hodgson, T.A., Ship, J.A., & Schiødt, M. (2007). Management of salivary hypofunction during and after radiotherapy. *Oral Surgery, Oral Medicine, Oral Pathology, Oral Radiology, and Endodontology, 103*(Suppl. 1), S66.e1–S66.e19. doi:10.1016/j.tripleo.2006.11.013

Smith, B.J. (2008). Oral health challenges of the vulnerable elderly: A new focus. *Dental Abstracts, 53*, 60–61. doi:10.1016/j.denabs.2008.01.002

Turner, M.D., & Ship, J.A. (2007). Dry mouth and its effects on the oral health of elderly people. *Journal of the American Dental Association, 138*(Suppl. 1), S15–S20.

von Bültzingslöwen, I., Sollecito, T.P., Fox, P.C., Daniels, T., Jonsson, R., Lockhart, P.B., … Schiødt, M. (2007). Salivary dysfunction associated with systemic diseases: Systematic review and clinical management recommendations. *Oral Surgery, Oral Medicine, Oral Pathology, Oral Radiology, and Endodontology, 103*(Suppl. 1), S57.e1–S57.e15. doi:10.1016/j.tripleo.2006.11.010

Warnakulasuriya, S., Sutherland, G., & Scully, C. (2005). Tobacco, oral cancer, and treatment of dependence. *Oral Oncology, 41*, 244–260. doi:10.1016/j.oraloncology.2004.08.010

Wiseman, M. (2006). The treatment of oral problems in the palliative patient. *Journal of the Canadian Dental Association, 72*, 453–456.

Withey, S., Pracy, P., Vaz, F., & Rhys-Evans, P. (2001). Sensory deprivation as a consequence of severe head and neck lymphoedema. *Journal of Laryngology and Otology, 115*, 62–64.

CHAPTER 15

Special Considerations in Pediatric Populations

Deborah L. McBride, RN, MSN, CPON®

Introduction

Over the past 30 years, multimodal therapies for pediatric cancers have produced a marked increase in survival rates. From 1999 to 2005, the five-year survival rate for childhood cancer was 81%, according to the National Cancer Institute's Surveillance, Epidemiology, and End Results Program (Horner et al., 2009). The therapies responsible for this survival rate produce unavoidable toxicities to normal cells. The mucosal lining, including the oral mucosa, is a prime target for treatment-related toxicity of cancer chemotherapy because of the high cellular turnover rate, the complex microflora, and repeated trauma related to normal oral function (Worthington, Clarkson, & Eden, 2007). Children with cancer are at an especially high risk because of their developmental status and because adverse long-term health outcomes may manifest months to years after completion of cancer treatment. The medical literature reports that 40% of adults and 90% of children develop some form of treatment-related oral complication (National Cancer Institute, 2009). Although the oral complications of cancer treatment reflect the tissue changes taking place throughout the gastrointestinal system, this chapter deals with the oral effects of chemotherapy and radiation treatments in children.

Cancer treatment for children differs from treatment for adults in several ways. One important difference is that cancer treatment for children often is more intense than that for adults because the dose-limiting toxicities of chemotherapy are reached at higher doses and children, therefore, are able to tolerate more intensive chemotherapy than adults. In addition, the toxic effects of chemotherapy have a more significant and longer-lasting effect on children than adults because of the developmental considerations during childhood. Finally, some types of supportive care used in adults may not be available to children because of the treatment toxicities associated with specific periods of childhood development.

Even the term *childhood* overlooks the differences across the childhood spectrum, from neonate to adolescent, related to survival and toxicities, which impact the treatment and supportive care provided to children. Different approaches based on the age of the child at the time of treatment will affect the outcomes related to the control of the disease and the quality of survivorship.

Oral Complications Associated With Cancer Treatment in Children

As with adults, the most common oral complications associated with cancer therapies in children are oral mucositis, infections, and salivary gland dysfunction. Secondary complications such as dehydration, taste distortion, and malnutrition may result. In addition, radiation of the head and neck can result in permanent damage to the oral mucosa, vasculature, muscle, and bone, resulting in xerostomia (dry mouth), dental caries, soft tissue necrosis and osteonecrosis, and inability to open the mouth secondary to damage to the trigeminal nerve. Finally, both chemotherapy and radiation therapy produce cosmetic and functional abnormalities of the teeth in children (van der Pas-van Voskuilen et al., 2009; Zarina & Nik-Hussein, 2005; Zwetchkenbaum & Oh, 2007).

Acute complications can be dose limiting, thus requiring a modification of the optimal therapy. Both dose and schedule modifications may be necessary to allow oral lesions to resolve. In severe cases, the patient may not be able to continue optimal therapy protocols, resulting in a reduction in survivorship.

Abnormalities of the Teeth Associated With Cancer Treatment

Dental abnormalities associated with cancer treatment occur primarily in children younger than three years of age who have not yet developed deciduous teeth. However, prepubertal children also can be at risk. Children younger than 12 years old may manifest abnormalities in the size and shape of teeth and in craniofacial development. Altered dental growth can lead to malformed teeth, including decreased crown size, shortened and conical-shaped roots, and microdontia. Complete agenesis also may occur. Tooth eruption may be delayed with an increased frequency of impacted maxillary canines. Deficient dental root development has been reported after conventional pediatric anti-cancer therapy (Barbería, Hernandez, Miralles, & Maroto, 2008; Maguire et al., 1987; Paulino, Koshy, & Howell, 2005). Recent research has demonstrated that disturbances of dental root growth always follow pediatric stem cell transplantation. Using root-crown ratios of fully developed permanent teeth of patients who were treated when they were younger than 10 years old, Hölttä, Hovi, Saarinen-Pihkala, Peltola, and Alaluusua (2005) found that 77% of the fully developed permanent teeth were affected by total body irradiation and stem cell transplantation. Children who were treated between the ages of three and five years had the most severe aberrations. High-dose chemotherapy alone harmed root growth, with 55% of the teeth having root-crown ratios outside plus or minus 2 standard deviations and 85% of patients treated with total body irradiation and high-dose chemotherapy outside the plus or minus 2 standard deviation range (Hölttä et al., 2005).

Developing teeth in pediatric patients are sensitive to the effects of specific drug toxicities. Abnormal tooth and root development has been associated with vincristine, actinomycin D, cyclophosphamide, 6-mercaptopurine, procarbazine, nitrogen mustard, and radiation (10 Gy is generally thought to destroy developing roots). The signs and symptoms of abnormal tooth and root development related to drug toxicities are pale enamel and small, uneven, and maloccluded teeth (Holmes, 1991).

Dental and skeletal growth and development alterations are complications of hematopoietic stem cell transplantation in pediatric patients. These complications include craniofacial growth and developmental abnormalities. Children irradiated for head and neck malignancies have significant alternation in some skeletal measurements indicative of treatment-induced asymmetry and potential deformity. Denys et al. (1998) found that deviation occurred in the cranial vault, the anterior and mid-interorbital distances, and lateral orbital wall length. Asymmetry existed in the medial and lateral orbital wall lengths and the zygomatic arches in children treated with radiation for head and neck cancers. Children in high-risk groups should be followed and given prophylactic treatment and intervention to reduce the consequences of the therapy (Dahllöf, 1998). Routine dental examinations every six months, with attention to caries, periodontal disease, and gingivitis, are recommended for childhood cancer survivors (National Cancer Institute, 2009; Paulino et al., 2005).

Treatment and Prevention of Oral Mucositis

Mucositis, a painful inflammation and ulceration of the mucous membrane, is one of the most common side effects of cancer treatment. Although the incidence and prevalence of mucositis in the pediatric oncology population are difficult to assess because of the lack of a universally used instrument for assessing mucositis in children, it is estimated that the prevalence ranges from 30% to 75% (Fulton, Middleton, & McPhail, 2002) depending on treatment. In aggressive myeloablative chemotherapy, it occurs in 90%–100% (Filicko, Lazarus, & Flomenberg, 2003). In about 50% of patients with mucositis, lesions can be severe, causing significant pain, interfering with nutrition, and requiring modification of the chemotherapy regimen (Sonis et al., 2004). Children are at a higher risk for developing oral mucositis than adults. The high prevalence may be related to the higher proliferating fraction of mucosal basal cells, variations in resistance, and immunologic status of children (Sonis & Sonis, 1979). In addition, the most common type of childhood cancer is hematologic, which is proposed to lead to higher rates of oral mucositis than solid tumors (Mahood et al., 1991). Mucositis may predispose a child to fungal, viral, and bacterial infections, which may lead to life-threatening systemic infection.

Parents and children should be informed of the importance of keeping the mouth clean and encouraged to practice good, basic oral hygiene. Although amifostine, allopurinol mouth rinse, ice chips, granulocyte macrophage–colony-stimulating factor, benzydamine, antibiotic pastilles/pastes, povidone-iodine, pilocarpine, and hydrolytic enzymes have been shown to be potentially beneficial for the prevention of mucositis in adult populations (Keefe et al., 2007), their use in children for the prevention of treatment-related mucositis needs further study. Allopurinol mouthwash is not recommended for children receiving cancer treatment other than 5-fluorouracil (5-FU). Although folinic acid may be used for the prevention of toxicity following treatment with methotrexate, it is not recommended for the routine prevention of chemotherapy- or radiotherapy-induced mucositis, as there is evidence that it may promote mucositis (United Kingdom Children's Cancer Study Group-Paediatric Oncology Nurses Forum [UKCCSG-PONF] Mouth Care Group, 2006).

No one standard treatment or drug is currently available that has shown consistent efficacy in preventing or treating mucositis in children. As a result, the guidelines for the prevention and treatment of mucositis vary from institution to institution. Many agents and protocols have been promoted for management or prevention of mucositis, but they have not been adequately supported by controlled clinical trials. Chlorhexidine has been cited as an agent that decreases the severity of mucositis, but the evidence is conflicting concerning its effectiveness. The American Academy of Pediatric Dentistry (2008–2009) and the Multinational Association for Supportive Care in Cancer (Rubenstein et al., 2004) reported that no studies demonstrated a prophylactic impact of chlorhexidine (Potting, Uitterhoeve, Op Reimer, & Van Achterberg, 2006) although there was a reduced colonization of *Candida* species in the mouth (Keefe et al., 2007). Chlorhexidine may provide antimicrobial activity during rinsing and for several hours thereafter. However, because the safety and efficacy of chlorhexidine in children has not yet been fully established, the benefits of its use should be weighed against the possible risks. Ingestion of 30 or 60 ml of chlorhexidine by a small child (10 kg or less body weight) might result in gastric distress, including nausea, or signs of alcohol intoxication. Medical attention should be sought if a small child ingests more than 120 ml of chlorhexidine or develops signs of alcohol intoxication. Cheng (2004) found that children preferred chlorhexidine over benzydamine in reducing mucositis.

No significant evidence of the effectiveness or tolerability of mixtures containing topical anesthetics has been found. In addition, lidocaine diminishes the taste and gag reflex and may cause a burning sensation in the mouth. Studies on the use of topical anesthetics for pain have not assessed the benefit and potential for toxicity in children. Topical anesthetics come in a liquid form that should be swished around the mouth and then spit out. Children who cannot follow directions to spit out the medication will swallow it. Children should avoid eating any food for an hour after the medication because the medication will numb the tongue and affect swallowing.

The UKCCSG-PONF Mouth Care Group (2006) guidelines found no evidence to support the use of the following for the treatment of chemotherapy- or radiotherapy-induced mucositis in children: benzydamine, chlorhexidine, sucralfate, tetrachlorodecaoxide, and "magic mouthwash" (lidocaine solution, diphenhydramine hydrochloride, and aluminum hydroxide suspension). However, the UKCCSG-PONF Mouth Care Group reported that the following have been shown to be potentially beneficial for the treatment of mucositis in adult populations: vitamin E, immunoglobulin, and allopurinol mouthwash. These guidelines are currently being updated.

In addition to the interventions already described, palifermin, also known as keratinocyte growth factor-1, and cryotherapy have been found to be effective in the treatment of mucositis (National Cancer Institute, 2009). The U.S. Food and Drug Administration approved palifermin in December 2004 to decrease the incidence and duration of severe oral mucositis in patients undergoing high-dose chemotherapy with or without radiation therapy followed by bone marrow transplantation for hematologic cancers. Langner et al. (2008) found that palifermin administered at 60 mcg/kg per day for three days reduced the severity and duration of oral mucositis from 12 to 6 days. The use of pain medications was also reduced from 378 to 150 morphine equivalents, but the duration of use was not shortened. Cryotherapy, the use of ice chips, is recommended as likely to be effective for bolus chemotherapy with a short half-life (bolus 5-FU or melphalan) to prevent mucositis (National Cancer Institute, 2009). Because 5-FU has a half-life of 5–20 minutes, patients should be instructed to swish ice chips in their mouth for 30 minutes beginning 5 minutes prior to 5-FU administration. Karagözo lu and Ulusoy (2005) reported that ice cubes decreased the severity and duration of mucositis in adult patients. According to Patient-Judged Mucositis Grading, the rate of mucositis was 36.7% in the study group and 90% in the control group ($p < 0.05$). The researchers speculated that administration of cryotherapy resulted in local vasoconstriction, which decreased blood flow in the oral mucosa and reduced the amount of drug distribution to cells.

Although efforts to treat mucositis have been less successful in the past, the advent of newer agents, including amifostine, keratinocyte growth factor, transforming growth factor-beta, and interleukin-11, provides hope that this toxicity will be significantly decreased in the near future. A recent study has shown that laser therapy can decrease the duration of chemotherapy-induced oral mucositis in children (Kuhn, Porto, Miraglia, & Brunetto, 2009). There is a continuing need for well-designed trials with a large number of participants to evaluate the effectiveness of new treatments and drugs for mucositis in children.

Pediatric Oral Assessment Tools

In an effort to standardize measurements of mucosal integrity, oral assessment scales have been developed to grade the level of mucositis in children. Specific instruments have been developed to evaluate the observable and functional dimensions of mucositis in pediatric patients (Sung et al., 2007; Tomlinson, Judd, Hendershot, Maloney, & Sung, 2008). The UKCCSG-PONF Mouth Care Group (2006) identified 27 individual oral assessment tools. Of the assessment scales evaluated, Oral Assessment Guide (OAG) (Eilers, Berger, & Petersen, 1988) was ranked as a valid, reliable, and clinically useful tool for assessing oral status of both adults and children (McGuire et al., 2002). The OAG is a combined scale that assesses the ability to swallow, the appearance of the lips, the corners of the mouth and the tongue, the quality of the saliva, the appearance of the mucous membrane and gingiva, teeth debris, and the ability to speak. Gibson et al. (2006) validated a modified OAG for children using a quantification process. In that study, the original OAG categories of teeth and voice were reported by nurses to cause confusion because babies do not have teeth, and changes to voice are difficult to ascertain in children too young to talk. The modified OAG gave children with no teeth a score of 1 under the teeth category and included crying when evaluating the voice quality of nonverbal children (UKCCSG-PONF Mouth Care Group, 2006). Before implementation, some form of training and reliability testing of the tool should be done in the clinical setting.

Infections Associated With Cancer Treatment

The oral cavity can also be a source of systemic infection in myelosuppressed patients, especially in children, who are a high-risk population. The most frequently documented source of sepsis in immunosuppressed patients with cancer is the mouth. Early and definitive dental intervention, including comprehensive oral hygiene measures, reduces the risk for oral and associated systemic complications (Little, Falace, Miller & Rhodus, 2008).

Candidiasis

Candidiasis is a yeast infection, most commonly caused by *Candida albicans*. Chemotherapy and radiation therapy may predispose a patient to candidiasis by altering immune status. In addition, changes to the oral cavity, such as mucositis, xerostomia, and poor hygiene, may increase a patient's risk of developing oral candidiasis. The most common form of oral candidiasis occurs on the buccal mucosa, dorsal tongue, and palate. It appears as a creamy, white to yellow, velvety covering that can be wiped off, leaving an erythematous, ulcerated surface. The affected area can increase in size and may lead to systemic infection. Oral candidiasis is a serious problem for children with cancer. The mortality rate for this infection has increased because of fungal septicemia, associated with a primarily buccal infection (González-García, Naval-Gías, Román-Romero, Sastre-Pérez, & Rodríguez-Campo, 2009).

Preventive therapy for oral candidiasis is not recommended for most patients. However, when choosing an antifungal agent for the prevention of candidiasis, one that is absorbed from the gastrointestinal tract is recommended (for example, fluconazole, itraconazole, or ketoconazole). Drug doses should be adjusted based on the weight of the child.

Oral antifungal agents have variable efficacy in treating fungal infection in immunocompromised patients. Several studies have demonstrated the inability of nystatin suspension to reduce the incidence of *Candida* infection in immunocompromised patients, but the practice continues in some centers. Clotrimazole troches and amphotericin oral solutions may have some efficacy in reducing colonization and treating *Candida* infections in immunocompromised patients. Levy-Polack, Sebelli, and Polack (1998) reported that pediatric patients with leukemia who followed a daily preventive protocol (plaque removal, chlorhexidine rinse, iodopovidone, and nystatin) experienced a significant decrease in moderate mucositis and candidiasis and had improved oral hygiene.

When systemic dissemination is possible, persistent fungal infection should be treated with systemic agents. Amphotericin B often is the drug of choice for treatment of systemic candidiasis.

Herpes Simplex Virus

Herpes simplex virus (HSV) infection can cause pain and blistering on the lips and around the mouth ranging from mild to serious conditions in patients receiving cancer treatment. HSV type 1 (HSV1) is the most common orofacial lesion. It is estimated that 80% of the population are asymptomatic carriers of the virus (Conference Consensus, 1989). The virus can lie dormant for many years after the primary infection until triggered by a stimulus such as sunlight, stress, the common cold, febrile illness, menstruation, or immunosuppression. Under immunosuppression, the virus can become activated and lead to severe oral and disseminated infections. Approximately 50%–90% of bone marrow transplant recipients who are seropositive for HSV will develop infections, usually within the first five weeks after transplantation. In addition, a high proportion of patients with acute leukemia or those receiving high-dose chemotherapy will develop HSV infections during the period when they are immunosuppressed (Conference Consensus, 1989). A recent study by Ramphal et al. (2007) found that 9% of the oral swabs of pediatric patients with cancer with febrile neutropenia tested positive for HSV, and oral HSV was associated with prolonged mucositis and poor response to initial therapy.

Acyclovir is effective at reducing the frequency of HSV infections in both adults and children. However, acyclovir is only recommended as a preventive strategy for HSV in patients undergoing high-dose chemotherapy with stem cell transplantation. Acyclovir is not recommended for routine prophylactic use because of the rarity of the problem and the cost.

Acyclovir is effective for the treatment of HSV in patients receiving chemotherapy or radiotherapy. Mild and nonprogressing lesions on the lip should be treated with topical acyclovir. Progressing and severe lesions on the lip should be treated with oral acyclovir. Intraoral lesions should be treated with oral acyclovir. When oral administration is not tolerated, IV acyclovir should be used.

Salivary Gland Dysfunction

Both chemotherapy and radiotherapy can cause salivary gland dysfunction. Chemotherapy drugs can affect both the flow and the composition of the saliva, causing xerostomia. Radiotherapy to the head and neck can cause damage to the salivary glands. The damage by radiotherapy develops soon after treatment starts, progresses during treatment, continues for some time after treatment stops, and may be permanent. Both salivary gland damage and xerostomia can cause discomfort, taste disturbances, difficulty chewing and swallowing, and speech problems, thereby having a negative impact on the patient's quality of life. In addition, the risk of infection, including oral candidiasis, is increased in patients with xerostomia and salivary gland damage.

Radiation damage can be caused by radiation greater than 40 Gy and more than 50% of a gland irradiated (Silverman, 2007). Dental examination, salivary flow studies, and attention to early caries and periodontal disease are diagnostic tests to identify decreased salivary gland function. Current management techniques include encouraging meticulous oral hygiene, saliva substitution, prophylactic fluoride, dietary counseling regarding avoiding fermentable carbohydrates, and pilocarpine (Paulino et al., 2005).

Saliva stimulants and artificial saliva may be beneficial for the treatment of postradiation xerostomia. Pilocarpine (5 mg three times a day) can reduce symptomatic xerostomia in adult patients with postradiation xerostomia; however, pilocarpine is not currently available in a form approved for children. Symptomatic treatments including saliva stimulants, artificial saliva, sugar-free gum, or frequent sips of water for the relief of dry mouth should be considered.

Oral and Dental Management

The management of oral care for children being treated for cancer can improve their quality of life; however, uncertainty exists as to what is appropriate oral care (Miller & Kearney, 2001). Regular oral assessment should be used to check that good basic oral hygiene is being maintained and that appropriate pain control and therapeutic interventions are available. The frequency with which a child's mouth is assessed will depend on the individual's oral status. Frequency should increase at the onset of mucositis or other oral complications.

All children should undergo a dental assessment at the time of cancer diagnosis and, if possible, before cancer treatment commences, according to the Association of Pediatric Hematology/Oncology Nurses (Kline, 2007) and the UKCCSG-PONF Mouth Care Group (2006). Ideally, the oncology team should include a pediatric dentist or a dental hygienist to undertake the initial assessment. If a dentally trained healthcare worker is not available, then a member of the oncology team should perform the assessment. Any required invasive dental treatment should be undertaken by a specialist pediatric dentist. A mechanism of notification should be set up between the oncology team and the pediatric dental units. For routine dental care, the community-based provider should be notified of the cancer diagnosis and arrangements before and during cancer treatment. Clear communication between the cancer center and the routine dental provider is important. The cancer center should provide appropriate training in oral assessment of pediatric patients with cancer for healthcare providers in collaboration with the dental team.

Oral Care After Cancer Treatment

Complications can develop during therapy or months to years after therapy. For pediatric patients, this creates a high burden of mortality and illness, with one-third of the survivors reporting severe or life-threatening complications 30 years after diagnosis of their primary cancer (Oeffinger, Hudson, & Landier, 2009). Unlike radiation therapy, which often results in permanent tissue damage, chemotherapy causes acute injury that resolves once the treatment has stopped.

Parents and children should be informed of the possible long-term dental and orofacial effects of childhood cancer and treatment. Children should continue to be monitored during the period of growth and development and referred back to their routine dental provider, who should be advised of the preventive regimen recommended by the consultant/specialist pediatric dental team and advised of future care arrangements and systems for referral as necessary.

Childhood cancer survivors, even those with the highest risk of abnormalities, visit the dentist less often than the American Dental Association's recommendation of once a year (Yeazel et al., 2004). The American Academy of Pediatric Dentistry recommends dental examination for childhood cancer survivors every six months with attention to early caries, periodontal disease, and gingivitis, with radiographic baseline taking place at age five to six years (American Academy of Pediatric Dentistry, 2008–2009).

Treatment of orthodontic problems for patients who have had treatment-related malocclusions or other alternations in dental growth and development appears to be increasing. However, specific guidelines for management have not been established for pediatric patients.

Compliance With Routine Oral Care

The success of an oral care protocol intervention is based on patient compliance. Data reveal that more than 90% of pediatric patients complied 100% with the oral care protocol (Dodd et al., 1996). Educating patients and families on oral care protocols needs to be emphasized, especially in the pediatric population, where family members are often assisting the patients with daily hygiene. Guidelines that are simple and realistic with a strong educational element for families will increase the compliance rate. A clinical team at Emory University Hospital posted a sign in patients' rooms itemizing the steps in oral care, which was found to increase adherence to the oral care protocol (Yeager, Webster, Crain, Kasow, & McGuire, 2000). The same study recommended giving families information both in writing and verbally to describe why oral care is an important part of their care, in order to overcome the large amount of information they receive at the beginning of their treatment. In addition, verbal advice regarding oral care may need to be repeated throughout therapy.

Routine Oral Hygiene Procedures

Although oral complications are common in children with cancer, it is clear that routine oral procedures are inadequate and that greater focus on oral care would prevent oral complications. The purpose of oral care is to maintain a functional and pain-free oral cavity, reducing bacterial activity to prevent systemic infections and enhance self-esteem.

In terms of frequency of care, Beck (1979) found that in patients receiving chemotherapy, performing oral care two to four times a day reduced incidence of infection by 50% compared to a control group. Concurrent dehydrating stressors (e.g., nasal oxygen, mouth breathing, restricted food or fluid intake) may necessitate increased frequency.

Patients should be advised to brush their teeth at least twice a day for two to three minutes with a mild-tasting fluoride toothpaste. The toothbrush should be for the sole use of the child, and the brush should be changed every two months or after an oral infection. A soft brush with a small head can be used if the child has a sore mouth. Rinsing the toothbrush in hot water for 15–30 seconds will soften the bristles, if needed. Allow the brush to air dry between brushings. If toothpaste irritates the mouth, the child can brush with a solution of 1 teaspoon of salt added to 4 cups of water. For children younger than six years old, parents should be instructed on how to brush their child's teeth. For babies without teeth, parents should clean the mouth with an oral sponge moistened with water. When it is not possible to brush a child's teeth, an oral sponge moistened with water or diluted chlorhexidine can be used.

Brushing is required to remove plaque and prevent periodontal disease. A small, soft toothbrush is the best tool for cleaning teeth. Some nurses prefer using foam sponge sticks, but studies have shown that only 20% of patients preferred the foam, and although foam sticks may be useful in cleansing soft tissues, they are ineffective at cleaning tooth surfaces (Howarth, 1977). Gentle tooth brushing should be used even in immunosuppressed patients. Gentle irrigation and mouthwashes may be all that can be tolerated based on the patient's oral condition.

Other type of aids, such as flossing and fluoride supplements, should be used based on a risk assessment by a member of the dental team. Sugary food and drink intake should be restricted because of the high risk for caries. This should include encouraging a noncariogenic diet, which limits dietary supplements high in carbohydrates and oral pediatric medications rich in sucrose (American Academy of Pediatric Dentistry, 2008–2009; National Cancer Institute, 2009). The child should see the dental team every six months during cancer treatment or at the onset of any oral problem.

Conclusion

Unfortunately, many pediatric patients with cancer encounter oral side effects, such as dental malformation, mucositis, infections, salivary gland dysfunction, and pain, during their treatment. With proper implementation of an effective oral protocol, bedside nurses can improve the care of their patients and reduce the incidence and severity of these complications. Compliance with routine oral care is key to maintaining a healthy mouth during cancer treatment. Therefore, patient education about the importance of oral care in minimizing complications and maximizing the treatment outcome is imperative. Bedside nurses are able to provide firsthand assessment and implementation of the oral protocol. In addition, some aspects of the oral protocol, such as tooth brushing and oral rinsing, are self-care activities that older children can do, allowing them to be more responsible for their health care. Nursing research is needed to fill in the gaps in knowledge required to improve the standards of care for pediatric patients with cancer.

References

American Academy of Pediatric Dentistry. (2008–2009). Guideline on dental management of pediatric patients receiving chemotherapy, hematopoietic cell transplantation, and/ or radiation. *Pediatric Dentistry, 30*(Suppl. 7), 219–225.

Barbería, E., Hernandez, C., Miralles, V., & Maroto, M. (2008). Paediatric patients receiving oncology therapy: Review of the literature and oral management guidelines. *European Journal of Paediatric Dentistry, 9,* 188–194.

Beck, S. (1979). Impact of a systematic oral care protocol on stomatitis after chemotherapy. *Cancer Nursing, 2,* 185–199.

Cheng, K.K. (2004). Children's acceptance and tolerance of chlorhexidine and benzydamine oral rinses in the treatment of chemotherapy-induced oropharyngeal mucositis. *European Journal of Oncology Nursing, 8,* 341–349. doi:10.1016/j.ejon.2004.04.002

Conference Consensus. (1989). Oral complications of cancer therapies: Diagnosis, prevention and treatment. National Institutes of Health. *Connecticut Medicine, 53,* 595–601.

Dahllöf, G. (1998). Craniofacial growth in children treated for malignant diseases. *Acta Ondontologica Scandinavica, 56,* 378–382.

Denys, D., Kaste, S.C., Kun, L.E., Chaudhary, M.A., Bowman, L.C., & Robbins, K.T. (1998). The effects of radiation on craniofacial skeletal growth: A quantitative study. *International Journal of Pediatric Otorhinolaryngology, 45,* 7–13. doi:10.1016/S0165-5876(98)00028-7

Dodd, M.J., Larson, P.J., Dibble, S.L., Miaskowski, C., Greenspan, D., MacPhail, L., … Shiba, D. (1996). Randomized clinical trial of chlorhexidine versus placebo for prevention of oral mucositis in patients receiving chemotherapy. *Oncology Nursing Forum, 23,* 921–927.

Eilers, J., Berger, A.M., & Petersen, M.C. (1988). Development, testing, and application of the oral assessment guide. *Oncology Nursing Forum, 15,* 325–330.

Filicko, J., Lazarus, H.M., & Flomenberg, N. (2003). Mucosal injury in patients undergoing hematopoietic progenitor cell transplantation: New approaches to prophylaxis and treatment. *Bone Marrow Transplantation, 31,* 1–10. doi:10.1038/sj.bmt.1703776

Fulton, J.S., Middleton, G.J., & McPhail, J.T. (2002). Management of oral complications. *Seminars in Oncology Nursing, 18,* 28–35. doi:10.1053/sonu.2002.30041

Gibson, F., Cargill, J., Allison, J., Begent, J., Cole, S., Stone, J., & Lucas, V. (2006). Establishing content validity of the oral assessment guide in children and young people. *European Journal of Cancer, 42,* 1817–1825. doi:10.1016/j.ejca.2006.02.018

González-García, R., Naval-Gías, L., Román-Romero, L., Sastre-Pérez, J., & Rodríguez-Campo, F.J. (2009). Local recurrences and second primary tumors from squamous cell carcinoma of the oral cavity: A retrospective analytic study of 500 patients. *Head and Neck, 31,* 1168–1180. doi:10.1002/hed.21088

Holmes, S. (1991). The oral complications of specific anticancer therapy. *International Journal of Nursing Studies, 28,* 343–360.

Hölttä, P., Hovi, L., Saarinen-Pihkala, U.M., Peltola, J., & Alaluusua, S. (2005). Disturbed root development of permanent teeth after pediatric stem cell transplantation: Dental root development after SCT. *Cancer, 103,* 1484–1493. doi:10.1002/cncr.20967

Horner, M.J., Ries, L.A.G., Krapcho, M., Neyman, N., Aminou, R., Howlader, N., … Edwards, B.K. (Eds.). (2009). SEER cancer statistics review, 1975–2006. Retrieved from http://seer.cancer.gov/csr/1975_2006

Howarth, H. (1977). Mouth care procedures for the very ill. *Nursing Times, 73,* 354–355.

Karagözo lu, S., & Ulusoy, M.F. (2005). Chemotherapy: The effect of oral cryotherapy on the development of mucositis. *Journal of Clinical Nursing, 14,* 754–765. doi:10.1111/j.1365-2702.2005.01128.x

Keefe, D.M., Schubert, M.M., Elting, L.S., Sonis, S.T., Epstein, J.B., Raber-Durlacher, J.E., … Peterson, D.E. (2007). Updated clinical practice guidelines for the prevention and treatment of mucositis. *Cancer, 109,* 820–831. doi:10.1002/cncr.22484

Kline, N.E. (Ed.). (2007). *The pediatric chemotherapy and biotherapy curriculum* (2nd ed.). Glenview, IL: Association of Pediatric Hematology/Oncology Nurses.

Kuhn, A., Porto, F.A., Miraglia, P., & Brunetto, A.L. (2009). Low-level infrared laser therapy in chemotherapy-induced oral mucositis: A randomized placebo-controlled trial in children. *Journal of Pediatric Hematology/Oncology, 31,* 33–37. doi:10.1097/MPH.0b013e318192cb8e

Langner, S., Staber, P., Schub, N., Gramatzki, M., Grothe, W., Behre, G., … Neumeister, P. (2008). Palifermin reduces incidence and severity of oral mucositis in allogeneic stem-cell transplant recipients. *Bone Marrow Transplantation, 42,* 275–279. doi:10.1038/bmt.2008.157

Levy-Polack, M.P., Sebelli, P., & Polack, N.L. (1998). Incidence of oral complications and application of a preventive protocol in children with acute leukemia. *Special Care in Dentistry, 18,* 189–193.

Little, J.W., Falace, D.A., Miller, C.S., & Rhodus, N.L. (2008). *Dental management of the medically compromised patient* (7th ed.). St. Louis, MO: Elsevier Mosby.

Maguire, A., Craft, A.W., Evans, R.G., Amineddine, H., Kernahan, J., Macleod R.I., … Welbury, R.R. (1987). The long-term effects of treatment on the dental condition of children surviving malignant disease. *Cancer, 60,* 2570–2575.

Mahood, D.J., Dose, A.M., Loprinzi, C.L., Veeder, M.H., Athmann, L.M., Therneau, T.M., … Gusa, N.L. (1991). Inhibition of fluorouracil-induced stomatitis by oral cryotherapy. *Journal of Clinical Oncology, 9,* 449–452.

McGuire, D.B., Peterson, D.E., Muller, S., Owen, D.C., Slemmons, M.F., & Schubert, M.M. (2002). The 20 item oral mucositis index: Reliability and validity in bone marrow and stem cell transplant patients. *Cancer Investigation, 20,* 893–903.

Miller, M., & Kearney, N. (2001). Oral care for patients with cancer: A review of the literature. *Cancer Nursing, 24,* 241–254.

National Cancer Institute. (2009, October 6). Oral complications of chemotherapy and head/neck radiation (PDQ®) [Health professional version]. Retrieved from http://www.cancer.gov/cancertopics/pdq/supportivecare/oralcomplications/HealthProfessional/page3

Oeffinger, K.C., Hudson, M.M., & Landier, W. (2009). Survivorship: Childhood cancer survivors. *Primary Care, 36,* 743–780. doi:10.1016/j.pop.2009.07.007

Paulino, A.C., Koshy, M., & Howell, D. (2005). Head and neck. In C.L. Schwartz, W.L. Hobbie, L.S. Constine, & K.S. Ruccione (Eds.), *Survivors of childhood and adolescent cancer: A multidisciplinary approach* (2nd ed., pp. 95–108). St. Louis, MO: Springer.

Potting, C.M., Uitterhoeve, R., Op Reimer, W.S., & Van Achterberg, T. (2006). The effectiveness of commonly used mouthwashes for the prevention of chemotherapy-induced oral mucositis: A systematic review. *European Journal of Cancer Care, 15,* 431–439. doi:10.1111/j.1365-2354.2006.00684.x

Ramphal, R., Grant, R.M., Dzolganovski, B., Constantin, J., Tellier, R., Allen, U., … Sung, L. (2007). Herpes simplex virus in febrile neutropenic children undergoing chemotherapy for cancer: A prospective cohort study. *Pediatric Infectious Disease Journal, 26,* 700–704. doi:10.1097/INF.0b013e31805cdc11

Rubenstein, E.B., Peterson, D.E., Schubert, M., Keefe, D., McGuire, D., Epstein, J., … Sonis, S.T. (2004). Clinical practice guidelines for the prevention and treatment of cancer therapy-induced oral and gastrointestinal mucositis. *Cancer, 100*(Suppl. 9), 2026–2046. doi:10.1002/cncr.20163

Silverman, S., Jr. (2007). Diagnosis and management of oral mucositis. *Journal of Supportive Oncology, 5*(2, Suppl. 1), 13–21.

Sonis, A., & Sonis, S. (1979). Oral complications of cancer chemotherapy in pediatric patients. *Journal of Pedodontics, 3,* 122–128.

Sonis, S.T., Elting, L.S., Keefe, D., Peterson, D.E., Schubert, M., Hauer-Jensen, M., … Rubenstein, E.B. (2004). Perspectives on cancer therapy-induced mucosal injury: Pathogenesis, measurement, epidemiology, and consequences for patients. *Cancer, 100*(Suppl. 9), 1995–2025.

Sung, L., Tomlinson, G.A., Greenberg, M.L., Koren, G., Judd, P., Ota, S., & Feldman, B.M. (2007). Validation of the oral mucositis assessment scale in pediatric cancer. *Pediatric Blood and Cancer, 49,* 149–153. doi:10.1002/pbc.20863

Tomlinson, D., Judd, P., Hendershot, E., Maloney, A.-M., & Sung, L. (2008). Establishing literature-based items for an oral mucositis assessment tool in children. *Journal of Pediatric Oncology Nursing, 25,* 139–147. doi:10.1177/1043454208317235

United Kingdom Children's Cancer Study Group-Paediatric Oncology Nurses Forum Mouth Care Group. (2006, February). *Mouth care for children and young people with cancer: Evidence-based guidelines* (Version 1.0). Retrieved from http://www.rcn.org.uk/__data/assets/pdf_file/0017/11276/mouth_care_cyp_cancer_guideline.pdf

van der Pas-van Voskuilen, I.G., Veerkamp, J.S., Raber-Durlacher, J.E., Bresters, D., van Wijk, A.J., Barasch, A., … Gortzak, R.A. (2009). Long-term adverse effects of hematopoietic stem cell transplantation on dental development in children. *Supportive Care in Cancer,* *17,* 1169–1175. doi:10.1007/s00520-008-0567-1

Worthington, H.V., Clarkson, J.E., & Eden, O.B. (2007). Interventions for preventing oral mucositis for patients with cancer receiving treatment. *Cochrane Database of Systematic Reviews* 2007, Issue 4. Art. No.: CD000978. doi:10.1002/14651858.CD000978.pub3

Yeager, K.A., Webster, J., Crain, J., Kasow, J., & McGuire, D.B. (2000). Implementation of an oral care standard for leukemia and transplantation patients. *Cancer Nursing, 23,* 40–47.

Yeazel, M.W., Gurney, J.G., Oeffinger, K.C., Mitby, P.A., Mertens, A.C., Hudson, M.M., & Robison, L.L. (2004). An examination of the dental utilization practices of adult survivors of childhood cancer: A report from the Childhood Cancer Survivor Study. *Journal of Public Health Dentistry, 64,* 50–54.

Zarina, R.S., & Nik-Hussein, N.N. (2005). Dental abnormalities of a long-term survivor of a childhood hematological malignancy: Literature review and report of a case. *Journal of Clinical Pediatric Dentistry, 29,* 167–174.

Zwetchkenbaum, S.R., & Oh, W.-S. (2007). Prosthodontic management of abnormal tooth development secondary to chemoradiotherapy: A clinical report. *Journal of Prosthetic Dentistry, 98,* 429–435. doi:10.1016/S0022-3913(07)60141-3

CHAPTER 16

Second Primary Cancers and Recurrence

Pamela Hallquist Viale, RN, MS, CS, ANP, AOCNP®

Introduction

New cases of cancers of the oral cavity and pharynx are expected to occur in 36,540 patients in 2010 (Jemal, Siegel, Xu, & Ward, 2010). The majority of these cases occur in men (25,420) compared to women (11,120), and the estimated number of deaths from these cancers is expected to be 7,880 for both sexes (Jemal et al., 2010). These tumors are diagnosed in the tongue, mouth, pharynx, or other oral cavity and carry a high risk of recurrence in comparison to other cancers (Day & Blot, 1992; Humphris et al., 2003). Studies have shown that most patients with squamous cell cancer of the head and neck die as a result of recurrent tumor in a locoregional site (Kotwall et al., 1987). The development of second primary cancers is a significant concern for patients initially treated for oral cancers. In fact, second primary tumors occur at an annual rate of 3%–7% in patients with head and neck squamous cell cancer (Khuri et al., 2001). This higher risk for second primary cancers is primarily attributed to tobacco smoking and alcohol use (Lin et al., 2005). Because of these factors, patients with oral cancer may suffer from psychological effects such as depression or even reduced quality of life (Hodges & Humphris, 2009).

Scope of the Problem

Patients with cancers of the oral cavity may receive treatment with radiation, chemotherapy, or a combination of both therapies. Once treatment is completed, surveillance is conducted to help identify recurrence and manage post-treatment toxicities or complications. Because of the high risk of recurrence in this patient population, identification of clinical and pathologic features that may help predict individuals who are at higher risk is important (González-García, Naval-Gías, Román-Romero, Sastre-Pérez, & Rodríguez-Campo, 2009) (see Figure 16-1). Additionally, the fear of recurrence may lead to depression or other effects that can affect the quality of life for patients with oral cancers.

Jones et al. (1995) examined the records of 3,436 patients with squamous cell carcinoma of the head and neck; 274 of these patients developed a second neoplasm. The median time to presentation for the second tumor was 36 months, and these tumors were more likely to occur in male patients younger than 60 years of age at the time of their initial diagnosis. Positive cervical lymph nodes predicted a greater chance of new tumor development as well. The most common sites for second primaries to develop were head and neck (50%) and lung (34%), and 86% of them were of squamous cell histology (Jones et al., 1995). A retrospective study by Kotwall et al. (1987) of 832 patients with head and neck cancer showed the overall incidence of metastases was 47% with the highest incidence of metastases at the hypopharynx (60%), then base of the tongue (53%) and anterior tongue (50%). The lung was the most commonly seen site of distant metastases (80%) (Kotwall et al., 1987). Other metastatic sites include the bone, liver, skin, mediastinum, and bone marrow (Ferlito, Shaha, Silver, Rinaldo, & Mondin, 2001).

A recently reported retrospective analytic study of 500 patients examined the incidence of local recurrences and second primary tumors from squamous cell carcinoma of the oral cavity (González-García et al., 2009). The patients were retrospectively analyzed for a possible association between different clinical and pathologic features and the presence of recurrence or second primaries. The patients were followed for a mean duration time period of 52.27 ± 49.52 months, and at the end of this period, 53.8% were alive without evidence of disease versus 31.48% who had died of disease. Second primaries had developed in 5.6% (28) of the patients, and 19% (95 patients) developed a local recurrence during the study period. The disease-specific five-year survival rate for the whole group of patients was 67.2% in comparison to 34.9% in patients who developed a local recurrence or second primary. Fac-

---

Figure 16-1. Possible Predictors of Recurrent Disease in Oral Cancers

- Lack of adequate surgical resection (Kos et al., 2008)
- Males younger than age 60; presence of cervical lymph nodes (Jones et al., 1995)
- Postoperative radiation therapy and bone involvement (González-García et al., 2009)
- Weight loss of greater than 5%, a poor Eastern Cooperative Oncology Group performance status (1 versus 0), presence of residual disease at primary tumor site, a primary tumor site other than oropharynx, prior radiation therapy, and well or moderate tumor cell differentiation (Argiris et al., 2004)
- Smoking and alcohol use (Zhang et al., 2000)
- Higher tumor stage, high alcohol consumption, and high-risk HPV infection (Rosenquist et al., 2007)

tors predicting risk of local recurrence included postoperative radiation therapy and bone involvement. On the basis of their findings, the authors of the study recommended aggressive surgical treatment following the appearance of a second primary or local recurrence (González-García et al., 2009). Elective neck dissection was shown to be an important factor in one retrospective trial of 154 patients with early-stage oral squamous cell carcinoma; the authors concluded that elective neck treatment should be considered even in patients with small primary tumors and negative clinical examinations because of the high incidence of metastases and the potential for regional recurrences (Capote et al., 2007).

Another trial looked at the effect of tumor characteristics and treatment modality on local recurrence and survival of patients with oral squamous cell carcinoma in a retrospective analysis of 67 patients who received surgery (n = 61), radiotherapy (n = 6), and a combination of both treatments (n = 28) (Kos, Łuczak, Brusco, & Engelke, 2008). The follow-up study period was an average of 40 months, and various relationships between independent variables were studied, including primary local advancement, tumor location, histologic grading, and the presence of lymph node metastases. The most significant independent prognostic parameter for disease-free survival and overall survival in this disease was determined to be a complete resection of the tumor (Kos et al., 2008). Argiris, Li, and Forastiere (2004) studied 399 patients over a median follow-up period of 4.7 years to determine prognostic factors and long-term survivorship when diagnosed with recurrent or metastatic carcinoma of the head and neck. The one-year overall survival rate for all patients was 32%, with independent unfavorable predictors of objective response determined to include

- Weight loss of more than 5%
- Poor Eastern Cooperative Oncology Group (ECOG) performance status (1 versus 0)
- Presence of residual disease at primary tumor site
- Primary tumor site other than oropharynx
- Prior radiation therapy
- Well or moderate tumor cell differentiation.

These factors were unfavorable for overall survival as well. Interestingly, the 49 patients (12%) who survived longer than two years were more likely to have achieved an objective response originally to chemotherapy, have poor tumor cell differentiation, be Caucasian, have an ECOG performance status of 0, and received no prior radiation therapy (Argiris et al., 2004).

One trial examined the impact of second primary tumors on survival in head and neck cancer and found a positive correlation between second primaries and stage I or II disease, low patient age, and initial tumors of the larynx and oral cavity (Rennemo, Zätterström, & Boysen, 2008). In an analysis of 2,063 cases, the authors noted that the patients with the highest risk of a second primary tumor were the younger patients (younger than age 60) with initial limited disease. A high proportion of patients who then developed a second primary were complete responders after therapy for the first tumor. Overall prognosis was poor after the actual diagnosis of the second primary (Rennemo et al., 2008).

Additionally, smoking and alcohol use have been implicated in the development of oral cancers. Cessation of these behaviors is recommended to reduce the risk of recurrent disease or the development of second primary tumors. Heavy users of tobacco have a 5-fold to 25-fold higher risk of developing head and neck cancers compared to nonsmokers (Marur & Forastiere, 2008). Alcohol use can be synergistic, further increasing the risk. In a European study reported in 2005, the authors noted that tobacco smoking affected survival of the 931 patients with laryngeal cancer and that alcohol drinking had an effect as well although the association was less apparent (Dikshit et al., 2005). The authors noted that high intake of vegetables, fiber, and vitamin C had a protective effect against mortality from the disease (Dikshit et al., 2005). Additionally, the mutation of tumor protein p53 (a tumor suppressor gene) has been linked to increased exposure to alcohol and tobacco (Ahrendt et al., 2000).

Rosenquist et al. (2007) studied recurrence in patients with oral and oropharyngeal squamous cell carcinoma, looking at human papillomavirus (HPV) and other risk factors. The researchers followed 128 consecutive cases to the first event of recurrence of second primary tumor and evaluated the competing risk of death in intercurrent disease. After a median follow time of 22 months, 30 recurrences and 2 second primaries were identified; 12 patients were lost to follow-up and 21 deaths occurred before either recurrence or second primary was observed. The significant variables identified as causing a higher risk of recurrence and second primaries were a higher tumor stage, high alcohol consumption, and high-risk HPV infection (Rosenquist et al., 2007).

Personalized medicine is of significant import for the science of oncology treatment today, and it is a goal of clinicians working to tailor appropriate therapies for various cancers. The identification of biomarkers that could predict tumor recurrence or patient survival is not yet a reality for oral and pharyngeal cancer; however, ongoing study of potential markers continues. In one study, the promoter methylation status of the DNA repair gene *MGMT* and the tumor suppressor genes *CDKN2A* and *RASSF1* was evaluated by methylation-specific polymerase chain reaction in 88 samples of primary oral and pharyngeal tumors, correlating them with survival and tumor recurrence (Taioli et al., 2009). The results of the study showed that 29.6% of the tumors had *MGMT* methylation, 11.5% showed *CDKN2A* methylation, and 12.1% showed *RASSF1* methylation. The samples with *MGMT* promoter methylation strongly predicted poorer overall and disease-free survival. A significant trend showing the amount of *MGMT* methylation (p_{trend} 0.002) and recurrence (p_{trend} 0.001) was also observed in the study, and the authors concluded that the results might indicate *MGMT* promoter methylation as a possible biomarker for oral and pharyngeal cancer prognosis.

Treatment of locally recurrent head and neck cancer is determined by whether the disease is resectable. A combination of surgery and possibly radiation therapy or chemotherapy may be used in patients who have not received prior radiation therapy (National Comprehensive Cancer Network [NCCN], 2010). For those who have received radiation therapy and have recurrence or a second primary cancer, the treatment involves possible surgery if resectable, or if unresectable, chemotherapy or possibly irradiation, if it is considered safe. Unfortunately, radiation therapy treatments to previously irradiated tissue can be difficult and carry a high incidence of significant toxicity (Wong, Machtay, & Li, 2006). Therefore, the current recommendation is that irradiation should be carried out in the context of a clinical trial (NCCN, 2010). Distant metastases is usually managed with clinical trial or standard chemotherapy; best supportive care is an option if appropriate as well (NCCN, 2010).

Chemoprevention

Great interest exists in reducing the risk of second primaries in patients with head and neck cancer. One of the most studied strategies for reduction of these second primary tumors is 13-cis-retinoic acid (Khuri et al., 2001). Khuri et al. (2001) conducted the Retinoid Head and Neck Second Primary Trial with 1,191 patients randomized and eligible; the study was launched in 1991 and closed to new patients in 1999. These patients were followed for survival, development of second primary, and index cancer recurrence. Results showed that smoking played a significant role in the development of second primaries, and stage of disease was important as well. The rate of recurrence was higher in patients initially diagnosed with stage II disease versus stage I. Retinoic acid was not found to be helpful in reducing second primary tumors in patients with early-stage head and neck cancer; however, the dose used was relatively low compared to previous studies (Freemantle, Dragnev, & Dmitrovsky, 2006; Khuri et al., 2006). A small trial reported in 2005 also found no significant difference in the occurrence of second primary disease ($p = 0.90$), the recurrence of primary disease ($p = 0.70$), or disease-free interval ($p = 0.80$) in the treatment and nontreatment arms of the study ($N = 151$) (Perry et al., 2005). Additional trials are under way; curcumin analogs, green tea extracts, and other substances such as aspirin and high vegetable intake are under study as well (Kapoor, 2008; Khuri & Shin, 2008).

A study reported in 2005 examined a clinical-based intervention for improvement of diet in patients with head and neck cancer at risk for a second primary tumor. High dietary intake of fruits and vegetables has been associated with a reduction in head and neck cancer. The authors aimed to study an intervention to increase consumption of these substances in patients with this tumor type (Falciglia, Whittle, Levin, & Steward, 2005). The study was a crossover-controlled design, and each patient served as his or her own control. A clinical-based intervention of a face-to-face counseling session, telephone call, and three mailings was conducted along with the usual surveillance care. Measurements of the participants' diet were taken at baseline and at 6 and 12 months. The study results showed that the intervention did increase their intake of fruits and vegetables, and an improvement in overall diet quality was determined (Falciglia et al., 2005).

Fear of Recurrence and Psychosocial Effect on Patients With Oral Cancer

Recurrent oral cancer has a poor prognosis and can create distress for both patients and caregivers (Griffiths, Humphris, Skirrow, & Rogers, 2008). Once diagnosed with recurrent cancer, patients may be discouraged and experience increased concerns about their demise (Mahon & Casperson, 1997). Humphris et al. (2003) examined two samples of patients prospectively to assess their fear of recurrence and psychological morbidity during follow-up. A total of 187 patients were studied at two different time periods, three months and seven months after initial therapy. The results of the study showed that more than 80% of the patients were concerned about the possibility of recurrence at three months after therapy; this level decreased to 72% at seven months (p = 0.06). About two-thirds of the sample patients were concerned at both of the assessment periods. Psychological morbidity was most significant at three months (probable anxiety 37%, and depression 28%), with women more likely than men to report anxiety at three months after treatment (p < 0.05). Interestingly, patients 65 years old or older had less concern regarding the threat of recurrence. The authors concluded that the positive association between psychological morbidity and fears of recurrence was present at most of the assessment periods (Humphris et al., 2003).

In a qualitative study, researchers recruited nine patients over a 13-month period and evaluated their psychosocial response to recurrence. They identified six themes: emotional reactions, reevaluation, active coping strategies, life changes, support, and improvement in relationships (Griffiths et al., 2008). The emotional reactions of the patients with recurrent disease included shock, devastation, fear, hopelessness, shame, and denial; however, some patients experienced positive experiences such as new feelings of openness and improvement in relationships (Griffiths et al., 2008). Some patients described changes in their perspective on life, a cognitive reappraisal in which the new diagnosis influenced a personal ability to cope with recurrence. Some of the study participants felt that resigning to their fate was a beneficial strategy and helped them come to terms with an inevitable outcome. Although the study was small, the authors pointed out that its content is very sensitive because recurrence is associated with a poor prognosis. They also noted that the study was one of the first of its type and thus contains significant information (Griffiths et al., 2008). Importantly, the study results showed the vulnerability of patients with recurrence and the need for healthcare providers to recognize their own distress in caring for very ill and distressed patients and families and the need for support for each faction, including healthcare workers.

Worry about disease recurrence is increasingly recognized as a significant stressor for patients with cancer; it can affect psychological morbidity and quality of life (Hodges & Humphris, 2009). A prospective trial of 101 patients with head and neck cancer and 101 caregivers was conducted to examine distress and illness concerns for both groups. Measurements were taken at two different time points, and the preliminary results showed that early fears and distress within the study participants affected the later reports for these symptoms; there was a weak association of influence from one attribute to another for some individuals in the study (Hodges & Humphris, 2009). On average, the caregivers scored higher on concerns regarding recurrence of disease compared to the patient group ($p < 0.001$). The authors concluded that intervention may be helpful to reduce the disease concern to a manageable level at an early stage in the disease process.

Nursing Implications

Because of the high risk for recurrence, oncology nurses should emphasize the importance of recognizing the signs and symptoms of oral cancer in patients who have completed therapy for this disease. Nurses who work in late effects or surveillance clinics should provide education regarding cessation of high-risk behaviors. The most significant known risk factors for oral and most second cancers are use of tobacco and alcohol, and nurses should counsel patients on the importance of avoiding these behaviors (Day & Blot, 1992). A study of 73 patients with oral and oropharyngeal cancer aimed to determine the role of psychological factors in understanding smoking behavior over a period of 12 months (Humphris & Rogers, 2004). The patients were assessed four times; 20 patients were consistent smokers, 37 abstained from smoking, 7 returned to smoking, and 9 stopped smoking by the final 15-month period. The smoking group of patients had a significantly higher level of distress at each assessment after baseline (Humphris & Rogers, 2004). The authors concluded that past and current smoking behavior is associated with psychological distress in patients with oral and oropharyngeal cancer in the first 15-month period following initial therapy and that fear of recurrence was weakly associated with smoking behavior (Humphris & Rogers, 2004). Oncology nurses can be pivotal in helping patients enroll in smoking cessation programs and can provide support during surveillance and ongoing care for patients who are having difficulty stopping this behavior. Education about the importance of limiting alcohol intake is crucial as well.

Improvements in dietary intake of fruits and vegetables may be beneficial for patients with head and neck cancers. Oncology nurses can implement interventions designed to assist patient with increasing their intake of desired substances (Falciglia et al., 2005).

Previous treatment for locoregional disease can produce significant acute and late toxicities. Therefore, healthcare professionals should carefully evaluate patients at subsequent clinic visits (Kurtin, 2009). These changes can create the formation of scars and irregular anatomy of oral structures, making full evaluation potentially more difficult (Fischer & Epstein, 2008). Careful and close surveillance is recommended for early identification of recurrence or second primary tumors. Patients who develop advanced recurrent or metastatic disease are generally classified into resectable or unresectable recurrent disease; treatment will vary according to previous therapies received and extent of tumor (Choong & Vokes, 2008; Marur & Forastiere, 2008) (see Table 16-1).

Table 16-1. Possible Treatment Strategies for Recurrent Disease	
Recurrence Type	**Possible Intervention**
Low-volume recurrence, particularly of larynx and nasopharynx (resectable or occurring in previously irradiated area)	Surgery or reirradiation; goal of therapy is cure.
Large-volume disease (unresectable or occurring in previously irradiated area)	Generally considered incurable; supportive care only; for select patients, chemotherapy or reirradiation with or without chemotherapy may be an option.
Distant disease	Generally considered incurable; clinical trial may be an option; combination chemotherapy or single-agent chemotherapy may be considered for select patients.
Note. Based on information from Marur & Forastiere, 2008; National Comprehensive Cancer Network, 2010; Wong et al., 2006.	

Conclusion

Most patients with squamous cell cancer of the head and neck die of recurrent locoregional disease (Kotwall et al., 1987). Recently, the incidence of second primary tumors after a diagnosis of squamous cell carcinoma of the oral cavity or oropharynx was estimated to be 13% over a five-year period and 21% over a 10-year period (van der Haring, Schaapveld, Roodenburg, & de Bock, 2009). Data from 917 consecutive patients with primary oral or oropharyngeal squamous cell carcinoma were reviewed; interestingly, no statistically significant risk factors were identified within the study population. The results indicated, however, that regular follow-up for more than 10 years is necessary for all patients treated for cancer of the oral cavity and oropharynx (van der Haring et al., 2009). Because of the potential for psychological distress during this period, healthcare providers and oncology nurses should be sensitive to the emotional changes that patients may experience during this time. If recurrence is diagnosed, patients and their caregivers may need assistance with coping and emotional stressors.

References

Ahrendt, S.A., Chow, J.T., Yang, S.C., Wu, L., Zhang, M.-J., Jen, J., & Sidransky, D. (2000). Alcohol consumption and cigarette smoking increase the frequency of p53 mutations in non-small cell lung cancer. *Cancer Research, 60,* 3155–3159.

Argiris, A., Li, Y., & Forastiere, A. (2004). Prognostic factors and long-term survivorship in patients with recurrent or metastatic carcinoma of the head and neck. *Cancer, 101,* 2222–2229. doi:10.1002/cncr.20640

Capote, A., Escorial, V., Muñoz-Guerra, M.F., Rodríguez-Campo, F.J., Gamallo, C., & Naval, L. (2007). Elective neck dissection in early-stage oral squamous cell carcinoma—Does it influence recurrence and survival? *Head and Neck, 29,* 3–11. doi:10.1002/hed.20482

Choong, N., & Vokes, E. (2008). Expanding role of the medical oncologist in the management of head and neck cancer. *CA: A Cancer Journal for Clinicians, 58,* 32–53. doi:10.3322/CA.2007.0004

Day, G.L., & Blot, W.J. (1992). Second primary tumors in patients with oral cancer. *Cancer, 70,* 14–19.

Dikshit, R.P., Boffetta, P., Bouchardy, C., Merletti, F., Crosignani, P., Cuchi, T., ... Brennan, P. (2005). Lifestyle habits as prognostic factors in survival of laryngeal and hypopharyngeal cancer: A multicentric European study. *International Journal of Cancer, 117,* 992–995. doi:10.1002/ijc.21244

Falciglia, G.A., Whittle, K.M., Levin, L.S., & Steward, D.L. (2005). A clinical-based intervention improves diet in patients with head and neck cancer at risk for second primary cancer. *Journal of the American Dietetic Association, 105,* 1609–1612. doi:10.1016/j.jada.2005.07.009

Ferlito, A., Shaha, A.R., Silver, C.E., Rinaldo, A., & Mondin, V. (2001). Incidence and sites of distant metastases from head and neck cancer. *ORL: Journal for Oto-Rhino-Laryngology and Its Related Specialties, 63,* 202–207. doi:10.1159/000055740

Fischer, D.J., & Epstein, J.B. (2008). Management of patients who have undergone head and neck cancer therapy. *Dental Clinics of North America, 52,* 39–60. doi:10.1016/j.oden.2007.09.004

Freemantle, S.J., Dragnev, K.H., & Dmitrovsky, E. (2006). The retinoic acid paradox in cancer prevention. *Journal of the National Cancer Institute, 98,* 426–427. doi:10.1093/jnci/djj116

González-García, R., Naval-Gías, L., Román-Romero, L., Sastre-Pérez, J., & Rodríguez-Campo, F.J. (2009). Local recurrences and second primary tumors from squamous cell carcinoma of the oral cavity: A retrospective analytic study of 500 patients. *Head and Neck, 31,* 1168–1180. doi:10.1002/hed.21088

Griffiths, M.J., Humphris, G.M., Skirrow, P.M., & Rogers, S.N. (2008). A qualitative evaluation of patient experiences when diagnosed with oral cancer recurrence. *Cancer Nursing, 31*(4), E11–E17. doi:10.1097/01.NCC.0000305750.50991.67

Hodges, L.J., & Humphris, G.M. (2009). Fear of recurrence and psychological distress in head and neck cancer patients and their carers. *Psycho-Oncology, 18,* 841–848. doi:10.1002/pon.1346

Humphris, G.M., & Rogers, S.N. (2004). The association of cigarette smoking and anxiety, depression and fears of recurrence in patients following treatment of oral and oropharyngeal malignancy. *European Journal of Cancer Care, 13,* 328–335. doi:10.1111/j.1365-2354.2004.00479.x

Humphris, G.M., Rogers, S., McNally, D., Lee-Jones, C., Brown, J., & Vaughan, D. (2003). Fear of recurrence and possible cases of anxiety and depression in orofacial cancer patients. *International Journal of Oral and Maxillofacial Surgery, 32,* 486–491.

Jemal, A., Siegel, R., Xu, J., & Ward, E. (2010). Cancer statistics, 2010. *CA: A Cancer Journal for Clinicians, 60*, 277–300. doi:10.3322/caac.20073

Jones, A.S., Morar, P., Phillips, D.E., Field, J.K., Husband, D., & Helliwell, T.R. (1995). Second primary tumors in patients with head and neck squamous cell carcinoma. *Cancer, 75*, 1343–1353.

Kapoor, S. (2008). Chemoprevention of head and neck cancers: Promising new biochemical prospects. *Journal of Clinical Oncology, 26*, 2417–2418. doi:10.1200/JCO.2008.16.3584

Khuri, F.R., Kim, E.S., Lee, J.J., Winn, R.J., Benner, S.E., Lippman, S.M., ... Hong, W.K. (2001). The impact of smoking status, disease stage, and index tumor site on second primary tumor incidence and tumor recurrence in the Head and Neck Retinoid Chemoprevention Trial. *Cancer Epidemiology, Biomarkers and Prevention, 10*, 823–829.

Khuri, F.R., Lee, J.J., Lippman, S.M., Kim, E.S., Cooper, J.S., Benner, S.E., ... Hong, W.K. (2006). Randomized phase III trial of low-dose isotretinoin for prevention of second primary tumors in stage I and II head and neck cancer patients. *Journal of the National Cancer Institute, 98*, 441–450. doi:10.1093/jnci/djj091

Khuri, F.R., & Shin, D.M. (2008). Head and neck cancer chemoprevention gets a shot in the arm. *Journal of Clinical Oncology, 26*, 345–347. doi:10.1200/JCO.2007.14.0913

Kos, M., Łuczak, K., Brusco, D., & Engelke, W. (2008). Impact of tumour characteristic and treatment modality on the local recurrence and the survival in patients with oral squamous cell carcinoma. *Otolaryngologia Polska: The Polish Otolaryngology, 62*, 722–726.

Kotwall, C., Sako, K., Razack, M.S., Rao, U., Bakamjian, V., & Shedd, D.P. (1987). Metastatic patterns in squamous cell cancer of the head and neck. *American Journal of Surgery, 154*, 439–442. doi:10.1016/0002-9610(89)90020-2

Kurtin, S.E. (2009). Systemic therapies for squamous cell carcinoma of the head and neck. *Seminars in Oncology Nursing, 25*, 183–192. doi:10.1016/j.soncn.2009.05.001

Lin, K., Patel, S.G., Chu, P.Y., Matsuo, J.M.S., Singh, B., Wong, R.J., ... Boyle, J.O. (2005). Second primary malignancy of the aerodigestive tract in patients treated for cancer of the oral cavity and larynx. *Head and Neck, 27*, 1042–1048. doi:10.1002/hed.20272

Mahon, S.M., & Casperson, D.M. (1997). Exploring the psychosocial meaning of recurrent cancer: A descriptive study. *Cancer Nursing, 20*, 178–186.

Marur, S., & Forastiere, A.A. (2008). Head and neck cancer: Changing epidemiology, diagnosis, and treatment. *Mayo Clinic Proceedings, 83*, 489–501. doi:10.4065/83.4.489

National Comprehensive Cancer Network. (2010, July 7). *NCCN Clinical Practice Guidelines in Oncology™: Head and neck cancers* [v.2.2010]. Retrieved from http://www.nccn.org/professionals/physician_gls/PDF/head-and-neck.pdf

Perry, C.F., Stevens, M., Rabie, I., Yarker, M.E., Cochrane, J., Perry, E., ... Coman, W. (2005). Chemoprevention of head and neck cancer with retinoids: A negative result. *Archives of Otolaryngology—Head and Neck Surgery, 131*, 198–203.

Rennemo, E., Zätterström, U., & Boysen, M. (2008). Impact of second primary tumors on survival in head and neck cancer: An analysis of 2,063 cases. *Laryngoscope, 118*, 1350–1356. doi:10.1097/MLG.0b013e318172ef9a

Rosenquist, K., Wennerberg, J., Annertz, K., Schildt, E.-B., Hansson, B.G., Bladström, A., & Andersson, G. (2007). Recurrence in patients with oral and oropharyngeal squamous cell carcinoma: Human papillomavirus and other risk factors. *Acta Oto-Laryngologica, 127*, 980–987. doi:10.1080/00016480601110162

Taioli, E., Ragin, C., Wang, X.H., Chen, J., Langevin, S.M., Brown, A.R., ... Sobol, R.W. (2009). Recurrence in oral and pharyngeal cancer is associated with quantitative MGMT promoter methylation. *BMC Cancer, 9*, 354. doi:10.1186/1471-2407-9-354

van der Haring, I.S., Schaapveld, M.S., Roodenburg, J.L., & de Bock, G.H. (2009). Second primary tumours after a squamous cell carcinoma of the oral cavity or oropharynx using the cumulative incidence method. *International Journal of Oral and Maxillofacial Surgery, 38*, 332–338. doi:10.1016/j.ijom.2008.12.015

Wong, S.J., Machtay, M., & Li, Y. (2006). Locally recurrent, previously irradiated head and neck cancer: Concurrent re-irradiation and chemotherapy, or chemotherapy alone? *Journal of Clinical Oncology, 24*, 2653–2658. doi:10.1200/JCO.2005.05.3850

Zhang, Z.-F., Morgenstern, H., Spitz, M.R., Tashkin, D.P., Yu, G-P., Hsu, T.C. & Schantz, S.P. (2000). Environmental tobacco smoking, mutagen sensitivity, and head and neck squamous cell carcinoma. *Cancer Epidemiology, Biomarkers and Prevention, 9,* 1043–1049.

CHAPTER 17

Oral Health Across the Continuum of Care: A Symptom Cluster Model

Patricia C. Buchsel, MSN, RN, OCN®, FAAN

Introduction

Oral health problems that occur across the continuum of care for patients with cancer and those treated with cancer therapies such as chemotherapy and radiation are now acknowledged as a serious concern that affect patients from the time of diagnosis to long-term care and beyond. It was not until the late 1980s that the term *oral mucositis* was described as a condition that caused chemotherapy- and radiotherapy-induced inflammation (Peterson, 1999). It has only been in recent years that cancer treatment has caused numerous other acute and long-term oral complications. The authors in this book have already addressed what is currently known concerning the clinical presentation, incidence, and economic implications in the management of the oral sequelae of cancer and its treatment.

This chapter has three purposes. The first is to present a brief summation of major advances in the management of oral complications that have significantly contributed to decreasing the debilitating consequences of oral complications. The second is to present the advantages of a symptom management model using the theory of symptom clusters. Finally, a case study is presented to illustrate an evidence-based approach to the symptom management of oral complications. The case study will focus on an unrelated stem cell transplant recipient, highlighting oral complications. Although this case study is taken from the hematopoietic stem cell transplantation (HSCT) setting, patients with head and neck cancers receiving highly toxic treatment regimens may manifest similar oral complications, with the exception of graft-versus-host disease (GVHD).

Major Advances in Treatment of Oral Problems in Cancer Treatments

It is well known that the oral cavity is a target area for complications occurring in patients whose disease is treated with high-dose chemotherapy or irradiation. The major complication is oral mucositis (Sonis, 2007). Accordingly, the majority of the literature about oral health in patients with cancer has centered on the toxic chemotherapy- and radiation-induced mucositis. More than 400,000 patients per year are affected by this painful and debilitating condition during cancer treatment (Posner & Haddard, 2007). The extent of mucositis and its sequelae can become a dose-limiting toxicity that leads to decreased doses or interruptions in treatment, placing the patient at risk for continued tumor burden (Keefe et al., 2007). The clinical, functional, and psychological consequences have been described extensively in the literature and earlier in this book (Berendt & D'Agostino, 2005; Eilers, 2004; Elting et al., 2003).

Pain is the cardinal clinical manifestation of oral mucositis and often requires the use of opioids (Sonis, 2007). Common sequelae are loss of critical functions such as eating, swallowing, and talking, while psychological complications include anger, depression, and poor quality of life (Dodd, Miaskowski, & Lee, 2004; Epstein et al., 1999; Murphy, 2007). However, it is interesting to note that Murphy (2007) suggested that attributing a decrease in the quality of life to a group of symptoms is difficult because symptom data generally are not powerful enough factors to influence overall quality of life.

The past decade has brought new understanding of the pathobiology and the clinical and economic consequences of oral mucositis, but prevention of this worrisome problem has eluded researchers (Sonis, 2007). A major exception is palifermin, which became the first agent that was approved by the U.S. Food and Drug Administration for the prevention of oral mucositis in the autologous HSCT population (National Cancer Institute [NCI], 2009a; Spielberger et al., 2004). Currently, based on a search by topic of the National Institutes of Health Web site clinicaltrials.gov, more than 50 clinical trials have been completed or are active on the effectiveness of the use of palifermin in the HCST setting. With future research, palifermin may be available to patients such as those with head and neck cancers receiving highly toxic treatment regimens, who are at equally high risk for oral mucositis.

Until such time that oral mucositis can be prevented or significantly diminished, robust research is needed. Pretreatment assessments by medical and dental healthcare providers, recognition of the timing and clinical manifestations of symptoms and their management, and patient and family education continue to be the mainstays of oral mucositis management.

Clinical and Functional Impairments

Numerous undesirable functional effects can arise from treatment regimens that contain high-dose cancer therapy (McGowan, 2008). These clinical consequences of cancer treatment are known to lead to a less than desirable quality of life (Epstein & Barasch, 2010; Epstein & Chow, 1999). Oral complications, such as taste alteration, odor, and smell, have only recently come to the attention of researchers. Most alterations are underdiagnosed and undertreated, causing significant barriers to optimal oral health. Hong et al. (2009), in a review article, summarized the common taste and odor disorders endured by patients treated with chemotherapy and irradiation. The investigators reviewed substantive studies to provide a clearer understanding of taste and odor dysfunction, which, left untreated, can lead to significant morbidity and mortality. Importantly, the review incorporated management strategies to improve taste and odor abnormalities. In a separate article, Halyard (2009) suggested that perhaps nutrition consultations before, during, and after treatment are paramount to avoid anorexia and subsequent weight loss. As more research emerges on the onset, characteristics, incidence, and severity of these subtle but significant oral complications, greater is the need to prevent, anticipate, and decrease their effects to improve quality of life in patients so afflicted (Elade, Epstein, Meyerowitz, Peterson, & Schubert, 2005; Epstein & Chow, 1999).

Prevention and Early Detection of Oral Complications

Perhaps the greatest strides made in the past decade have occurred in the prevention and early pretreatment recognition of periodontal disease and dental caries and in the management of oral complications in patients with cancer and those treated with highly toxic regimens. In the past, oral complications of therapy were tolerated as inevitable and treated only when they appeared (Sonis, 2000). However, pretreatment dental assessments, screening, and treatment prior to therapy can identify risks that herald serious problems that arise during treatment (Barker & Barker, 2001). Dental and medical teams working with patients at risk for oral complications have contributed to the increased awareness of the early dental problems that may place the patient at risk for oral complications. Pretreatment examinations are critical in preventing or diminishing the severity, intensity, and duration of problems and in ensuring that sources of dental infection and trauma can be eliminated (Stevens, 2004). The Multinational Association of Supportive Care in Cancer (MASCC), the International Society for Oral Oncology, and the National Comprehensive Cancer Network have made recommendations for those receiving high-dose chemotherapy agents to receive a complete dental consultation prior to treatment (Keefe et al., 2007; MASCC/International Society for Oral Oncology, 2005).

Multidisciplinary research among professional organizations has advanced the knowledge of oral complications. Two international organizations have contributed to the understanding of a variety of oral complications. The formation of the Oral Care Study Group of the MASCC Study Group has led to international efforts to enhance the knowledge and clinical management of the wide range of oral complications from cancer and its therapies. The objectives of the group are to understand the clinical impact of oral complications, such as xerostomia, dysgeusia, dysphagia, oral pain, fungal infection, viral infection, osteoradionecrosis, osteonecrosis from bisphosphonates, dental disease, and trismus, and to develop and coordinate new evidence-based management guidelines. For example, revised guidelines put forth by this group include the use of a soft-bristle toothbrush with regular flossing, rinsing, and moistening (see Table 17-1). Further areas of interest include conducting multiple systematic reviews of the incidence, prevalence, management guidelines, quality of life, and economic impact of oral complications from cancer therapy.

Prevention and early detection of long-term oral complications are essential to the overall success of treatment (Barker & Barker, 2001; Buchsel, 2009). Often, patients are referred home to a primary healthcare team who are unaware of potential adverse effects in the oral cavity. Secondary cancers of the head and neck can appear, and long-term survivors of HSCT for childhood cancers have demonstrated craniofacial growth abnormalities that require the expertise of dental medicine teams familiar with people who have undergone HSCT (Majorana, Schubert, Porta, Ugazio, & Sapelli, 2000). It is critical that patients are referred to long-term clinics or have access to the facilities where they received their treatment (Buchsel, Leum, & Randolph, 1996).

Oral Care Protocols

The importance of patient and family education cannot be overstated (Daniel, Damato, & Johnson, 2004). Numerous misunderstandings and myths about the components of oral care protocols have been dismissed over the past few years. The era of evidence-based practice to prevent or diminish the consequences of oral problems has guided practitioners in managing painful and debilitating sequelae that accompany cancer and its therapies (Harris, Eilers, Harriman, Cashavelly, & Maxwell, 2008; Potting et al., 2009). Guidelines from MASCC (2005) and NCI have given clear directions on best practices that include evidence-based care for the management of oral complications (NCI, 2009b).

Table 17-1. Summary of Evidence-Based Clinical Practice Guidelines for Care of Patients with Oral and Gastrointestinal Mucositis (2005 Update)

Previous Guideline	Updated or New Guideline
ORAL MUCOSITIS	

Foundations of Care

The panel suggests that oral care protocols that include patient education be used to attempt to reduce the severity of mucositis from chemotherapy or radiation therapy.	The panel suggests multidisciplinary development and evaluation of oral care protocols, and patient and staff education in the use of such protocols to reduce the severity of oral mucositis from chemotherapy and/or radiation therapy. As part of the protocols, the panel suggests the use of a soft toothbrush that is replaced on a regular basis. Elements of good clinical practice should include the use of validated tools to regularly assess oral pain and oral cavity health. The inclusion of dental professionals is vital throughout the treatment and follow-up phases.
The panel recommends patient-controlled analgesia with morphine as the treatment of choice for oral mucositis pain in patients undergoing hematopoietic stem cell transplantation (HSCT).	The panel recommends patient-controlled analgesia with morphine as the treatment of choice for oral mucositis pain in patients undergoing HSCT. Regular oral pain assessment using validated instruments for self-reporting is essential.

Radiation Therapy—Prevention

None	The panel recommends that sucralfate not be used for the prevention of radiation-induced oral mucositis.
None	The panel recommends that antimicrobial lozenges not be used for the prevention of radiation-induced oral mucositis.
The panel recommends the use of midline radiation blocks and three-dimensional radiation treatment to reduce mucosal injury.	No change
The panel recommends benzydamine for prevention of radiation-induced mucositis in patients with head and neck cancer receiving moderate-dose radiation therapy.	No change
The panel recommends that chlorhexidine not be used to prevent oral mucositis in patients with solid tumors of the head and neck who are undergoing radiotherapy.	No change

(Continued on next page)

Table 17-1. Summary of Evidence-Based Clinical Practice Guidelines for Care of Patients with Oral and Gastrointestinal Mucositis (2005 Update) *(Continued)*

Previous Guideline	Updated or New Guideline
Standard-Dose Chemotherapy—Prevention	
The panel recommends that patients receiving bolus 5-fluorouracil (5-FU) chemotherapy undergo 30 minutes of oral cryotherapy to prevent oral mucositis. The panel suggests that 20–30 minutes of oral cryotherapy be used to attempt to decrease mucositis in patients treated with bolus doses of edatrexate.	No change
The panel recommends that acyclovir and its analogues not be used routinely to prevent mucositis.	No change
Standard-Dose Chemotherapy—Treatment	
The panel recommends that chlorhexidine not be used to treat established oral mucositis.	No change
High-Dose Chemotherapy With or Without Total Body Irradiation Plus Hematopoietic Cell Transplantation—Prevention	
None	In patients with hematological malignancies receiving high-dose chemotherapy and total body irradiation with autologous stem cell transplant, the panel recommends the use of keratinocyte growth factor-1 (Palifermin) in a dose of 60 µg/kg/day for 3 days prior to conditioning treatment and for 3 days post-transplant for the prevention of oral mucositis.
None	The panel suggests the use of cryotherapy to prevent oral mucositis in patients receiving high-dose melphalan.
The panel does not recommend the use of pentoxifylline to prevent mucositis in patients undergoing HSCT.	No change
None	The panel suggests that granulocyte macrophage–colony-stimulating factor mouthwashes not be used for the prevention of oral mucositis in patients undergoing HSCT.

(Continued on next page)

Table 17-1. Summary of Evidence-Based Clinical Practice Guidelines for Care of Patients with Oral and Gastrointestinal Mucositis (2005 Update) *(Continued)*

Previous Guideline	Updated or New Guideline
High-Dose Chemotherapy With or Without Total Body Irradiation Plus Hematopoietic Cell Transplantation—Prevention *(Cont.)*	
Low-level laser therapy (LLLT) requires expensive equipment and specialized training. Because of interoperator variability, clinical trials are difficult to conduct, and their results are difficult to compare; nevertheless, the panel is encouraged by the accumulating evidence in support of LLLT. The panel suggests that, for centers able to support the necessary technology and training, LLLT be used to attempt to reduce the incidence of oral mucositis and its associated pain in patients receiving high-dose chemotherapy or chemoradiotherapy before HSCT.	No change
GASTROINTESTINAL MUCOSITIS	
Basic Bowel Care and Good Clinical Practices	
None	The panel suggests that basic bowel care should include the maintenance of adequate hydration, and that consideration should be given to the potential for transient lactose intolerance and the presence of bacterial pathogens.
Radiation Therapy—Prevention	
None	It is suggested that amifostine in a dose of at least 340 mg/m^2 may prevent radiation proctitis in those receiving standard-dose radiation therapy for rectal cancer.
The panel suggests that 500 mg sulfasalazine orally twice daily be used to help reduce the incidence and severity of radiation-induced enteropathy in patients receiving external beam radiotherapy to the pelvis.	No change
Oral sucralfate does not prevent acute diarrhea in patients with pelvic malignancies undergoing external beam radiotherapy, and compared with placebo it is associated with more gastrointestinal side effects, including rectal bleeding; consequently, the panel recommends that oral sucralfate not be used.	No change

(Continued on next page)

Table 17-1. Summary of Evidence-Based Clinical Practice Guidelines for Care of Patients with Oral and Gastrointestinal Mucositis (2005 Update) *(Continued)*

Previous Guideline	Updated or New Guideline
Radiation Therapy—Prevention *(Cont.)*	
The panel recommends that 5-amino salicylic acid and its related compounds mesalazine and olsalazine not be used to prevent gastrointestinal mucositis.	No change
Radiation Therapy—Treatment	
The panel suggests that sucralfate enemas be used to help manage chronic radiation-induced proctitis in patients who have rectal bleeding.	No change
Standard-Dose and High-Dose Chemotherapy—Prevention	
The panel recommends either ranitidine or omeprazole for the prevention of epigastric pain following treatment with cyclophosphamide, methotrexate, and 5-FU or treatment with 5-FU with or without folinic acid chemotherapy.	No change
None	The panel recommends that systemic glutamine not be used for the prevention of gastrointestinal mucositis.
Standard-Dose and High-Dose Chemotherapy—Treatment	
When loperamide fails to control diarrhea induced by standard-dose or high-dose chemotherapy associated with HSCT, the panel recommends octreotide at a dose of at least 100 μg subcutaneously twice daily.	No change
Combined Chemotherapy and Radiation Therapy—Prevention	
The panel suggests that amifostine be used to reduce esophagitis induced by concomitant chemotherapy and radiotherapy in patients with non–small cell lung cancer.	No change

Note. From Multinational Association of Supportive Care in Cancer/International Society for Oral Oncology (MASCC/ISOO) Guidelines and Assessment Tools. Retrieved from http://data.memberclicks. com/site/mascc/Guidelines_mucositis.pdf. Copyright 2005 by Multinational Association of Supportive Care in Cancer. Reprinted with permission.

Symptom Clusters

The ultimate goal of cancer therapy is to cure the patient. In that trajectory toward cure, patients endure multiple symptoms that dramatically affect their quality of life. Because cure is not always possible, robust and evidence-based management of various symptoms is mandated. Recognition of the onset, duration, and intensity of symptoms is a major step in supporting patients through their treatments.

The past decade has seen important research recognizing that a group or cluster of symptoms most often accompanies cancer and its treatment (Barsevick, 2007; Barsevick, Whitmer, Nail, Beck, & Dudley, 2006; Dodd et al., 1996; Miaskowski et al., 2006). Early work by a number of research scientists has led to the concept of "symptom clusters." Symptom clusters are defined as two or more concurrent symptoms that are related to one another but are not necessarily of the same etiology (Dodd, Miaskowski, & Paul, 2001; Miaskowski, Dodd, & Lee, 2004). One query of great interest to these researchers was that if symptom clusters could be identified, could the cluster perhaps indicate possible morbidity? For example, conditions such as ulcerative lesions, bleeding, and pain lead to difficulty in eating, weight loss, speech problems, depression, and decreased quality of life (Miaskowski et al., 2004).

Research by Borbasi et al. (2002) indicated that patients with oral mucositis reported, "I'd say mucositis was the worst thing that happened" and having oral and gastric discomfort described as "the burn of caustic soda" and "the slice of razor blades" (p. 1054). These comments underscore the title of the research article, "More Than a Sore Mouth." A multicenter study by So et al. (2009) studied 215 women treated for breast cancer and identified a symptom cluster of anxiety, fatigue, depression, and pain. Honea, Brant, and Beck (2007) found that patients who received radiotherapy to the head and neck region shared the common experiences of dry mouth and difficulty in swallowing that triggers nighttime awakening. Other investigators have studied the validity of using several symptom symptom assessment tools. Henoch, Ploner, and Tishelman (2009) studied symptom clusters among a homogenous group of patients (N = 145) with inoperable lung cancer. The investigators found three symptom clusters: a pain cluster, a mood cluster, and a respiratory cluster. Of particular interest in this study is that the researchers used different instruments and analytical methods to test the validity of the measures. As more research is conducted in the symptom cluster model, it will be important to identify the timing of symptom measures and the results of symptom interventions. As the growth of outpatient care continues and with patients living far from research centers, reliable patient self-report symptom measures will be imperative to identify specific symptom clusters relative to clinical conditions (Dodd et al., 2004). A rich source of inquiry would be in the long-term effects of oral complications in patients who have received high-dose antineoplastic agents for their treatment.

Case Study in an Allogeneic Hematologic Stem Cell Transplant Recipient

HSCT is a long process complicated by profound immunosuppression, life-threatening infections, and insults to every body system. The purpose of this case study is to present an exemplar of the effects of this treatment on the oral cavity and its sequelae.

Patient Jones is a 12-year-old girl diagnosed with acute lymphocytic leukemia in second relapse. She arrives at a medical center in the northwest United States for an unrelated allogeneic HSCT. Her pretreatment evaluation includes examinations by the transplantation oncologist, radiation oncologist, dietary staff, and dental staff to ensure that she will sustain minimal complications. Although the acute and chronic complications are well known, an integrated team approach throughout the HSCT process is optimal to reduce pretransplantation conditions that can be prevented.

The dental medicine team notes that the patient has upper and lower orthodontic braces. Two dental caries are revealed as well. The dental caries are treated, and the patient and her mother are advised that the dental appliances need to be removed because of the risk for mechanical trauma, secondary infections, and radiation scatter. Although disappointed to have two years of orthodontic work interrupted, the patient is assured that once her immune system is stable after the HCST, the orthodontic treatment can be resumed.

Two weeks later, the patient is admitted for high-dose cyclophosphamide and total body irradiation. Patient and family teaching include the need for extensive and vigorous oral care to remove oral debris and microorganisms, provide mucosal hydration, and decrease oral pain that will occur with xerostomia, oral mucositis, and oral infections. The transplantation team reassures the patient that she will have 24-hour intensive supportive care. As anticipated, on day 8 she is profoundly immunosuppressed but is supported with blood products, antimicrobials, total parenteral nutrition, and psychological support. Her complete blood count (CBC) shows a white blood cell count of $900/mm^3$, hemoglobin 7.5 g/dl, and platelet count of $75,000/mm^3$. On day 10, she complains of xerostomia and a burning sensation in the oral cavity. On examination, mild mucosal edema, erythema, and pseudomembrane formation is noted. On day 12, further examination by the dental team reports that the patient has worsening mucosal edema and erythema, ulceration, and slight oral hemorrhage, and the patient complains of severe oral pain. The dental medicine team, using the NCI Cancer Therapy Evaluation Program's (2009) Common Terminology Criteria for Adverse Events oral mucositis grading scale, determines that she has grade 3 mucositis (see Table 17-2). The patient is supported by the nursing staff and her mother in vigorous mouth care, especially in the use of cryotherapy. The patient finds the most relief from the use of ice chips.

Table 17-2. Oral Mucositis Grading Scale	
Grade	Description
1	Asymptomatic or mild symptoms; intervention not indicated
2	Moderate pain; not interfering with oral intake; modified diet indicated
3	Severe pain; interfering with oral intake
4	Life-threatening consequences; urgent intervention indicated
5	Death

Note. From *Common Terminology Criteria for Adverse Events* [v.4.0], by National Cancer Institute Cancer Therapy Evaluation Program, 2009. Retrieved from http://evs.nci.nih.gov/ftp1/CTCAE/CTCAE_4.03_2010-06-14_QuickReference_5x7.pdf.

Additionally, the dental team is concerned that dry, raised, yellowish-brown plaques are present on the buccal mucosa, which upon culture show a gram-positive staphylococcal infection. The patient is started on appropriate systemic antibiotics. She requires parenteral opioids and is unable to eat. Her weight is decreased by five pounds; she is started on total parenteral nutrition. She has increasing episodes of diarrhea.

Her body develops a maculopapular rash and erythroderma with desquamation, and her liver function levels rise. She is diagnosed with acute GVHD (see Table 17-3), and her immunosuppressive medications of methotrexate in combination with cyclosporine are increased in dosage. She reports to the nursing staff that she is extremely fatigued and cannot eat or drink, swallow, or talk. She tells her mother that she hates being ugly and does not want any of her friends to visit her.

Although challenged with this profound medical picture, the patient endures and understands that soon she will progress into the healing part of her therapy. The encouraging news is that her day 7, 12, and 21 bone marrow aspiration and biopsy examinations determine that she has engraftment and remission. On day 28 after HSCT, the patient's CBC shows a white blood cell count of $2,100/mm^3$, hemoglobin of 12.2 g/dl, and platelets at $125,000/mm^3$. She is free of infections, the marrow aspiration and biopsies show her disease to be in remission and established engraftment, and the oral mucositis has resolved. On day 35, her symptoms were such that she is discharged to the outpatient clinic until her 100-day evaluation by the referring oncologist.

Her outpatient course is unremarkable, and she and her mother look forward to returning home. A 100-day evaluation is performed to determine the patient's clinical course. A lip biopsy reveals that she has chronic GVHD of the mouth and skin. Although the patient was placed on a prophylactic GVHD regimen, she now continues on a chronic GVHD treatment with alternating cyclosporine and prednisone. Even though xerostomia is the only presenting symptom on biopsy, the patient is educated about the consequences of chronic GVHD symptoms of pain, weight loss, and dental caries, caused by the lack of salivary IgA (immunoglobulin A). The dental team advises close follow-up with a dentist familiar with the treatment of patients who have undergone chemotherapy and irradiation for cancer. Often, radiation-induced xerostomia mimics candidiasis in the presence of chronic GVHD of the mouth. If left untreated, the patient is at risk for worsening chronic GVHD. She is also made aware that her future dental examinations must include surveillance for oral cancer because of the high-dose therapy she has received.

Table 17-3. Clinical Staging and Grading of Acute Graft-Versus-Host Disease		
Staging by Organ		
Organ	Stage	Parameters
Rash		
Skin	I	< 25% BSA
	II	25%–50% BSA
	III	Generalized erythroderma
	IV	Bullae and desquamation
Total Bilirubin (mg/dl)		
Liver	I	2–3.5
	II	3.5–8
	III	8–15
	IV	> 15
Volume of Diarrhea (ml/24 hr)		
Gut	I	Adult: 500–1,000 ml/day Pediatric: 10–15 ml/kg/day
	II	Adult: 1,000–1500 ml/day Pediatric: 15–20 ml/kg/day
	III	Adult: 1,500–2000 ml/day Pediatric: 20–30 ml/kg/day
	IV	Adult: > 2,000 ml/day Pediatric: > 30 ml/kg/day

(Continued on next page)

**Table 17-3. Clinical Staging and Grading of
Acute Graft-Versus-Host Disease *(Continued)***

Overall Clinical Grade	
Grade	Description
0	Stage I clinical skin GVHD
I	Stage II clinical skin GVHD
II	Stage II–III clinical skin GVHD and stage II–IV clinical liver and/or gut GVHD; only one system stage III or greater
III	Stage II–IV clinical skin GVHD (with grade 2 or higher histology) and stage II–IV clinical liver and and/or gut GVHD; only one system stage III or greater
IV	Stage II–IV clinical skin GVHD (with grade 2 or higher histology) and stage II–IV clinical liver and/or gut GVHD; two or more systems stage III or higher

BSA—body surface area; GVHD—graft-versus-host disease

Note. Based on information from Chao, 1999; Ferrara & Antin, 1999; Kapustay & Buchsel, 2000; Shapiro et al., 1997.

From "Nursing Implications of Hematopoietic Stem Cell Transplantation," by T.W. Shapiro in J.K. Itano and K.N. Taoka (Eds.), *Core Curriculum for Oncology Nursing* (4th ed., p. 824). Copyright 2005 by Elsevier. Reprinted with permission.

The patient returns to the transplantation center for her annual follow-up examination. When asked about her experiences during HSCT, she reports that oral mucositis was the most painful experience she endured and that scrupulous mouth care was difficult. Although the experience was painful, she attributes her endurance through this treatment to the transplantation team, who managed her symptoms in a manner she could sustain. She remains in remission, her chronic GVHD medication tapers have been successful, and she is doing well in high school.

As illustrated in this case study, insults to the oral cavity subsequent to high-dose therapy are the cause of significant morbidity. The patient's experience is not unique but is mirrored in anecdotal patient reports and in a vast amount of publications. Preventive approaches were exercised to diminish the possible complications stemming from trauma to the oral cavity; this is paramount to successful HSCT. During treatment, despite the use of aggressive supportive care, the patient experienced the commonly reported symptom cluster associated with oral mucositis. The conditions of oral mucositis, oral infections, and acute GVHD created a spiraling symptom burden of nausea, vomiting, diarrhea, fatigue, pain, infection, and depression.

Conclusion

Oral complications of high-dose chemotherapy and irradiation can cause considerable morbidity and mortality. Those most susceptible to severe problems are patients receiving radiation for head and neck cancers and recipients of HSCT. These therapies may disrupt the integrity of the oral mucosa, creating an open portal for bacteria, fungus, and viruses to become a systemic problem. Symptom clusters of pain; depression; loss of functional activities of eating, swallowing, and talking; fatigue; and poor self-image have been reported extensively in the literature. The long-term effects of these therapies are underreported.

Significant strides have been made in new knowledge of the complexity of oral complications. Pretreatment consultations by medical dental teams are known to decrease the occurrence and consequences of oral infections, dental trauma, and dental caries. Evidence-based mouth care protocols have emerged to promote excellence in oral care (Shih, Miaskowski, Dodd, Stotts, & MacPhail, 2002). The complex pathophysiology of mucositis has resulted in identification of products that, when used in concert during the various phases of mucositis, can decrease its intensity (Keefe et al., 2007). Research in a new model of symptom management called *symptom clusters* is emerging not only for oral complications but also for other areas of cancer treatment. Vigorous research continues to prevent or diminish the occurrence, intensity, and duration of problems that greatly affect the quality of life of patients and their families. The close collaboration of an interdisciplinary team consisting of oncologists, oral medicine dentists, oncology nurses, dental hygienists, pharmacists, dietitians, and patients and their families is essential to supporting patients through the journey of treatment.

References

Barker, B.F., & Barker, G.J. (2001). Oral management of the patient with cancer in the head and neck region. *Journal of the California Dental Association, 29,* 619–623.

Barsevick, A.M. (2007). Introduction. *Seminars in Oncology Nursing, 23,* 87–88. doi:10.1016/j.soncn.2007.01.010

Barsevick, A., Whitmer, K., Nail, L., Beck, S., & Dudley, N. (2006). Symptom clusters: Research, conceptual design, measurement and analysis. *Journal of Pain and Symptom Management, 31,* 85–95. doi:10.1016/j.jpainsymman.2005.05.015

Berendt, M., & D'Agostino, S. (2005). Alterations in nutrition. In J.K. Itano & K.N. Taoka (Eds.), *Core curriculum for oncology nursing* (4th ed., pp. 277–317). St. Louis, MO: Elsevier Saunders.

Borbasi, S., Cameron, K., Quested, B., Olver, I., To, B., & Evans, D. (2002). More than a sore mouth: Patients' experience of oral mucositis. *Oncology Nursing Forum, 29,* 1051–1057. doi:10.1188/02.ONF.1051–1057

Buchsel, P.C. (2009). Survivorship issues in hematopoietic stem cell transplantation. *Seminars in Oncology Nursing, 25,* 159–169. doi:10.1016/j.soncn.2009.03.003

Buchsel, P.C., Leum, E.W., & Randolph, S.R. (1996). Delayed complications of bone marrow transplantation: An update. *Oncology Nursing Forum, 23,* 1267–1291.

Chao, N. (Ed.). (1999). *Graft versus host disease.* Austin, TX: R.G. Landis Co.

Daniel, B.T., Damato, K.L., & Johnson, J. (2004). Educational issues in oral care. *Seminars in Oncology Nursing, 20,* 48–52.

Dodd, M., Dibble, S., Miaskowski, C., Paul, S., Cho, M., MacPhail, L., & Greenspan, D.L. (1996). Comparison of the affected state and quality of life of chemotherapy patients who do and do not develop chemotherapy induced oral mucositis. *Journal of Pain and Symptom Management, 21,* 498–505.

Dodd, M.J., Miaskowski, C., & Lee, K.A. (2004). Occurrence of symptom clusters. *Journal of the National Cancer Institute Monographs, 2004*(32), 76–78. doi:10.1093/jncimonographs/lgh008

Dodd, M.J., Miaskowski, C., & Paul, S.M. (2001). Symptom clusters and their effect on the functional status of patients with cancer. *Oncology Nursing Forum, 28,* 465–470.

Elade, S., Epstein J., Meyerowitz, C., Peterson, D., & Schubert, M. (2005). Oral and dental management for cancer patients. In P.C. Buchsel & C.H. Yarbro (Eds.), *Oncology nursing in the ambulatory care setting: Issues and models of care* (2nd ed., pp. 279–301). Sudbury, MA: Jones and Bartlett.

Eilers, J. (2004). Nursing interventions and supportive care for the prevention of and treatment of oral mucositis associated with cancer treatment. *Oncology Nursing Forum, 31*(Suppl. 4), 13–23. 10.1188/04.ONF.S4.13-23

Elting, L.S., Cooksley, C., Chambers, M., Cantor, S.B., Manzullo, E., & Rubinstein, E.B. (2003). The burdens of cancer therapy: Clinical and economic outcomes of chemotherapy-induced mucositis. *Cancer, 98,* 1531–1539. doi:10.1002/cncr.11671

Epstein, J.B., & Barasch, A. (2010). Taste disorders in cancer patients: Pathogenesis, and approach to assessment and management. *Oral Oncology, 46,* 77–81. doi:10.1016/j.oraloncology.2009.11.008

Epstein, J.B., & Chow, A.W. (1999). Oral complications associated with immunosuppression and cancer therapies. *Infectious Disease Clinics of North America, 13,* 901–923. doi:10.1016/S0891-5520(05)70115-X

Epstein, J.B., Emerton, S., Kolbinson, D.A., Le, N.D., Phillips, N., Stevenson-Moore, P., & Osoba, D. (1999). Quality of life and oral function following radiotherapy for head and neck cancer. *Head and Neck, 21,* 1–11. doi:10.1002/(SICI)1097-0347(199901)21:1<1::AID-HED1>3.0.CO;2-4

Ferrara, J.L.M., & Antin, J.H. (1999). The pathophysiology of graft versus host disease. In E.D. Thomas, K.G. Blume, & S.J. Forman (Eds.), *Hematopoietic cell transplantation* (2nd ed., pp. 305–315). Malden, MA: Blackwell Science.

Halyard, M.Y. (2009). Taste and smell alterations in cancer patients—Real problems with few solutions. *Journal of Supportive Oncology, 7,* 68–69.

Harris, D.J., Eilers, J., Harriman, A., Cashavelly, B.J., & Maxwell, C. (2008). Putting evidence into practice: Evidence-based interventions for the management of oral mucositis. *Clinical Journal of Oncology Nursing, 12,* 141–152. doi:10.1188/08.CJON.141-152

Henoch, I., Ploner, A., & Tishelman, C. (2009). Increasing stringency in symptom cluster research: A methodological exploration of symptom clusters in patients with inoperable lung cancer [Online exclusive]. *Oncology Nursing Forum, 36,* E282–E292. doi:10.1188/09.ONF.E283-E292

Honea, N., Brant, J., & Beck, S.L. (2007). Treatment-related symptom clusters. *Seminars in Oncology Nursing, 23,* 142–151. doi:10.1016/j.soncn.2007.01.002

Hong, J.H., Omur-Ozbek, P., Stanek, B.T., Dietrich, A.M., Duncan, S.E., Lee, Y.W., & Lesser, G. (2009). Taste and odor abnormalities in cancer patients. *Journal of Supportive Oncology, 7,* 58–65.

Kapustay, P.M., & Buchsel, P.C. (2000). Process, complications, and management of peripheral blood stem cell transplantation. In P.C. Buchsel & P.M. Kapustay (Eds.), *Stem cell transplantation: A clinical textbook* (pp. 5.1–5.28). Pittsburgh, PA: Oncology Nursing Society.

Keefe, D.M, Schubert, M.M, Elting, L.S., Sonis, S.T., Epstein, J.B., Raber-Durlacher, J.E., … Peterson, D.E. (2007). Updated clinical practice guidelines for the prevention and treatment of mucositis. *Cancer, 109,* 820–831. doi:10.1002/cncr.22484

Majorana, A., Schubert, M.M., Porta, F., Ugazio, A.G., & Sapelli, P.L. (2000). Oral complications of pediatric hematopoietic cell transplantation: Diagnosis and management.
Supportive Care in Cancer, 8, 353–365. doi:10.1007/s005200050003

McGowan, D. (2008). Chemotherapy-induced oral dysfunction: A literature review. *British
Journal of Nursing, 17,* 1422–1426.

Miaskowski, C., Dodd, M., & Lee, K. (2004). Symptom clusters: The new frontier in symptom management research. *Journal of the National Cancer Institute Monographs, 2004*(32),
17–21. doi:10.1093/jncimonographs/lgh023

Miaskowski, C., Cooper, B.A., Paul, S.M., Dodd, M., Lee, K., Aouizerat, B.E., … Bank, A.
(2006). Subgroups of patients with cancer with different symptom experiences and
quality-of-life outcomes: A symptom cluster analysis [Online exclusive]. *Oncology Nursing
Forum, 33,* E79–E89. doi:10.1188/06.ONF.E79-E89

Multinational Association of Supportive Care in Cancer/International Society for Oral Oncology.
(2005). Guidelines and assessment tools: Summary of evidence-based clinical practice guidelines for care of patients with oral and gastrointestinal mucositis (2005 update). Retrieved
from http://data.memberclicks.com/site/mascc/Guidelines_mucositis.pdf

Murphy, B.A. (2007). Clinical and economic consequences of mucositis induced by chemotherapy and/or radiation therapy. *Journal of Supportive Oncology, 5*(9, Suppl. 4), 13–21.

National Cancer Institute. (2009a, March 2). Cancer drug information: Palifermin. Retrieved
from http://www.cancer.gov/cancertopics/druginfo/palifermin

National Cancer Institute. (2009b, October 6). Oral complications of chemotherapy and head/
neck radiation (PDQ®) [Health professional version]. Retrieved from http://www.cancer
.gov/cancertopics/pdq/supportivecare/oralcomplications/HealthProfessional/page1

National Cancer Institute Cancer Therapy Evaluation Program. (2009). *Common terminology
criteria for adverse events* [v.4.0]. Retrieved from http://evs.nci.nih.gov/ftp1/CTCAE/
CTCAE_4.02_2009-09-15_QuickReference_5x7.pdf

Peterson, D.E. (1999). Research advances in oral mucositis. *Current Opinion in Oncology,
11,* 261–266.

Posner, M.R., & Haddard, R.I. (2007). Novel agents for the treatment of mucositis. *Journal
of Supportive Oncology, 5*(9, Suppl. 4), 33–39.

Potting, C., Mistiaen, P., Poot, E., Blijlevens, N., Donnelly, P., & van Achterberg, T. (2009).
A review of quality assessment of the methodology used in guidelines and systematic
reviews on oral mucositis. *Journal of Clinical Nursing, 18,* 3–12. doi:10.1111/j.1365-
2702.2008.02493.x

Shapiro, T.W., Davison, D.B., & Rust, D.M. (Eds.). (1997). *A clinical guide to stem cell and bone
marrow transplantation.* Sudbury, MA: Jones and Bartlett.

Shih, A., Miaskowski, C., Dodd, M.J., Stotts, N.A., & MacPhail, L. (2002). A research
review of the current treatments for radiation-induced oral mucositis in patients
with head and neck cancer. *Oncology Nursing Forum, 29,* 1063–1076. doi:10.1188/02.
ONF.1063-1080

So, W.K.W., Marsh, G., Ling, W.M., Leung, F.Y., Lo, J.C.K., Yeung, M., & Li, G.K.H. (2009).
The symptom cluster of fatigue, pain, anxiety, and depression and the effect on the quality of life of women receiving treatment for breast cancer: A multicenter study [Online
exclusive]. *Oncology Nursing Forum, 36,* E205–E214. doi:10.1188/09.ONF.E205-E214

Sonis, S.T. (2000). Oral complications. In R.C. Bast Jr., D.W. Kufe, R.E. Pollock, R.R.
Weichselbaum, J.F. Holland, & E. Frei III (Eds.), *Holland-Frei cancer medicine* (5th ed.).
Hamilton, Ontario, Canada: BC Decker. Retrieved from http://www.ncbi.nlm.nih.gov/
bookshelf/br.fcgi?book=cmed&part=A40626

Sonis, S.T. (2007). Pathobiology of oral mucositis: Novel insights and opportunities. *Journal
of Supportive Oncology, 5*(9, Suppl. 4), 3–11.

Spielberger, R., Stiff, P., Bensinger, W., Gentile, T., Weisdorf, D., Kewalramani, T., …
Emmanouilides, C. (2004). Palifermin for oral mucositis after intense therapy for
hematologic cancers. *New England Journal of Medicine, 351,* 2590–2598. doi:10.1056/
NEJMoa040125

Stevens, M.M. (2004). Gastrointestinal complications of hematopoietic stem cell transplantation. In S. Ezzone (Ed.), *Hematopoietic stem cell transplantation: A manual for nursing practice* (pp. 147–165). Pittsburgh, PA: Oncology Nursing Society.

Index

The letter f *after a page number indicates that relevant content appears in a figure; the letter* t, *in a table.*

A

acetaminophen, 129t, 131t
acromegaly, 15
actinomycin D, 239
acupuncture
  for pain management, 139
  for xerostomia, 55, 168–169
acute graft-versus-host disease, 55, 273–275, 274t–275t
acute pain, 127
acute side effects, definition of, 47, 110
acyclovir, 243–244
addiction
  behaviors associated with, 142
  fear of, 140
Addison disease, 15
ageusia, 7, 58, 187. *See also* taste alterations/loss
AIDS, 17
alcohol use/abuse, 10, 18, 107–108, 211, 217, 225, 251
allogeneic bone marrow transplant
  case study of, 272–275, 273t–275t
  oral manifestations of, 40t–41t, 55–56
allopurinol, 4t, 240
aloe vera, 162–163
alternative treatments, definition of, 159. *See also* complementary and alternative medicine
American Academy of Pediatric Dentistry, 240
American Academy of Pediatrics, 9
American Cancer Society, 210, 210t, 216

American Dietetic Association, 99
American Psychosocial Oncology Society, 217
amifostine (Ethyol®)
  adverse effects of, 116–117
  dosing/administration of, 116
  for oral mucositis, 51, 240
  for taste protection, 58
  for xerostomia, 42, 54, 103, 105, 114–118
amiloride, 4t
ampicillin, 3t
analgesics, oral manifestations of, 3t, 104
anatomy, of oral cavity, 5–7, 6f
anemia, 16
anesthetics, oral manifestations of, 3t
angiotensin-converting enzyme inhibitors, oral manifestations of, 3t, 12
angular cheilitis, 13, 13f
anorexia, 19–20
antiarrhythmics, oral manifestations of, 3t
antibiotics, oral manifestations of, 3t
anticholinergics, oral manifestations of, 4t, 19
anticoagulation therapy, oral manifestations of, 3t, 12, 14, 16
anticonvulsants, for pain management, 134, 135t–136t
antidepressants
  oral manifestations of, 19, 104
  for pain management, 134, 135t
antidiarrheals, oral manifestations of, 3t
antiemetics, 117

antihistamines, oral manifestations of, 3*t*, 104

antihypertensives, oral manifestations of, 3*t*–4*t*, 12, 104

anti-inflammatory agents, oral manifestations of, 4*t*

antilipidemics, oral manifestations of, 4*t*

antineoplastics, oral manifestations of, 4*t*, 16, 19. *See also* chemotherapy/chemotherapeutic agents

antiparkinsonians, oral manifestations of, 4*t*, 19

antipyretics, oral manifestations of, 4*t*

anti-reflux medications, oral manifestations of, 4*t*

antithyroids, oral manifestations of, 4*t*

anxiolytics, oral manifestations of, 4*t*

aphasia, 151

aphthous ulcers, 16, 161

armamentarium, for oral examination, 26, 27*f*

arthritic conditions, oral manifestations of, 12

artificial saliva products, 53–54, 59, 106, 197, 244

aspiration, 148, 150, 154

aspiration pneumonia, 14, 20

aspirin, 3*t*, 130

assessment. *See* oral assessment

Association of Community Cancer Centers, 159, 194

atraumatic tooth brushing, 39

autoimmune disorders, oral manifestations of, 14, 19, 54

B

baby teeth. *See* primary teeth

baclofen, 4*t*, 137*t*

bacterial infections, 18, 20, 39, 40*t*, 42–43, 187–188, 198

bacterial testing, 32–33

Ban Lan Gen, 161–162

barbiturates, 3*t*

Bell's palsy, 19

benzocaine, 3*t*

benzodiazepines, oral manifestations of, 4*t*

benzydamine hydrochloride, for OM pain, 51

beta-blockers, oral manifestations of, 3*t*, 12

BETTER model, for sexual health assessment, 190

biopsy, 33

Biotene® products, 53, 53*t*, 105–106, 183

bismuth, 3*t*

bisphosphonate-associated osteonecrosis (BON), 63, 194

bisphosphonates
  osteonecrosis from, 63, 194
  for pain management, 137*t*

body image, 208–209, 211

bone disorders, oral manifestations of, 12

bone marrow suppression, 43

bone marrow transplantation (BMT), oral manifestations of, 40*t*–41*t*, 55–56

bone metastasis, pain with, 135–137

breakthrough pain, 127–128, 132*f*, 134–135

Brief Pain Inventory, 127

BRUSHED Assessment Model, 86

brushing, 21, 39, 183, 246–247

bulimia, 19–20

bumps, differential diagnosis of, 36*t*, 38*f*

buprenorphine, 130

butorphanol tartrate, 130

C

calcitonin, for pain management, 137*t*

calcium channel blockers, 3*t*, 12

calcium channel ligands, 134

Canadian Cancer Society Research Institute assessment tools, 72

Cancer Care for the Whole Patient, 205, 212

Candida albicans, 17*f*, 17–18, 33, 40*t*

candidiasis
  in children, 242–243
  oral, 17*f*, 17–18, 33, 62, 99–100, 163–164, 187–188

canker sores, 16

cannabinoids, 134

Caphosol® rinse, for OM pain, 50–51, 133

capsaicin, for pain management, 51, 134, 165

captopril, 4*t*

carbamazepine, 3*t*, 135*t*

carbimazole, 4*t*

carboplatin, taste changes from, 58

cardiac disease, oral manifestations of, 12

cardiac transplantation, oral manifestations with, 3*t*, 12

caries. *See* dental caries
carious lesions, 198
celecoxib, 130
celiac disease, 16
cementum, of teeth, 5
cerebrovascular accident (CVA), 13, 13*f*
cerebrovascular diseases, 13*f*, 13–14
cetuximab, 109
cevimeline hydrochloride (Evoxac®), for xerostomia, 42, 54, 107
chamomile, 165–166
chemoprevention, 255–256
chemotherapy/chemotherapeutic agents
  dental work before, 56
  diet following, 193–194
  for oral cancers, 109–110
  oral examination before/after, 27. *See also* oral examination
  oral manifestations of, 4*t*, 16, 19, 40*t*–41*t*
  oral mucositis from, 40*t*–41*t*, 48–49, 94, 126
  speech impairments from, 148
  taste changes from, 57–58
  xerostomia from, 104, 110
chicken pox, 17
children
  cancers in, 237–238
  dental/craniofacial abnormalities in, 41*t*, 238–239
  infections in, 242–244
  oral assessment for, 85–86, 242
  oral complications in, 238–241
  oral health/hygiene in, 8–9, 244–247
  oral mucositis in, 239–241
  stem cell transplants in, 194–195
  xerostomia in, 244
Children's International Mucositis Evaluation Scale (ChIMES), 85–86
chloramphenicol, 3*t*
chlorhexidine, 3*t*, 107, 240
chlorzoxazone, 4*t*
cholestyramine, 4*t*
chronic graft-versus-host disease, 55–56, 195–196, 206–207
chronic obstructive pulmonary disease, 20
chronic pain, 127
chronic side effects, definition of, 47
cimetidine, 4*t*
ciprofloxacin, 3*t*
cirrhosis, 18
cisplatin, 126

oral mucositis from, 49
  taste changes from, 58
citrus flavors, for taste alterations, 160
Clinacanthus mutans, 161
clindamycin, 3*t*
clinical examination, 26–31, 28*f*–31*f*, 150
clofibrate, 4*t*
clonazepam, for pain management, 136*t*
clonidine, for pain management, 137*t*
clotrimazole, for fungal infections, 62
cocaine, 11
codeine, 128, 130, 131*t*
  oral manifestations of, 3*t*
cognition evaluation, 151
cognitive-behavioral pain management, 139, 165
cognitive-behavioral therapy, 216
colchicines, oral manifestations of, 4*t*
cold/heat application, for pain management, 138
collagen-vascular disorders, oral manifestations of, 14
Common Terminology Criteria for Adverse Events (CTCAE), 34, 72, 74*t*, 78–79, 97, 177, 178*t*
complementary and alternative medicine (CAM), 86–87, 157–159
  definitions of, 159
  evidence for use, 159
  for oral mucositis, 160–168
  for xerostomia, 168–170
complementary, definition of, 159
computer-based communication systems, 152
condition-specific tools, 71–72, 74*t*–75*t*. *See also* oral assessment
Consensus Auditory-Perceptual Evaluation of Voice (CAPE-V) assessment, 150
constipation, from opioids, 133
continuous-infusion opioids, for OM pain, 51
corticosteroids
  oral manifestations of, 4*t*, 20
  for pain management, 134–135, 136*t*
cranial nerve IX, 6–7
cranial nerve V, 6, 19
cranial nerve VII, 7
cranial nerve X, 7
craniofacial abnormalities
  in pediatric patients, 41*t*
  in survivorship, 208, 211
craniofacial complex, 2

cryotherapy, for OM management, 160–161, 241
cultural competence, 141–142
Cushing disease, 15
cyclophosphamide, 58, 110, 126, 239
cyclosporine, 4t, 12
cytarabine, 49, 126
cytomegalovirus, 17, 40t
cytoprotection, 103, 114–118
    with amifostine, 42, 51, 54, 58, 103, 105, 114–118, 240

D

daily saline sprays, 177–181, 179t, 180f
dapsone, 3t
deciduous teeth. See primary teeth
dehydration, 117
dementia, oral manifestations with, 19
dental care. See also oral health/hygiene
    barriers to, 43–44
    in patients with cancer, 39–43, 40t–41t, 105, 138, 176, 182–183
    in children, 244–247
    in older adults, 222–223
dental caries, 5, 8f, 8–9, 9f, 30f, 40t
    nutrition concerns with, 100, 198–199
    with periodontal disease, 56–57
    from radiation, 198
    with xerostomia, 39–42
dental flossing, 21, 39, 53t, 247
dental plaque, 9–10, 21
dental radiography, 32, 32f
dental work/extractions, 56
dentin, of teeth, 5
dentition, 29, 30f. See also teeth
dentures, 31, 188
dermatologic conditions, oral manifestations of, 14–15
dermatomyositis-polymyositis, 14
desipramine, for pain management, 135t
dexamethasone, 117
    oral manifestations of, 4t
    for pain management, 136t
dezocine, 130
diabetes mellitus, oral manifestations of, 15
diagnostic tools, 32f, 32–34, 34t–36t, 71–72, 73t–77t. See also oral assessment
dialysis, 20
diclofenac, 130

differential diagnosis, of oral diseases, 34, 35t–36t, 36f–38f
diltiazem, 4t
diphenhydramine, 133
disease-specific tools, 71–72, 74t–75t. See also oral assessment
distress. See psychosocial effects
distress thermometer, 212–214, 213f, 218
diuretics, oral manifestations of, 3t, 12, 104
doxorubicin, taste changes from, 58
dry mouth. See xerostomia
dry socket, 20
duloxetine, for pain management, 135t
Dynasplint® Trismus System, 61, 207
dysgeusia, 7, 98. See also taste alterations/loss
dysphagia, 14, 60, 148
    in end-of-life care, 154
    evaluation of, 150, 178t
    exercise interventions for, 151–153, 182, 182f
    nutrition interventions for, 95t, 99, 151, 199–200
    in older adults, 227–228
    in survivorship, 208

E

Eastern Cooperative Oncology Group, 109
Easy-to-Swallow, Easy-to-Chew Cookbook, 153
eating disorders, 19–20
economic challenges, 209–212
edentulism, 198–199, 223
Eilers' oral assessment tool, 71
employment concerns, 211
enalapril, 4t
enamel, of teeth, 5
endocrine disorders, oral manifestations of, 15
end-of-life care, 153–154
enteral nutrition, 100
epirubicin, 110
Epstein-Barr virus, 17, 40t
erythema multiforme, 14–15
erythematous lesions, differential diagnosis of, 35t, 36f
erythromycin, 3t
esophageal stage, of swallowing, 6–7
ethnicity, and pain experience, 141–142
etodolac, 129t, 130
etoposide, 49, 126

European Organisation for Research and Treatment of Cancer (EORTC) toxicity scales, 72, 73*t*, 75*t*, 78–79, 83–84
evidence-based practice, 70
exercises, 182, 182*f*
  for dysphagia, 151–153
  for pain management, 138–139
  for psychosocial issues, 216
  for trismus, 61, 138–139, 153
Extending Medicare Coverage for Preventive and Other Services (2000), 43
extraoral examination, 27–28, 28*f*–29*f*
E-Z Flex® system, for trismus, 61

F

facial disfigurement, 41*t*, 208, 211
facial nerve, 7
factor VIII, 16
fauces, 6*f*
fenoprofen calcium, 129*t*
fentanyl, 128, 130, 131*t*, 132
financial assistance, 210, 210*t*
financial challenges, 209–212
5-fluorouracil (5-FU), 110, 126
  oral mucositis from, 48–49
  taste changes from, 58
5-HT$_3$ antagonists, 117
flossing, 21, 39, 53*t*, 247
fluconazole (Diflucan®), for fungal infections, 62
fluoride
  oral supplementation of, 9, 53*t*, 105, 107, 247
  in toothpaste, 21, 246
  in water, 1
fluorouracil, 110, 126
  oral mucositis from, 48–49
  taste changes from, 58
folate deficiency, 16
folinic acid, 240
frenulum, 6*f*
frontal bossing, 15
full agonist opioids, 130, 131*t*
Functional Assessment of Cancer Therapy—General (FACT), 207
Functional Assessment of Cancer Therapy—Head and Neck Cancer (FACT-H&N), 71–72, 118, 215
fungal infections, 17*f*, 17–18, 20, 33, 40*t*, 42–43, 62

G

gabapentin, for pain management, 134, 136*t*
gastroesophageal reflux disease (GERD), 16
gastrointestinal disorders, oral manifestations of, 16
gastrointestinal mucositis, care protocols for, 269*t*–270*t*
Gaucher disease, 15
Gelclair® gel, for OM pain, 50, 133, 161
general profile instruments, 71, 73*t*
genetic disorders, oral manifestations of, 15–16
Gilda's Club, 216
gingivae, 6*f*, 29, 30*f*
gingival hyperplasia, 20
gingival stomatitis, 21
gingivitis, 9–10, 10*f*
glossopalatine arch, 6*f*
glossopharyngeal nerve, 6–7
glutamine, 86–87, 97
glutamine interleukin-15, 114
gluten-sensitive enteropathy, 16
glycyrrhizic acid, for OM management, 161
gonadal dysgenesis, 15
gonorrhea, 18
graft-versus-host disease (GVHD)
  case study of, 273–275, 274*t*–275*t*
  oral manifestations of, 16, 55–56, 195–196
Graves disease, 15
Great Ormond Street Hospital Oral Assessment Guide (GOSH OAG), 85
gustation. *See* taste

H

hairy leukoplakia, 17
hard palate, 6*f*
hard tissue, examination of, 29–31, 30*f*–31*f*
head and neck cancers, types of, 18
health insurance, dental care coverage by, 43
hearing evaluation, 150
heat/cold application, for pain management, 138
hematologic disorders, oral manifestations of, 16

hematopoietic growth factors, for OM
    pain, 51
hematopoietic stem cell transplantation
    (HSCT), 52, 194–196, 206–207
    case study of, 272–275, 273*t*–275*t*
hemodialysis, 20
hemophilia A, 16
herpes simplex virus (HSV), 17, 33, 40*t*,
    161, 187–188, 243–244
history taking, 25–31, 27*f*–31*f*
HIV, 17
homeopathy, 166–167
honey, 163–164
Hospital Anxiety and Depression Scale
    (HADS), 214, 218
human papillomavirus (HPV), 108–109,
    187
hydralazine, 3*t*
hydration, 117
hydrocodone, 130, 131*t*
hydrocortisone, 4*t*
hydromorphone, 130, 131*t*, 132
hydroxyurea, 126
hyperadrenalism, 15
hyperbaric oxygen (HBO) therapy, for
    osteoradionecrosis, 63
hypertension, oral manifestations of, 12
hyperthyroidism, 15
hypnosis, for xerostomia, 169–170
hypoadrenalism, 15
hypogeusia, 59, 98. *See also* taste altera-
    tions/loss
hypoglycemics, oral manifestations of, 4*t*
hyposalivation. *See* xerostomia
hyposmia, 59
hypothyroidism, 15

I

ibuprofen, 129*t*, 130
ice chewing, for OM management, 160–
    161, 241
image-guided radiotherapy, 111
imagery, 164
immobilization, for pain management,
    138–139
immunosuppressants, oral manifesta-
    tions of, 4*t*, 12, 18, 20
incisional tissue biopsy, 33
indigowood root, 161–162
infancy, oral health in, 8–9
infections

bacterial, 18, 20, 39, 40*t*, 42–43, 187–
    188, 198
    in children, 242–244
    effect on sexuality, 187–188
    fungal, 17*f*, 17–18, 20, 33, 40*t*, 42–43, 62
    in older adults, 229–230
    viral, 17, 33, 40*t*, 42–43, 187
infectious diseases, oral manifestations
    of, 17*f*, 17–18
Institute of Medicine
    on dental care, 43
    on psychosocial services, 205, 212
integrative treatments, definition of, 159.
    See also complementary and alter-
    native medicine
intensity-modulated radiotherapy
    (IMRT), 58, 104, 111–114
International Society for Oral Oncolo-
    gy, 266
intraoral examination, 28–31, 30*f*–31*f*
intubated patients, oral assessment for,
    85. *See also* tube feeding
iron-deficiency anemia, 16
Isatis indigotica Fort., 161–162
ischemic heart disease, oral manifesta-
    tions of, 12
isoniazid, 3*t*

J

jaw. *See also* osteonecrosis; trismus
    exercises for, 61, 138–139, 153
    immobilization of, 138–139

K

kaolin, 133
Kaposi sarcoma, 17*f*, 17–18
Kaposi-sarcoma-associated herpes virus, 17
keratinocyte growth factor, 51, 114, 241
ketamine, for OM pain, 51
ketoprofen, 129*t*, 130
ketorolac tromethamine, 129*t*, 130
kidney transplantation, oral manifesta-
    tions with, 20

L

labial frenulum, 6*f*
Lactobacillus infection, 18, 198

Lance Armstrong Foundation, 210, 210*t*
language evaluation, 151
laser therapy, 241
late complications, of radiation therapy, 110
lemon juice, for taste alterations, 160
lesions, differential diagnosis of, 35*t*, 36*f*–37*f*
leukemia, 16
Leukemia and Lymphoma Foundation, 216
levamisole
    oral manifestations of, 4*t*
    taste changes from, 58
levodopa, 4*t*, 19
levorphanol, 130
L-glutamine, 167–168
lichenoid lesions, 55
lichen planus, 14
licorice, for OM management, 161
lidocaine
    for OM pain, 50, 134, 136*t*, 240
    oral manifestations of, 3*t*
lingual frenulum, 6*f*
lithium carbonate, 4*t*
liver disease, oral manifestations of, 18
liver transplantation, oral manifestation with, 18
Livestrong, 210, 210*t*
local anesthetics
    for OM pain, 50, 133–134, 240–241
    oral manifestations of, 3*t*
    for pain management, 136*t*
lorazepam, 117
lumps, differential diagnosis of, 36*t*, 38*f*
lupus, 14
lymphedema, in older adults, 229
lymph nodes, 28, 29*f*

M

MacDibbs Mouth Assessment, 81–83
macroglossia, 15
"magic" mouthwashes, for OM pain, 50
magnesium salicylate, 130
major salivary glands, 7, 28, 52, 83, 104, 113
malnutrition, in patients with cancer, 93–94
mandibular teeth, 5
mandibular tori, 31
manganese superoxide dismutase plasmid, liposome (SOD2-PL), 114

Marfan syndrome, 15
massage, for pain management, 138
maternal periodontal disease, 21
Matricaria recutita L., 165–166
maxillary teeth, 5
maxillary tori, 31, 31*f*
MD Anderson Symptom Inventory—Head and Neck (MDASI-HN), 72, 75*t*
medical food supplement drinks, 96*f*, 100
medical insurance, dental care coverage by, 43
Medicare, 43
medications, oral manifestations of, 3*t*–5*t*, 104. *See also* chemotherapy/chemotherapeutic agents
melatonin, 114
Memorial Symptom Assessment Scale, 110
menopause, oral manifestations during, 21
menses, 20
meperidine, 133
methadone, 130, 132–133
methimazole, 4*t*
"meth mouth," 11
methotrexate, 110, 126
    oral mucositis from, 49
    taste changes from, 58
methylphenidate, for pain management, 137*t*
methylthiouracil, 4*t*
metoclopramide, 117
metronidazole, 3*t*
mexiletine, 134, 136*t*
microbiology testing, in oral assessment, 32–33
milk of magnesia, 133
minocycline, 3*t*
minor salivary glands, 7, 52, 104, 113
minoxidil, 4*t*
mixed agonist-antagonist opioids, 130–131
mononucleosis, 17
morphine, 51, 128, 130, 131*t*, 132–133
motor functions, of oral cavity, 6
Mouth and Throat Soreness (MTS) questionnaire, 188
Mouth Kote®, 106
mouth mirror, 26, 27*f*
mouth rinses, 39, 53*t*, 133, 183
mucositis
    gastrointestinal, 269*t*–270*t*
    oral. *See* oral mucositis

Mucotrol®, for OM pain, 133
mucous component, of saliva, 52–53, 104
Multicultural Personality Questionnaire, 141–142
multileaf collimator, 58
Multinational Association for Supportive Care in Cancer, 240, 265–266
multiple sclerosis, 19
muscle relaxants, oral manifestations of, 4*t*
muscles of mastication, 28
myasthenia gravis, 19
Mycobacterium tuberculosis, 20
myocardial infarction, oral manifestations of, 12

N

nalbuphine hydrochloride, 130
naproxen, 129*t*, 130
narcotic patches, for OM pain, 51
nasopharyngeal carcinoma, 17
National Cancer Institute
    CTCAE scoring system, 34, 34*t*, 72, 74*t*, 78–79, 97, 177
    financial assistance, 210*t*
National Center for Complementary and Alternative Medicine (NCCAM), 158
National Comprehensive Cancer Network (NCCN), 138, 212
National Dysphagia Diet, 99, 194, 195*t*
National Institutes of Health, 158
National Survey of Households Affected by Cancer, 205
nausea/vomiting, 39, 40*t*, 117
neck muscles, 27, 28*f*
NeedyMeds, 210*t*
Neisseria gonorrhoeae, 18
nerve blocks, 135–137
neurologic diseases, oral manifestations of, 19
neuropathic pain, 126–127, 133–134
neutropenia, oral mucositis with, 52
niacin deficiency, 16
nifedipine, 4*t*
nitrogen mustard, 239
nitroglycerin, 5*t*
N-methyl-D-aspartate receptor antagonists, 134
nociceptive pain, 126
non-Hodgkin lymphoma, 106

noniatrogenic xerostomia, 106
nonsteroidal anti-inflammatory drugs (NSAIDs), 128, 129*t*, 129–135
    drug interactions with, 130
    oral manifestations of, 3*t*
    side effects of, 130
nortriptyline, for pain management, 135*t*
nose clips, 152
nutrition support/interventions, 100, 181, 181*f*
    after chemotherapy, 193–194
    after radiation therapy, 196–199
    for dysphagia, 95*t*, 99
    for oral mucositis, 94–97, 95*t*, 96*f*, 97*t*
    for taste changes, 95*t*–96*t*, 98–99, 197–198
    for trismus, 100, 153, 198
    for xerostomia, 96*t*, 97–98, 196–197

O

objective pain behaviors, 127
older adults, 142, 221–222
    assessment/interventions for, 231–232
    oral health in, 222–225
    oral manifestations in, 223–230
omega-3 fatty acids, 114
Oncology Nursing Society (ONS)
    on CAM/integrative therapies, 159
    Patient Outcomes Survey, 88
    Radiation Therapy Patient Care Record, 79
ondansetron, 117
one-way speaking valve, 152
opioids, 130–133, 131*t*, 132*f*
    for breakthrough pain, 134–135
    for neuropathic pain, 134
    for OM pain, 51
    principles of administration, 132*f*
    side effects of, 133
opportunistic infections
    bacterial, 18, 20, 39, 40*t*, 42–43, 187–188, 198
    fungal, 17*f*, 17–18, 20, 33, 40*t*, 42–43, 62
    viral, 17, 33, 40*t*, 42–43, 187
oral aphthous ulcers, 16
oral assessment, 69–70, 176–182, 178*t*–179*t*, 180*f*–182*f*
    history taking during, 25–31, 27*f*–31*f*
    in special populations, 85–86
    tools for, 32*f*, 32–34, 34*t*–36*t*, 71–72, 73*t*–77*t*, 214–217

Oral Assessment Guide (OAG), 72, 74*t*, 79–81, 83–85, 87, 242
oral bleeding, 40*t*, 183
oral cancers, 107–109
  incidence/mortality of, 108
  signs/symptoms of, 107–108
  treatments for, 109–110
oral candidiasis, 17*f*, 17–18, 33, 62, 99–100, 163–164, 187–188, 242–243
oral cavity
  anatomy of, 5–7, 6*f*
  functions of, 5–6
oral contraceptives, 20
oral cryotherapy, for OM prevention, 51
oral diseases
  common types, 8–11, 8*f*–11*f*
  differential diagnosis of, 34, 35*t*–36*t*, 36*f*–38*f*
  epidemiology of, 2, 3*t*–5*t*
Oral Exam Guide, 72, 80
oral examination, 26–31, 28*f*–31*f*
  armamentarium for, 26, 27*f*
oral health/hygiene
  barriers to, 43–44
  in cancer patients, 39–43, 40*t*–41*t*, 105, 138, 176, 182–183
  in childhood, 8–9, 244–247
  definition of, 1
  and general health, 11–12
  history of, 1–2
  maintenance of, 21
  in older adults, 222–225
  patient education on, 183
  protocols for, 266, 267*t*–270*t*
  with xerostomia, 53, 53*t*
oral lubricants, 170
oral manifestations. *See also specific conditions*
  of cancer therapy, 4*t*, 16, 19, 40*t*–41*t*
  of medications, 3*t*–5*t*, 104
  in older adults, 223–230
  prevention/early detection of, 265–266, 267*t*–270*t*
  recent treatment advances for, 264–265
  in survivorship, 207–209
  of systemic medical diseases, 12–20
oral moisturizers, 170
oral mucosa, examination of, 29
oral mucositis (OM), 47–52, 48*f*–49*f*, 264
  from allogeneic bone marrow transplant, 40*t*–41*t*
  CAM interventions for, 160–168
  care protocols for, 267*t*–269*t*

from chemotherapy, 40*t*–41*t*, 48–49, 94, 126
  in children, 239–241
  duration of, 94
  effect on sexuality, 186–187
  incidence of, 48
  management of, 50–51, 133
  nutrition interventions for, 94–97, 95*t*, 96*f*, 97*t*
  pathobiology of, 49*f*, 49–50
  prevention of, 51
  from radiation therapy, 40*t*–41*t*, 49, 94
  research needs in, 264–265
  risk factors for, 48*f*, 48–49, 160
  scoring systems for, 33–34, 34*t*, 71–72, 73*t*–77*f*, 81–83, 178*t*, 273*t*
  signs/symptoms of, 50–51
  speech impairment with, 148
Oral Mucositis Assessment Scale (OMAS), 71–72, 76*t*, 81–82, 87
Oral Mucositis Daily Questionnaire (OMDQ), 188
Oral Mucositis Index (OMI-20), 71–72, 76*t*, 81–82
oral opioids, for OM pain, 51
oral pain. *See* pain
oral piercing, 10
oral preparatory stage, of swallowing, 6
oral prostheses, 31
oral sprays, 170
oral stage, of swallowing, 6
oral stomatitis, 17
OraStretch® device, 207
Orbit® gum, 53
Oren-gedoku-to, 166
oropharyngeal cancers, 108
orthodontic appliances, 31
osteoarthritis, oral manifestations of, 12
osteonecrosis, 63–64, 126, 139, 229. *See also* postradiation jaw osteonecrosis
osteopetrosis, 15–16
osteoradionecrosis (ORN), 62–63, 100, 126, 139, 199
oxycodone, 128, 130, 131*t*, 132
oxymorphone, 131*t*

P

pain
  assessment of, 127–128, 178*t*
  beliefs/perceptions about, 140–142

with bone metastasis, 135–137
breakthrough, 127–128, 132*f*, 134–135
causes of, 125–127
effect on sexuality, 187
management of. *See* pain management
neuropathic, 126–127
nociceptive, 126
in older adults, 228
with oral mucositis, 50–51, 126, 133–134, 264
orofacial, 168
in survivorship, 207–209
pain management
with adjuvant drugs, 135*t*–137*t*, 135–139
barriers to, 140–142
cognitive-behavioral, 139
nonpharmacologic, 138–139
by nonsteroidal anti-inflammatory drugs, 129*t*, 129–135
with oral mucositis, 50–51, 126, 133–134
patient education on, 128
palatine tonsils, 6*f*
palifermin (Kepivance®), for OM prevention, 51, 114, 241
pamidronate
osteonecrosis from, 63, 194
for pain management, 137
parenteral nutrition, 100
with oral mucositis, 95–97
Parkinson disease, 19
parotiditis, 53
parotid salivary glands, 7, 28, 52, 83, 104
lymphomas of, 106
sparing of, 111–114
partial agonist opioids, 130
pathology testing, in oral assessment, 32–33
patient-controlled analgesia (PCA), for OM pain, 51
patient education, 217
on dental care, 183
on pain management, 128
on sexuality changes, 190
on speech/voice changes, 149
payayor, 161
pediatric patients
cancers in, 237–238
craniofacial/dental abnormalities in, 41*t*, 238–239
infections in, 242–244
oral assessment in, 85–86, 242

oral complications in, 238–241
oral health/hygiene in, 8–9, 244–247
oral mucositis in, 239–241
stem cell transplants in, 194–195
xerostomia in, 244
pellagra, 16
pemphigus vulgaris, 14
penicillin, 3*t*
pentazocine, 130
perimenopause, 21
periodontal disease, 9–10, 10*f*–11*f*, 14
from bacterial infection, 18
dental caries with, 56
with diabetes mellitus, 15
with HIV infection, 17
during pregnancy, 21
periodontal pockets, 10
periodontitis, 9–10, 11*f*
periodontium, examination of, 29, 30*f*
peritoneal dialysis, 20
pharyngeal stage, of swallowing, 6–7
pharyngopalatine arch, 6*f*
phenothiazines, oral manifestations of, 4*t*
phenytoin
oral manifestations of, 3*t*
for pain management, 136*t*
pilocarpine (Salagen®) saliva stimulant, 54, 103–107, 117–118, 244
pituitary gland, diseases of, 15
plaque. *See* dental plaque
Plummer-Vinson syndrome, 16
Porphyromonas gingivalis, 18
postmenopause, 21
postradiation jaw osteonecrosis (PRON), 39, 41*t*, 42. *See also* osteonecrosis
prednisone, for pain management, 136*t*
pregabalin, for pain management, 136*t*
pregnancy gingivitis, 21
pressure, for pain management, 138
primary teeth, 5, 8
probiotics, 100
problem-solving techniques, 216
procainamide, 3*t*
procaine hydrochloride, 3*t*
procarbazine, 126, 239
prochlorperazine, 117
propylthiouracil, 4*t*
prostheses, 31
Pseudomonas infection, 40*t*
psychosocial effects, 205–207, 206*f*
assessment of, 212–214, 213*f*, 215*f*
of cancer recurrence, 251–252, 256–257

financial challenges and, 209–212, 210*t*

interventions for, 216

resources on, 217–218

in survivorship, 207–209

psychotropics, oral manifestations of, 4*t*

puberty, oral manifestations during, 19–20

pulmonary diseases, oral manifestations of, 20

pulp, of teeth, 5

Q

Qingre Liyan decoction (QRLYD), 162

QOL SF-36 assessment tool, 71

quality of life, 118, 207. *See also* psychosocial effects

Quality of Life Questionnaire (QL-Q), 71–72, 73*t*, 84, 215

Quality of Life Scale (University of Washington), 118, 215

Quick Reference for Oncology Clinicians, 217

R

radiation caries, 198

radiation therapy

advances in, 58, 104, 111–114

in children, 239

dental extractions before, 56

diet following, 196–199

for oral cancers, 109

oral complications of, 19, 40*t*–41*t*, 110

oral mucositis from, 40*t*–41*t*, 49, 94

speech impairments from, 148

taste changes from, 57–58

trismus from, 60–61

xerostomia from, 53, 83, 104

Radiation Therapy Oncology Group (RTOG), 72, 75*t*, 78–79

0129 clinical trial, 108–109

Acute Radiation Morbidity Scoring Criteria, 79

oral mucositis scales, 34, 34*t*

radiofrequency ablation, for pain management, 137

radiographic examination, 32, 32*f*

radioprotection. *See* cytoprotection

ratanhia, 164

receptor cells, in taste buds, 7

recreational drug use, 10–11

recurrence

fear of, 251–252, 256–257

nursing implications of, 257–258, 258*t*

red lesions, differential diagnosis of, 35*t*, 38*f*

registered dietitians, 93

relaxation techniques, for pain management, 139, 165

religion, and pain experience, 141

renal diseases, oral manifestations of, 20

repositioning, for pain management, 138–139

rheumatoid arthritis, oral manifestations of, 12

riboflavin deficiency, 16

risk factors

for oral diseases, 2, 3*t*–5*t*

for oral mucositis, 48*f*, 48–49, 160

for taste alterations, 7, 57–59

rituximab, 107

Rotterdam Symptom Checklist, 71

S

safe sex practices, 187

salicylates, oral manifestations of, 4*t*

saline sprays, 177–181, 179*t*, 180*f*

saliva, 7, 52–53

thick, 96*t*, 98, 197

salivary glands, 7, 28, 52–53, 83, 104, 113

Salivary Hypofunction Questionnaire, 72

saliva stimulants, 54, 59, 103–107, 117–118, 244

saliva substitutes, 53–54, 59, 106, 197, 244

sarcoidosis, 14

scleroderma, 14

screening tools, 71, 214–217. *See also* oral assessment

secondary malignancies, 41*t*, 251–255, 252*f*

chemoprevention of, 255–256

selegiline, 19

sensory functions, of oral cavity, 6

serotonin norepinephrine reuptake inhibitors (SNRIs), for neuropathic pain, 134

serous component, of saliva, 52

sexuality/sexual health

assessment of, 188–191

factors in, 185–186, 186*f*

interventions for, 189–191

oral complications and, 186–187

sexually transmitted diseases, oral mani-
    festations of, 18
shingles, 17
sialogogues, 53–54, 59, 106, 197, 244
6-mercaptopurine, 239
Sjögren syndrome, 14, 54, 104, 106–107,
    223
slippery elm, 166
smoking. *See* tobacco use
Society for Integrative Oncology, 159
soft foods, 97*t*, 99, 153
soft palate, 6*f*
soft tissue, examination of, 29, 30*f*
speaking valve, 152
speech impairments, 148, 152
speech pathologists
    and end-of-life care, 153–154
    evaluation by, 149–151
    pretreatment session, 149
    role of, 147–148
    treatment by, 151–154
"spray-and-weigh" programs, 175–176. *See
    also* oral assessment
    daily saline sprays in, 177–181, 179*t*,
        180*f*
    equipment for, 179*t*, 179–181, 180*f*
Staphylococcus aureus, 18
Staphylococcus veridians, 18
sternocleidomastoid muscle, 27, 28*f*
stimulated whole saliva (SWS) flow rate,
    33
stomatitis. *See* mucositis
Streptococcus mutans, 18, 198
Streptococcus viridans, 39
stress-reduction exercises, 216
stroke, oral manifestations with, 13–14
sublingual salivary glands, 6*f*, 7, 28, 52, 83
submandibular salivary glands, 6*f*, 7, 28,
    52, 83
    surgical transfer of, 105
substance abuse, history of, 142
sucralfate, 50, 133
sulfa antibiotics, oral manifestations of,
    3*t*
sulfasalazine, 3*t*
sulfonylureas, oral manifestations of, 4*t*
Surgeon General's Report on Oral
    Health (2000), 1–2, 21
surgery
    diet following, 199–200
    oral complications of, 18–19
surgical transfer
    of submandibular salivary glands, 105

survivorship
    in older adults, 230
    oral complications in, 207–209, 211
swallowing
    dysfunction in, 20. *See also* dysphagia
    evaluation of, 150
    stages of, 6–7
symptom clusters, 271
Syousaikotou, 166
syphilis, 18
systemic analgesics, for OM pain, 51

T

tardive dyskinesia, 19
targeted therapies, for oral cancers, 109–
    110
taste, 7, 57
taste alterations/loss, 7, 57–59
    assessment scales for, 71–72, 73*t*–77*t*,
        78–87
    CAM interventions for, 160
    effect on sexuality, 187
    management of, 58–59
    nutrition interventions for, 95*t*–96*t*,
        98–99, 197–198
    in older adults, 230
    risk factors for, 7, 57–59
    in survivorship, 207–208
taste buds, 7, 57
taste receptors, 7
taste sensations, 7
teeth, 5, 6*f*. *See also* dental caries
    examination of, 29, 30*f*
    loss of, 198–199, 223
temporomandibular joint (TMJ), 5, 12,
    27, 28*f*, 207, 228
tetracyclines, oral manifestations of, 3*t*
Therabite® Jaw Motion Rehabilitation
    System, 61, 207–208
therapeutic communication, 190–191
thiazide diuretics, oral manifestations of,
    3*t*, 12
thick saliva, 96*t*, 98, 197
third molars, 5, 20
three-dimensional conformal radiation
    therapy, 58, 111
three-finger test, for trismus, 61
thrombocytopenia, toothbrushing with, 39
thyroid gland, diseases of, 15
tobacco use, 10, 18, 20, 107–108, 217,
    225, 251

tongue, 6*f*
tongue blade, 26
tongue lesions, 55
tonsils, 6*f*
tooth brushing, 21, 39, 183, 246–247
tooth enamel, 5
toothpaste, 21, 39, 183, 246
topical anesthetics
    for OM pain, 50, 133–134, 240–241
    oral manifestations of, 3*t*
    for pain management, 136*t*
total parenteral nutrition (TPN), 52
tracheostomy, 150, 152
traditional Chinese medicine (TCM),
    161–162
tramadol, 128, 131*t*, 134
transcutaneous electrical nerve stimula-
    tion (TENS), 139
transforming growth factor-beta, 114
transplantation
    bone marrow, 40*t*–41*t*, 55–56
    cardiac, 3*t*, 12
    hematopoietic stem cell, 52, 194–196,
        272–275, 273*t*–275*t*
    liver, 18
    renal, 20
trapezius muscle, 27, 28*f*
Traumeel S®, 86–87, 166–167
Treponema denticola, 18
Treponema pallidum, 18
tricyclic antidepressants, for neuropath-
    ic pain, 134
trigeminal nerve, 6
trigeminal neuralgia, 19
trismus, 41*t*, 42, 60–61
    assessment of, 151
    effect on sexuality, 187
    management of, 61, 138–139, 153
    nutrition concerns with, 100, 153,
        198
    in older adults, 228–229
    pain with, 127
    in survivorship, 207–208
tube feeding, 100, 208
    with oral mucositis, 95–97
tuberculosis, 20
Turner syndrome, 15

U

UKCCSG-PONF Mouth Care Group,
    241–242, 245

ulceration
    differential diagnosis of, 35*t*, 37*f*
    with GVHD, 56
Ulmus fulva, 166
Ulmus rubra, 166
unstimulated whole saliva (UWS) flow
    rate, 33
uremic stomatitis, 20
U.S. Preventive Services Task Force, 9
uvula, 6*f*

V

vagus nerve, 7
valproate, for pain management, 135*t*
varicella zoster, 17, 40*t*
vasodilators, oral manifestations of, 5*t*
venlafaxine, for pain management, 135*t*
verapamil, 4*t*
vibration, for pain management, 138
videofluoroscopic swallowing studies,
    150, 153
vinblastine, 126
vincristine, 126, 239
viral infections, 17, 33, 40*t*, 42–43, 187
vitamin deficiencies, 16
voice impairments, 148–150, 152
Von Willebrand disease, 16

W

weight monitoring, 181, 181*f*. *See also*
    "spray-and-weigh" programs
Wellness Community, 216
Western Consortium for Cancer Nursing
    Research (WCCNR), Stomatitis
    Staging System, 72, 77*t*, 81–82
white blood cell disorders, 16
white lesions, differential diagnosis of,
    35*t*, 37*f*
wisdom teeth, 5, 20
workplace concerns, 211
World Health Assembly (2007), 2
World Health Organization (WHO)
    analgesic pain ladder, 128–129
    Global Oral Health Programme
        (2008), 2
    oral mucositis scoring system, 33–34,
        34*t*, 72, 76*t*, 81–82
    Report on Oral Health (2003), 2, 21
    sexual health definition, 185

X

xerostomia, 2, 14, 40*t*, 52–55, 53*t*, 103–106
  assessment of, 151
  assessment scales for, 71–72, 73*t*–77*t*,
    83–84, 178*t*
  CAM interventions for, 168–170
  dental caries and, 39–42
  effect on sexuality, 187
  management of, 53–55, 104–105
  medications causing, 104, 110
  during menopause, 21
  noniatrogenic, 106
  nutrition interventions for, 96*t*, 97–98,
    196–197
  objective measurement of, 33
  in older adults, 223–224, 227
  oral hygiene with, 53, 53*t*
  prevention of, 111–114
  in survivorship, 207
  voice impairments with, 148

Xerostomia Questionnaire (XQ), 71–72,
  77*t*, 83–84
Xylifresh® gum, 53
xylitol gum, 53, 170

Y

Yangyin Humo decoction (YHD), 162

Z

zinc
  deficiency of, 16
  supplementation of, 59, 97–99, 165
  and taste perception, 59
zoledronic acid
  osteonecrosis from, 63, 194
  for pain management, 137*t*